RESPONSIBLE CONDUCT OF

RESEARCH

RESPONSIBLE CONDUCT OF

RESEARCH

Adil E. Shamoo and David B. Resnik

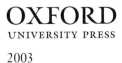

OXFORD
UNIVERSITY PRESS

2003

OXFORD
UNIVERSITY PRESS

Oxford   New York
Auckland   Bangkok   Buenos Aires   Cape Town   Chennai
Dar es Salaam   Delhi   Hong Kong   Istanbul   Karachi   Kolkata
Kuala Lumpur   Madrid   Melbourne   Mexico City   Mumbai   Nairobi
São Paulo   Shanghai   Taipei   Tokyo   Toronto

Published by Oxford University Press, Inc.
198 Madison Avenue, New York, New York 10016

www.oup.com

Oxford is a registered trademark of Oxford University Press

Library of Congress Cataloging-in-Publication Data
Shamoo, Adil E.
   Responsible conduct of research / by Adil E. Shamoo, David B. Resnik.
      p. cm.
   Includes bibliographical references and index.
   ISBN 0-19-514845-2; 0-19-514846-0 (pbk)
      1. Medicine—Research—Moral and ethical aspects.   2. Medical ethics.   3. Bioethics.
4. Human experimentation in medicine—Moral and ethical aspects.   I. Resnik, David B.
II. Title.
R852 .S47 2002
174'2—dc21   2001055428

9 8 7 6 5 4 3 2 1

Printed in the United States of America
on acid free paper

To
Abe, Zach, and Jessica
and
Susan, Peter, and Michael

Preface

In the last decades of the twentieth century, media headlines featuring research misconduct in American universities focused public attention on the dramatic ethical problems that can arise in research. In some instances, investigators have been accused and occasionally found guilty of falsifying, fabricating, or plagiarizing data. Other cases have involved such allegations as the theft of ideas from grant applications and the abuse of human subjects in research protocols. There is widespread concern that public confidence in the scientific research establishment has been undermined. In the current atmosphere of accountability, the once-exempt research enterprise is now under increased scrutiny by the media, congress, and the public. In response to these pressures, there have been congressional hearings, legislative remedies, policies to manage conflicts of interest, policies to deal with research misconduct, national conferences on a variety of themes, the creation of the U.S. Commission on Research Integrity, the Office of Research Integrity (or ORI), and a proliferation of university-based research ethics courses and other less formal academic experiences.

Aside from concerns about research misconduct, the economic and commercial aspects of research have increased ethical problems and dilemmas in research and have heightened public awareness. Research and development (R&D) has become a big business with huge financial investments at stake. Money spent on public and private R&D in the United States alone now exceeds $200 billion per year, and the 2001 federal budget requests call for $95 billion per year in R&D spending. With all of this money at stake, conflicts of interest, sharing data, and intellectual property are prominent in R&D, whether conducted in a private laboratory or at a public university. The lines between academia and industry have blurred, as universities have entered into various agreements and arrangements with private companies. These public–private partnerships can have profound effects on the intellectual and moral climate of the university and can undermine protections for human and animal subjects.

New ethical issues dilemmas arise in research almost daily due to rapid and breathtaking advances in biotechnology and biomedicine, such as genetic engineering of plants and animals, genetic testing, gene therapy, in vitro fertilization, surrogate pregnancy, prenatal testing, preimplantation, genetic diagnosis, mammalian cloning, stem cell research, gene patenting, and the sequencing and mapping of the human genome. These breakthroughs raise important ethical, theological, and political questions for researchers and clinicians, as well as for society at large.

For some years, all trainees (students, fellows, and others) on grants from the National Institutes of Health (NIH) have been required to have some exposure to issues related to research ethics. In the fall of 2000, the ORI announced its long-awaited mandate for training and education in responsible conduct of research (RCR). The agency recommended that all personnel involved in research funded by U.S. Public Health Service (PHS) grants or contracts, including principal investigators, postdoctoral students, graduate students, technicians, and staff, receive some education in RCR. The ORI also outlined nine core areas for RCR education—all of which are covered in this book—and recommended that institutions also provide ongoing education in RCR. Although the ORI mandate was suspended when the Bush administration took control of the executive branch of government in January 2001, it is likely that some form of RCR training will be mandated for all research personnel who conduct research under the auspices of the PHS, which includes the NIH and other agencies. It is also likely, in our opinion, that other agencies, such as the National Science Foundation (NSF), will follow this example.

The academic community has yet to fully respond to the need for didactic materials that provide support to courses or to other experiences related to research ethics. Our textbook, *Responsible Conduct of Research*, presents a comprehensive introduction to the ethical issues at stake in the conduct of research. A total of 12 chapters range in scope from the broad issues relating to social responsibility, research funding, and freedom of inquiry to more narrow topics such as the ethical aspects of entering data into lab notebooks, designing experiments, citing published works, and deciding authorship matters. The chapters also contain questions for discussion and case studies. Because this book deals with ethical issues in the use of humans and animals in research, and because its content parallels the recommendations of the ORI, its primary focus is on biomedical research. However, the chapters on such topics as intellectual property, authorship, peer review, and conflict of interest make this text suitable for most research-focused disciplines.

To understand problems and questions in research ethics, one must understand the historical, economic, cultural, political, legal, and philosophical aspects of research, since these factors play a key role in influencing and legitimizing the norms of research. Thus, our book includes some introductory discussions of these social and contextual features of research. We include these discussions to help students get a better grasp of the ethical issues in research, and we apologize in advance for presenting materials that may be considered overly simplistic by historians, philosophers, social scientists, and other science studies scholars. We also apologize for any errors or oversights in this first edition. Please feel free to send us your comments and suggestions: Adil E. Shamoo, Ph.D., Department of Biochemistry and Molecular Biology, University of Maryland School of Medicine, 108 North Greene Street, Baltimore, Maryland 21201-1503; e-mail: ashamoo@umaryland.edu.

Acknowledgments

We are grateful to Dr. James T. Rule, professor emeritus at the University of Maryland School of Dentistry, for his invaluable contributions to chapters on conflict of interest and scientific misconduct. Dr. Shamoo is also grateful for all of the students and guest lecturers in his research ethics classes since 1991 for their input and discussions. For useful discussions and insight about ethics in research, Dr. Resnik is especially grateful to Dr. Loretta Kopelman, Dr. Kenneth De Ville, Dr. Thomas Feldbush, Dr. John Bradfield, Dr. Jeremy Sugarman, Frank Grassner, John Doll, and students and co-instructors in his research ethics classes taught in 1999 and 2001 at the Brody School of Medicine. Finally, we thank the many anonymous reviewers of the prospectus during the publisher's review process for their considerable and valued suggestions for improving the textbook in content and style.

Contents

RESPONSIBLE CONDUCT OF

RESEARCH

1

Scientific Research and Ethics

There is a growing recognition among scientists, government officials, and research institutions that ethical conduct is an important part of research. Ethical conduct is important in research because science is a cooperative enterprise that takes place within a social context. Modern science can be viewed as a profession akin to medicine or law. Standards of conduct in research play a key role in advancing the goals of science; in promoting cooperation, collaboration, and trust among researchers; and in attaining the public's trust and support. This chapter discusses the importance of ethics in research, the nature of scientific professionalism, some important concepts, theories, and principles of ethics, a method for ethical decision making, some principles for ethical conduct in research, and the value of ethics education and ethical leadership in research.

Ethical problems, issues, and dilemmas occur for most people on a daily basis. Whenever we ask the question, "What should I do?" there is a good chance that an ethical issue or concern lurks in the background. In everyday life, such questions frequently arise as we make choices among different interests and commitments, such as career, family, community, church, society, prestige, and money. Professional researchers—scientists, engineers, and scholars—also frequently face ethical problems, issues, and dilemmas. Consider the following cases:

Case 1

You are graduate student in pharmacology at a large university working under the direction of a senior researcher. You notice, on reading a paper on the pharmacology of a new serotonin reuptake inhibitor, which your senior director published in a top journal in your field, that there is a problem with the diagrams in the paper. You cannot seem to reconcile the diagrams with the published data. You approach her with this problem and she shrugs it off, saying that you do not understand the research well enough to make a judgment about it. What should you do?

Case 2

You are a postdoctoral student in computer science working on some artificial intelligence programs for use in chemical manufacturing. Two other graduate students are working with you on the project, which is directed by a senior researcher. You have just received an e-mail from a research team at another university asking you for some preliminary data and designs related to your project. They are working on a similar project and said that they are interested in collaborating. It is likely that your research will have significant economic value and will result in patented products. What should you do?

Case 3

You are Associate Professor of Anthropology planning to teach a course on herbal medicine in the world's cultures. There are several books in the field that you could use in teaching your course and you have just published a book, which you believe to be the best in the field. Before the course begins, one of your teaching assistants asks you whether the students will object to having to buy your book. What should you do?

Case 4

You are the director of the Department of Comparative Medicine at a medical school associated with a university medical center. You are also the chair of your institution's animal care and use committee, which oversees animal research. The group People for the Ethical Treatment of Animals (PETA) has staged some protests recently in your community. A local reporter calls you on the phone and wants to do an interview with you about animal research and animal rights. What should you do?

Case 5

You are Professor of Pediatrics and an expert on child abuse. You have been asked to serve as an expert witness for the defense in a case. The prosecutors have hired two experts who are prepared to testify that child abuse probably occurred. You know these experts from professional meetings and from their published work, and you have a great deal of respect for them. After examining the x-rays, photographs, and other data, you are not convinced that child abuse has occurred, and you could offer testimony that supports the defense in this case. As a long-standing advocate of child welfare and rights, you would have a hard time testifying for the defense and contradicting the testimony offered by your colleagues. You want to protect your reputation in any case. The defense will find another expert if you refuse their request. What should you do?

Each case above presents researchers with complex and difficult choices relating to the conduct of research and raises ethical, social, and legal issues. To make well-informed, reasonable, and responsible choices in cases like these, as well to guide conduct in simpler cases, researchers need some understanding of the ethical and social dimensions of research. The purpose of this book is to provide researchers with some of the education that is required for the responsible conduct of research (RCR).

In recent years universities, research organizations, professional societies, funding agencies, politicians, the media, and most scientists have come to realize that ensuring ethical conduct is an essential part of basic, applied, and clinical research. Little more than a few decades ago, many scientists would not have accepted this statement. According to a view that has held sway among scientists, humanists, and the general public for centuries, science is objective (Snow 1964) and ethics are subjective—hence, scientists need not deal with ethical issues and concerns when conducting research. Ethical and social questions, according to this view, occur in the applications of science, but these questions have little to do with conducting research. Humanists, politicians, and the public can grapple with the ethical (or moral) aspects of research; the main task of the scientist is to do research for its own sake (Rescher 1965). (Note that, although some scholars distinguish between "ethics" and "morality," in this book we use these terms interchangeably.)

While it is important for scientists to strive for objectivity, this does not mean that ethical questions, problems, and concerns have no place in research conduct. The idea that ethics is an important part of research is by no means new. Charles Babbage (1830 [1970]) wrote about the lack of ethics, honesty, and integrity in British science. During the Nuremberg trials after World War II, researchers became painfully aware of the need for ethical reflection on research when the world learned about the horrors of Nazi research on human beings. Such physicists as Albert Einstein and Robert Oppenheimer came to terms with their moral responsibilities in the war effort, both as supporters of research on atomic weapons during the war and as advocates for the peaceful use of atomic energy after the war (Zuckerman 1966).

In the 1960s, ecologist Rachel Carson published *Silent Spring* (1961), which alerted the public to the dangers of pesticides and helped to launch the environmentalist movement. Clinical researcher Henry Beecher (1966) published an influential essay in the *New England Journal of Medicine* that exposed unethical or questionable research involving human subjects, including the now infamous Willowbrook experiments, where children were exposed to hepatitus virus. In 1972, the public learned about the Tuskegee syphilis study, and congressional investigations exposed many ethical problems, including violations of informed consent and failure to provide subjects with adequate medical care (Jones 1981). (Chapter 9 discusses this case in depth.)

Today, however, there are many reasons why scientists need to pay special attention to research ethics in their own work and in teaching students about how to conduct research (Shamoo 1989, Sigma Xi 1986, Shamoo and Dunigan 2000). First, modern research is not a solitary activity. Scientists collaborate with students and colleagues in their own institutions as well as with other scientists in other institutions (Merton 1973, Ziman 1984). Although Isaac Newton was able to develop his laws of motion with little help from other physicists, today's physicists work together in research teams. It is not uncommon for more than a hundred researchers from across the world to collaborate on a single experiment in high-energy physics. Collaboration is also important in the evaluation of research proposals and projects that occurs in peer review. Peer review functions as a gate-keeping mechanism to ensure that published research or research proposals meet certain research standards. Because scientists must collaborate in conducting research and in peer review, they need to adhere to standards of conduct that promote the goals of research as well as effective collaboration (Hull 1988). Thus, ethical concepts and principles, such as honesty, integrity, trust, accountability, respect, confidentiality, and fairness, play a key role in shaping research conduct within science (Resnik

1998a, Macrina 2000, Panel on Scientific Responsibility 1992, National Academy of Sciences 1994, LaFollette 1992, AAAS-ABA 1988).

Second, research always takes place within a social context. Various social, economic, cultural, religious, and political interests influence research goals, resources, and practices. Most universities and research organizations would not exist without an ample supply of public and private funds. Money plays a crucial role in deciding whether a particular problem will be studied, who will study it, how it will be studied, and even whether the results will be published. For example, many illnesses are not sufficiently studied because of a lack of funding, which in the private sector is a function of how profitable it would be to develop a treatment for the illness. Pharmaceutical companies tend to invest heavily in studying diseases that afflict many people, such as heart disease or hypertension, while virtually ignoring illnesses that affect fewer people, such as personality disorders and malnutrition. Cultural and political interests, not just economic interests, can also influence the research process. For example, research in HIV/AIDS languished during the 1980s but took off during the 1990s, due in large part to intense lobbying efforts by AIDS activists. U.S. government funding for AIDS research is now over $1 billion annually, outpacing even cancer research. In contrast, anti-abortion activists pushed for a ban on the use of fetal tissue in federally funded research. Although there have been some changes and interpretations in this regulation, it still poses a significant barrier to research on embryonic stem cells. One of the biggest challenges facing scientists today is how to conduct objective research despite its economic, political, social, cultural, and religious aspects (Resnik 1998a, Longino 1990, Ziman 1984).

Because science takes place within society, scientists must strive to earn the public's support and trust. We use the results of research to address practical problems in medicine, engineering, agriculture, industry, and public policy. If these results are erroneous or unreliable, then people may be killed or harmed, money and resources may be misused or wasted, and we may enact misguided laws or policies. Research results also play an important role in public education. School-age children, as well as adults, learn about science every day, and science can have a profound impact on how they view the world. Because science can influence how we relate to each other, to society, and to nature, it is important for research results to be reliable and relevant. Together, these applications and implications of science entail duties of public responsibility and accountability (Resnik 1998a,b, National Academy of Sciences 1994, Shrader-Frechette 1994).

A third reason why scientists should pay special attention to research ethics involves the highly publicized and politically charged events that have called special attention to the importance of ethics, both within the research community and in science's interactions with society:

- Allegations of fraud in a paper coauthored by Nobel Laureate David Baltimore on foreign genes and antibody formation, as well as cold fusion research, in the National Surgical Breast and Bowel Project, and in the Strategic Defense Initiative (SDI)

- Priority disputes, such as the debate between Robert Gallo and Luc Montagnier over the discovery of HIV
- Questions about authorship and the ownership of intellectual property, including disputes about biotechnology and information technology patents
- Conflicts of interest in research and in access to data
- Poor record keeping or incompetence in the Federal Bureau of Investigation's crime lab
- Debates over clinical trials research, such as HIV research, fetal tissue research, stem cell research, and research on the mentally ill
- Moral questions about the use of animals in research
- Revelations of secret government radiation experiments
- New developments in human genetics and reproduction, such as genetic testing and diagnosis, DNA typing, gene therapy, and cloning
- New developments in agricultural biotechnology, such as genetically modified foods and genetically engineered animals
- IQ research, including Herrnstein and Murray's controversial book *The Bell Curve* (1994)
- Important policy debates involving scientific research, such as global warming, population control, public health, gun control, passive smoking, alternative medicine, and the regulation of foods, drugs, and nutraceuticals

And the list goes on (Broad and Wade 1982 [1993], LaFollette 1992, 1994a,b, Pascal 2000, Steneck 1999, Shamoo and Dunigan 2000, Advisory Committee 1995, Resnik 1998a,b, Kevles 1998, American Association for the Advancement of Science 1991).

Fourth, science's evolving relationship with private industry has raised many ethical issues in research, because the academic values of objectivity and openness frequently clash with the business interests of profit and competitiveness. Science–industry collaborations can create issues concerning conflicts of interest, biases, secrecy, insider trading, and social responsibility as well as intellectual property disputes (Bowie 1994, Spier 1995, Rule and Shamoo, 1997, Resnik 1998a). These issues have become increasingly important as private investments in research and development have skyrocketed in recent years: in the United States, total private funding of research and development (R&D) rose from $50 billion annually in 1980 to $100 billion annually in 1995. As we begin the twenty-first century, private funding of R&D is probably more than $200 billion per year. Private funding of R&D now accounts for more than 60% of all R&D funding (Shamoo 1989, Jaffe 1996, National Science Foundation, 1997).

For these reasons and many others, universities, funding agencies, research institutions, professional societies, and scientists are now very much aware of the importance of ethics in research. There have been a variety of responses to these ethical concerns, including workshops and conferences; books, journals articles, and edited volumes; debates about the definition of "research misconduct"; investigations of misconduct in research; revisions of journal policies; drafts and revisions of professional codes of ethics in research; and education in research ethics, including formal courses and seminars.

SCIENCE AS A PROFESSION

In discussions of ethics in research among scientists, science scholars, ethicists, and policy analysts, there has been a broad and emerging consensus that research ethics can be understood according to the professional model (Resnik 1998a, Shrader-Frechette 1994). According to this approach, most contemporary science is a profession like medicine, law, accounting, or engineering. Professions have some common social and moral characteristics (Davis 1995a). First, a profession is more than an occupation; it is a career or vocation. The first people to be recognized as professionals were physicians and ministers, who viewed themselves as being "called" to serve and devoted their lives to doing good works for society. Second, because professionals provide valuable goods and services, they have public responsibilities and can be held publicly accountable. Physicians, for example, have professional duties to promote not only the health of their patients but also the public's health. Third, although professionals have public responsibilities, they are also granted a great deal of autonomy; society allows professionals to be self-regulating. Professionals can make their own standards and rules, provided that they obey the law and fulfill the public responsibilities. Physicians, for example, set their own standard of care and determine what it takes to become a qualified member of the profession. Fourth, ethical standards play a key role in professional conduct by promoting self-regulation and public responsibility. Most professions have developed codes of ethics (or codes of conduct) as a public expression of their commitment to ethical behavior. Ever since the time of Hippocrates (circa 460–377 BC), physicians have sworn allegiance to a code of conduct. Although modern codes of conduct in health care differ from the Hippocratic Oath, they still play a key role in governing professional conduct. Finally, professionals are recognized as having expertise. Physicians, for example, have expertise when it comes to diagnosing, treating, and preventing diseases (Bayles 1988).

Prior to the Scientific Revolution of the 1500s through the 1700s, science was more of an avocation than a vocation. Scientists often worked in isolation and financed their own research. They did not publish very frequently—the printing press was not invented until the mid 1400s—and when they did, their works were not peer reviewed. There were no professional scientific societies or journals until the mid 1600s. Universities taught only a small number of scientific subjects, and many scientists could master several different subjects. For example, Newton made contributions in mechanics, astronomy, optics, and mathematics (Newton 1687 [1995]). Private businesses and governments saw little reason to invest in research. Science also did not have a great deal of social status or impact: the church and the state battled for social influence and power (Ziman 1984, Burke 1995).

But all of that changed in the 1800s and 1900s. Now at the turn of the twenty-first century there are thousands of scientific societies and professional journals. Peer review plays a key role in funding and publications decisions. As noted above, scientists now work in research groups, which may include laboratory assistants and data analysts as well as postdoctoral, graduate, and undergraduate students. Universities now offer study in hundreds of different scientific subjects, and it is virtually impossible to achieve scientific expertise without specialization. Governments and private corporations now invest billions of dollars each year in science. Science has become the most influential social institution in society (Ziman 1984). Most of the technologies and many of the ideas in our modern world are the direct or indirect result of scientific research. Scientists now publish millions of articles a year, and the information boom continues to increase. Scientists give expert testimony to congressional committees and government agencies, and they provide advice to presidents, governors, generals, and corporate executives. Children learn about science in school, and most professional careers require some type of scientific and technical knowledge.

Science is now also a sizable part of the world's economy: total (private and public) R&D investments account for about 2.5% of the gross domestic product (GDP) in developed countries such as the United States, United Kingdom, and Germany (May 1998). As we enter the twenty-first century and move into the information economy, investments in R&D are likely to continue an upward trend that began in World War II (Dickson 1988). Literally millions of scientists are employed in universities, research institutions, private laboratories, or other organizations that conduct research (National Science Foundation 1997). It is estimated that there are more scientists alive today than all of the scientists who have lived during the past 2,500 years of human history (Dickson 1988).

For better or worse, the modern age is a scientific age. These increases in science's power carry added social responsibilities, and science should now be regarded as a profession, of which science has all the characteristics: it is a career, entails public responsibilities, is self-regulating, and has ethical standards, and scientists have expertise and intellectual authority. Ethical standards can play an important role in research by promoting the goals of science, such as pursuing objective knowledge and solving practical problems; by promoting cooperation and collaboration among scientists; and by helping to boost the public's trust in science. Many scientific disciplines have developed codes of ethics to express their commitment to ethics (Resnik 1998a). To understand professional conduct in science, we therefore need to have a better understanding of ethics.

WHAT IS ETHICS?

Although there are many different definitions of "ethics," for our purposes we will focus on four senses of the term: (1) ethics as standards of conduct that distinguish between right and wrong, good and bad, and so on; (2) ethics as an academic discipline that studies standards of conduct; (3) ethics as an approach to decision making; and (4) ethics as a state of character. This book focuses on 1, 2, and 4, but we also briefly mention some important points about item 3.

Ethics as an academic discipline is a branch of philosophy (moral philosophy) that is concerned with answering age-old questions about duty, honor, integrity, virtue, justice, the good life, and so on. The questions asked by moral philosophy are normative (rather than descriptive) in that they have to do with how one ought to live or how society ought to be structured. Several disciplines in the human sciences, such as psychology, sociology, anthropology, and political science, take a descriptive approach to ethical questions in that they attempt to describe and explain ethical beliefs, attitudes, and behaviors. Although facts pertaining to beliefs, attitudes, and behaviors can have some bearing on these normative questions, they cannot, by themselves, solve ethical questions because solving these problems requires some assessment of values.

The study of ethics can be subdivided into theoretical (or normative) ethics, which studies general theories, concepts, and principles of ethics; meta-ethics, which studies the meaning and justification of ethical words, concepts, and principles; and applied (or practical) ethics, which studies ethical questions that arise in specific situations or areas of conduct, such as medicine, business, and so on (Frankena 1973). Research ethics is a branch of applied ethics that studies the ethical problems, dilemmas, and issues that arise in the conduct of research.

In this book we do not explore meta-ethical issues in great depth, but we mention one issue that has some relevance for research ethics. One of the key questions of meta-ethics is whether ethical standards are universal (Pojman 1995, Frankena 1973). According to one school of thought known as objectivism, the same ethical (or moral) standards apply to all people at all times in all situations. A contrasting school of thought known as relativism holds that different ethical standards apply to different people in different situations: there are no universal moral rules or values. We mention this issue here because there are some situations in research ethics where one must take a stand on the relativism/objectivism dispute (Angell 1997a,b, Resnik 1998b; Emanuel et al. 2000). For example, different countries have different views about human rights, including the right to informed consent and the right to medical care. Should a researcher in a developing nation conduct research that violates Western standards pertaining to informed consent or that provides subjects with less than the Western standard of care? Although we believe that there are some universal standards of research ethics, we recognize that difficult problems and issues can arise in applying those standards to particular situations.

Returning to our focus on the first sense of ethics, ethics as a standard of conduct, it is important to compare and contrast ethics and the law. Laws, or legal standards of conduct, are like ethical standards in several ways. First, laws, like ethics, tell people how they ought to behave. Second, ethical and legal standards share many concepts and terms, such as duty, responsibility, negligence, rights, benefits, harms, and so forth. Third, the methods of reasoning used in law and ethics are quite similar: both disciplines give arguments and counterarguments, analyze concepts and principles, and discuss cases and examples.

However, ethics differ from laws in several important ways as well. First, actions or policies that are legal may still be unethical. For instance, it may be perfectly legal to not give credit to someone who makes a major contribution to a research project, but this action would still be unethical because it would violate principles of fairness and honesty. Because laws must be enforceable, and they are usually based on some type of social consensus, they tend to set a minimal standard of conduct. Ethical standards, on the other hand, often deal with moral ideals as well as specific insights or commitments. Hence, ethical standards often transcend legal ones. Second, even laws can be evaluated from an ethical perspective; a law may be unethical. If we consider a law to be unethical, then we may be morally obligated to change the law or perhaps even disobey it. For example, many people who considered South Africa's system of Apartheid to be unethical fought to change the system. Some of them made a conscious decision to protest Apartheid laws and engaged in kind of law breaking known as civil disobedience. Finally, ethical standards tend to be more informal and less arcane and convoluted than legal standards; ethical standards are not usually legalistic. Because ethics and the law are not the same, scientists must consider and weigh both legal and ethical obligations when making ethical decisions (more on this later).

It is also important to distinguish between ethics and politics. Politics, like ethics, deals with norms or standards for human conduct. However, political questions tend to focus on broad issues having to do with the structure of society and group dynamics, whereas ethical questions tend to focus on narrower issues pertaining to the conduct of individuals within society (Rawls 1971). Many of the controversial areas of human conduct have both ethical and political dimensions. For instance, abortion is an ethical issue for a woman trying to decide whether to have an abortion, but it is a political issue for legislators and judges who must decide whether laws against abortion would unjustly invade a woman's sphere of private choice. Thus, distinction between ethics and politics is not absolute (Rawls 1971). Although this book focuses on the ethics of research, many of the issues it covers have political dimensions as well, for example, funding for stem cell research.

The distinction between ethics and religion is also important for our purposes. Ethical theories and religious traditions have much in common in that they both propose standards of human conduct and provide some account of the meaning and value of life. Many people use religious teachings, texts, and practices (such as prayer) for ethical guidance. We do not intend to devalue or belittle the importance of religion in inspiring and influencing ethical conduct. However, we stress that ethics is not the same as religion. First, people from different religious backgrounds can agree on some basic ethical principles and concepts. Christians, Jews, Muslims, Hindus, and Buddhists can all agree on the importance of honesty, integrity, justice, benevolence, respect for human life, and many other ethical values despite their theological disagreements. Second, the study of ethics, or moral philosophy, is a secular discipline that relies on human reasoning to analyze and interpret ethical concepts and principles. Although some ethicists adopt a theological approach to moral questions and issues, most use secular methods and theories and reason about arguments and conclusions. While our book focuses on research ethics, many of the issues it addresses have religious aspects as well. For instance, throughout history different religions have opposed specific scientific ideas, such as heliocentric astronomy and the theory of evolution. Today, various churches have taken developed opinions on specific issues in research, such as cloning, assisted reproduction, DNA patenting, and genetic engineering.

ETHICAL CONCEPTS, THEORIES, AND PRINCIPLES

For a better understanding of some of the different approaches to ethics, it is useful to provide a rough overview of some key ethical theories, concepts, and principles. Philosophers, theologians, and others have defended a number of different ethical theories, concepts, and principles. What these theories have in common is that they provide an overall framework for specifying ethical norms and interpreting ethical concepts. No theory, in our opinion, is the "single true theory," although different theories capture important moral insights and intuitions. Thus, we encourage you not to analyze all problems from a single theoretical point of view, but rather to consider different theoretical perspectives. The theories we mention throughout this text are as follows:

Kantianism

Kantianism is a theory developed by the German Enlightenment philosopher Immanuel Kant (1724–1804), which has been revised and fine-tuned by modern-day Kantians, such as Korsgaard (1996). The basic insight of Kantianism is that ethical conduct is a matter of choosing to live one's life according to moral principles or rules. The concept of a moral agent plays an important role in Kant's theory: a moral agent is someone who can distinguish between right and wrong and can make and follow moral laws. Moral agents (or persons) are autonomous (or self-governing) insofar as they can choose to live according to moral rules. For Kant, the motives of agents (or reasons for action) matter a great deal. One should do the right action for the right reason (Pojman 1995). What is the right thing to do? According to Kant (1753 [1981]), the right thing to do is embodied in a principle known as the categorical imperative (CI), which has several versions. The universality version of CI, which some have argued is simply a more sophisticated version of the Golden Rule, holds that one should act in such as way that one's conduct could become a universal law for all people. In making a moral decision, one needs to ask, "What if everybody did this?" According to the respect-for-humanity version of CI, one should treat humanity, whether in one's own person or in other persons, always as an end in itself, never only as a means. The basic insight here is that human beings have inherent (or intrinsic) moral dignity or worth:

we should not abuse, manipulate, harm, exploit, or deceive people in order to achieve specific goals. As we discuss later, this concept has important applications in the ethics of human research.

Utilitarianism

English philosopher/reformists Jeremy Bentham (1748–1832) and John Stuart Mill (1806–1873) developed the theory of utilitarianism in the 1800s. The basic insight of utilitarianism is that the right thing to do is to produce the best overall consequences for the most people (Pojman 1995, Frankena 1973). Philosophers have introduced the term "consequentialism" to describe theories such as utilitarianism that evaluate actions and policies in terms of their outcomes or consequences (good or bad). "Deontological" theories, on the other hand, judge actions or policies insofar as they conform to rules or principles; these theories do not appeal to consequences directly. For instance, Kantianism is a deontological theory because it holds that actions are morally correct insofar as they result from moral motives and conform to moral laws. Different theorists emphasize different types of consequences. Mill and Bentham thought that the consequences that mattered were happiness and unhappiness. According to Mill's Greatest Happiness Principle, one should produce the greatest balance of happiness for the most people (Mill 1861 [1979]). Different theorists also stress different types of evaluation. For instance, act-utilitarians argue that individual actions should be judged according to their utility, whereas rule-utilitarians believe that we should assess the utility of rules, not actions. A number of different approaches to social problems are similar to utilitarianism in that they address the consequences of actions and policies. Cost–benefit analysis examines economic costs and benefits, and risk-assessment theory addresses risks and benefits. All consequentialist theories, including utilitarianism, depend on empirical evidence relating to the probable outcomes. In this book, we discuss how many important ethical questions in research and science policy can be analyzed from a utilitarian perspective.

Natural Law

The natural law approach has a long tradition dating back to the time of the ancient Greeks. The Stoics and Aristotle (384–322 bc) both adopted natural law approaches. According to this view, some things, such as life, happiness, health, and pleasure, are naturally good, while other things, such as death, suffering, disease, and pain, are naturally evil (Pojman 1995). Our basic ethical duty is to perform actions that promote or enhance those things that are natural goods and to avoid doing things that result in natural evils. One of the most influential natural law theorists, Thomas Aquinas (1225–1274), developed a theological approach to the natural law theory and argued that the natural law is based on God's will. Most natural laws theorists hold that moral rules are objective, because they are based on natural or divine order, not on human ideas or interests. Natural law theorists, like Kantians, also believe that motives matter in morality. Thus, a concept that plays a key role in natural law theory is the concept of double effect: we may be held morally responsible for the intended or foreseeable effects of our actions but not for the unintended or unforeseeable effects. For example, suppose a physician gives a dying patient morphine in order to relieve his pain and suffering, and the patient dies. The physician would not be condemned for killing the patient if he did not intend to bring about the patient's death or could not have foreseen that death would result from the dose of morphine. One of the important challenges for the natural law theorist is how to respond to developments in science and technology, such as medicine, genetic engineering and assisted reproduction, that can overturn the natural order.

Virtue Ethics

The virtue ethics approach also has a long history dating to antiquity. Virtue theorists, unlike Kantians and utilitarians, focus on the fourth sense of "ethics" mentioned earlier, developing good character traits. Their key insight is that ethical conduct has to do with living a life marked by excellence and virtue (Aristotle 330 BC? [1984], Pojman 1995). One develops morally good character traits by practicing them: a person who acts honestly develops the virtue of honesty, a person who performs courageous acts develops the virtue of courage, and so on. Although virtue theorists do not emphasize the importance of moral duties, we cannot become virtuous if we routinely fail to fulfill our moral obligations or duties. Some of the frequently mentioned virtues include honesty, honor, courage, benevolence, fairness, humility, and temperance.

Integrity, according to this approach, is a kind of meta-virtue: we have the virtue of integrity insofar as our character traits, beliefs, decisions, and actions form a coherent, consistent whole. If we have integrity, our actions reflect our beliefs and attitudes; we "talk the talk" and "walk the walk." Moreover, if we have integrity, we are sincere in that our actions and decision reflect deeply held convictions. However, because we can develop our beliefs, attitudes, and character traits over the course of our lifetime, integrity is more than simply sticking to our convictions, come what may. But changes in beliefs, attitudes, and traits of character should maintain the integrity of the whole person (Whitbeck 1998). Integrity has become an important concept in research ethics. Although many people use it as simply another word for "honesty," "honor," "ethics," it has its own meaning.

Natural Rights

The natural rights approach emerged with the development of property rights in Europe during the 1600s. The British philosopher John Locke (1632–1704) founded this approach, and it is has been refined by many different theorists in the twentieth century. According to this view, all people have some basic rights to life, liberty, property, freedom of thought and expression, freedom of religion, and so on (Locke 1784 [1980]). These rights are "natural" in that they do not depend on any other duties, obligations, or values. The U.S. Constitution, with its emphasis on rights, reflects the natural rights approach to ethics and politics. Although most theorists agree that it is important to protect individual interests and well-being, there is an inherent tension in ethical and policy analysis between respecting individual rights (or interests) and promoting what is best for society. The harm principle is a widely accepted policy for restricting individual rights (Feinberg 1973). According to this rule, society may restrict individual rights in order to prevent harms (or unreasonable risks of harm) to other people. A more controversial restriction on individual rights is known as paternalism. According to this principle, society may restrict individual rights in order to promote the best interests of individuals. Drug regulations are paternalistic in that they are designed to protect individuals, as well as society, from harm (Feinberg 1973).

Social Contract Theory

Social contract theory began with the English philosopher Thomas Hobbes (1588–1679); it was later developed by the French philosopher Jean-Jacques Rousseau (1712–1778) and helped to inspire the French Revolution. The key insight provided by this theory is that moral standards are conventions or rules that people adopt in forming a just society (Rawls 1971). People accept moral and political rules because they recognize them as mutually advantageous. According to Hobbes, people form civil society because life without society is "a war of all against all" and is "solitary, poor, nasty, brutish, and short" (Hobbes 1651 [1962], p. 100). We discuss in this book how this Hobbesian insight also applies to science: many of the rules of scientific ethics are conventions designed to promote effective collaboration and cooperation in research (Resnik 1998a).

Divine Command Theory

The divine command theory can trace its history to the beginning of human civilization. As long as they have worshipped deities, people have believed that they should follow the commands of the deities. Many religious texts, such as the Bible, contain claims about divine commandments as well as stories about sin (disobeying God's commands) and redemption from sin. As we discussed above, many natural law theorists base moral laws on divine commands. Many theologians and philosophers other than Thomas Aquinas have also defended the divine command approach to ethics. Although we do not criticize the divine command theory here, we note that many philosophers have challenged the connection between morality and religion. Religion may inspire ethical conduct even if it is not the foundation for moral concepts and principles (Pojman 1995). Moreover, many of the ethical commands that one finds in religious texts, such as Jesus' command to love your neighbor as yourself, can be accepted by people from different religious backgrounds.

In addition to these different theories, ethicists have developed some basic moral principles. Most of these principles are supported by more than one ethical theory and agree with commonsense intuitions (National Commission 1979, Beauchamp and Childress 1994, Fox and DeMarco 1990). We may also consider them to be prima facie principles: although they have strong theoretical and intuitive support, they are not absolute rules (Ross 1930). Although we should follow these principles, they may conflict, and we may have to choose between them sometimes:

1. Nonmaleficence: Do not inflict unjustified harm to ourselves or other people. The word "unjustified" is important here because some harms can be justified in relation to their benefits: the harms associated with a visit to the dentist can be justified in relation to the long-term benefit to our dental health.

2. Beneficence: Promote one's own well-being and benefit others. Two interrelated concepts that play a large role in applying these first two principles are the concepts of "harm" and "benefit." According to a standard view, benefits and harms can be understood in terms of interests: to benefit someone is to promote or advance their interests; to harm someone is to undermine or threaten their interests. An interest is something that any rational person would want or need, such as food, shelter, health, love, self-esteem, freedom from pain or suffering, and so forth.

3. Autonomy: Allow rational individuals to make their own decisions and act on them. A rational individual is someone who is capable of making an informed, responsible choice.

4. Justice: "Justice" is a complex concept that we will not analyze here. We will simply note that there are formal as well as material principles of justice. Formal principles, such as "Treat equals equally, unequals, unequally," and "Give people what they deserve," merely set logical conditions for applying principles that have more definite content, such as, "Allocate resources fairly." Some of the approaches to resource distribution include equality ("distribute equally"), need ("distribute according to need"), merit ("distribute according to desert or merit"), chance ("distribute randomly"), and utility ("distribute resources so as to promote utility").

These four moral principles, one could argue, also imply a variety of subsidiary obligations, such as duties of honesty, fidelity, respect for privacy, respect for human dignity, and obligations not to lie, cheat, steal, kill, maim, coerce, deceive, exploit, and so on.

ETHICAL DECISION MAKING

Having described some important ethical theories, concepts, and principles, we are now prepared to discuss ethical decision making. An ethical decision (or choice) occurs in a situation where there are at least two different options, and the options are not ethically neutral; that is, the choice is morally significant. For example, selecting apples at the grocery store is probably not an ethical decision. However, deciding whether or not to give blood probably is an ethical decision, because several moral theories and principles would recommend that you should help others by giving blood.

Ethical decisions that are particularly vexing and uncomfortable are known as ethical dilemmas. An ethical dilemma is a situation where there are at least two different options that appear to be just as good (or bad) from a moral point of view (Fox and DeMarco 1990). That is, different principles or theories may recommend different options; the principles or theories may conflict in this particular situation. For example, suppose that a person, Alice, is faced with giving blood or honoring a prior obligation to attend a committee meeting. The principle of beneficence (or the moral theory known as utilitarianism) may recommend giving blood, but by doing so, she would break a promise or display a lack of honor or integrity. What should she do? Better yet, how should she decide what to do? There are many different ways of making decisions: we can take an economic, legal, or political perspective on the decision. We can consult an astrologer or seer. But if our goal is to make an ethical choice or decision, then we should choose the option that is, all things considered, the best or right thing to do. Ethical reasoning is impartial in that it takes all of the relevant interests, facts, and values into account, examines different aspects of the issue, and attempts to arrive at an optimal solution. The following is a basic method for ethical decision making (Resnik 1998a, Swazey and Bird 1997, Weil 1993, Fox and DeMarco 1990):

Step 1: State or define the problem. For Alice, the problem could be, "Should I give blood or attend the committee meeting?"

Step 2: Gather relevant information. Alice may want to know the needs for blood in general or her type in particular, her medical status for giving blood (e.g., is she well enough to give blood?), the nature of the meeting (e.g., how important is the meeting?), her role in the meeting (e.g., how important is it for her to be there?), and so forth. It is always important to gather relevant information, because ignorance of the relevant facts often leads to poor decision making.

Step 3: Delineate or construct different options. Alice needs to know what she can do. The obvious actions are "give blood" or "go to the meeting." But she needs to consider or imagine alternative choices, such as going to the meeting but giving blood at some other time, rescheduling the meeting, and so forth.

Step 4: Relate the different options to the different values or principles that are at stake. In Alice's case, "help others" supports the option "give blood"; "honor your commitments" supports the option "go to the meeting." Both principles may support a third option, such as "give blood at another time and go to the meeting." In some cases, the values or principles that have some bearing on the situation may include legal, economic, institutional, professional, personal, or other considerations.

Step 5: Evaluate the different options in light of different values or principles as well as the relevant facts. Here Alice must take everything into account, carefully and critically examine the different options, and decide what is the best thing to do. This is often the most difficult part of making a decision because we may have to prioritize different values or principles in the situation. For instance, if it is impossible for Alice to give blood and go to the meeting, she may need to decide that honoring her commitments takes precedence in this case. Facts can play a key role in deciding what is the "best" option. For instance, if the meeting is not very important and Alice can afford to miss it, and if there is an urgent need for her blood type, then she may decide to skip the meeting, provided that she notifies people that she will not be there.

Step 6: Make a decision and act.

We recommend this procedure as a useful method for decision making, although we recognize that real-world decisions sometimes deviate from this stepwise progression. For example, sometimes we may go from step 1 to step 2 to step 3 and realize that the problem is not the same as we first thought or that a new problem has arisen. So then we may restate the problem or define a new problem. Perhaps we progress to step 5 and then realize that we need more information. We could even proceed through steps 1–6 in a very short time without being aware that our reasoning process conforms to these steps.

We also recommend that people faced with difficult choices seek advice or guidance from friends, peers, mentors, or other people who have faced similar situations. It is often helpful to obtain an outside opinion in order to overcome our own biases or shortcomings. Although we emphasize reasoning as the best way to make decisions, we recognize that reason has its limitations. If reasoning does not lead to a clear answer, the wisest course of action may be to appeal to other sources of guidance, such as intuition (or emotion), spiritual guidance, or chance.

Because this approach to decision making deals with possible conflicts of values or principles, it reintroduces the issue of relativism mentioned above. Step 5 requires the decision maker to prioritize values or principles, and it is possible that different values or principles may have different priorities in different situations. If this is the case, then one could argue that all moral decisions depend on factors inherent in the situation. Thus, the right thing to do varies from one situation to the next; there are no universal values or principles. The view that what makes something right or wrong depends on factors inherent in the given situation is known as situation ethics. Although we acknowledge that ethical decision making is situational (or situation specific), we do not endorse situation ethics, primarily because we believe it is not consistent with a commitment to integrity, for two reasons.

First, when people make an ethical decision, they may be held accountable for their choices and methods. That is, they may be asked to defend their decisions to peers, supervisors, students, the media, or even before a court of law. In justifying decisions, they must be able to give reasons for them. Chief among these reasons would be the relevant facts as well as important principles or values. A person with integrity is someone whose beliefs, attitudes, and actions form a coherent whole. One may show a lack of integrity by being inconsistent or insincere. A person who cites values or principles that have no bearing on the decision would lack integrity by being insincere. Acting with integrity in justifying a decision requires a sincere commitment to standards that transcend that decision.

Second, situation ethics lead to policies that lack integrity. To justify a public policy, such as a regulation or law, we also need to appeal reasons, which include facts as well as values and principles. If every policy decision is made on its own merits without appealing to values or principles that transcend particular situations, then it is likely that these decisions will be inconsistent. For example, imagine a university admissions committee that decided every candidate on his or her own qualifications, without appealing to any criteria for admission. The committee's decisions could be very inconsistent: a person with low standardized test scores may be denied admission in one situation but not another. To avoid inconsistency and promote integrity, the committee needs to adopt and employ criteria that apply to different decisions; they cannot make decisions on a purely situational basis.

PRINCIPLES FOR ETHICAL CONDUCT IN RESEARCH

We now briefly describe some principles for ethical conduct in research. The principles we describe here, like the principles mentioned above, are prima facie rules. Each of these principles can be justified from a theoretical and intuitive point of view, and researchers should follow them, provided that they do not conflict with other principles (Resnik 1996a, 1998a,b). Other things being equal, follow these principles. When the principles conflict in a practical decision, use the decision-making method described above to settle conflicts.

Although we believe these principles make intuitive sense to most researchers, we also offer a theoretical justification for them (Resnik 1996a, 1998a). First, many of these principles are justified because they have a direct bearing on the goals of research, including developing objective knowledge, solving practical problems, providing an understanding of nature, and making successful predictions. It would be virtually impossible to achieve these goals without a strong commitment to honesty in research, one of the most important principles of research ethics. Second, many of the principles can be justified because they promote cooperation, collaboration, and trust among researchers, which help promote the goals of science (Resnik 1996a, Hull 1988). For instance, researchers need principles for allocating credit ensure that selfish researchers do not take advantage of altruistic colleagues and so that researchers may be held accountable for mistakes or misdeeds. Third, many of the principles can be justified on the grounds that they promote social responsibility and the public's support for science (Shrader-Frechette 1994). For instance, scientists should make an effort to educate and inform the public to promote the public's understanding of science, which can promote public support for science. Fourth, many of the principles can be justified insofar as they meet legal requirements (Panel on Scientific Responsibility 1992). For example, a researcher who lies on a federal grant application would be violating federal laws that prohibit fraud. Fifth, many of the principles can be justified on broader moral or ethical grounds (Gert 1993, Pellegrino 1992, Resnik 1996a, 1998a). For example, the moral principles of autonomy, beneficence, non-maleficence, and justice all support rules for protecting human subjects in research (Levine 1988, Emanuel et al. 2000).

Guidelines for Ethical Research Conduct

Honesty: Strive for honesty in all scientific communications. Honestly report data, results, methods and procedures, publication status, research contributions, and potential conflicts of interest. Do not fabricate, falsify, or misrepresent data.

Objectivity: Strive for objectivity in experimental design, data analysis, data interpretation, peer review, personnel decisions, grant writing, expert testimony, and other aspects of research where objectivity is expected or required. Avoid or minimize bias.

Integrity: Act with integrity in all aspects of the research process.

Carefulness: Avoid careless errors and negligence; carefully and critically examine your own work and the work of your peers. Keep good records of research activities, such as data collection, research design, and correspondence with agencies or journals.

Openness: Share data, results, ideas, tools, and resources. Be open to criticism and new ideas.

Confidentiality: Protect confidential communications, such as papers or grants submitted for publication, personnel records, trade or military secrets, and patient records.

Respect for Colleagues: Respect your colleagues and students; avoid harming them and promote their well-being. Treat your colleagues fairly.

Respect for Intellectual Property: Honor patents, copyrights, and other forms of intellectual property. Do not use unpublished data, methods, or results without permission. Give credit where credit is due but not where it is not due.

Freedom: Institutions, governments, and researchers should promote freedom of thought and inquiry.

Social Responsibility: Strive to promote social good and prevent or mitigate social harms through research, public education, and advocacy.

Efficiency: Make efficient use of human, financial, and technological resources.

Education: Help to educate, mentor, and advise the next generation of scientists.

Competence: Maintain and improve your own professional competence and expertise through lifelong education and learning; take steps to promote competence in science as a whole.

Equality of Opportunity: Promote equality of opportunity for science students and colleagues; avoid discrimination in admissions decisions, personnel decisions, and peer review decisions.

Legality: Know and obey relevant laws and governmental policies.

Animal Care: Show proper respect and care for animals when using them in research. Do not conduct unnecessary or poorly designed animal experiments.

Human Subjects Protection: When conducting research on human subjects, minimize harms and risks and maximize benefits; respect human dignity, privacy, and autonomy; take special precautions with vulnerable populations; and strive to distribute fairly the benefits and burdens of research.

Many of these principles may seem familiar to readers who have some experience with professional codes of ethics in research, government funding requirements, or journal policies. We recognize that there are now many useful sources of ethical guidance for researchers; our principles should complement but not undermine existing ethics codes and policies. Some readers may wonder whether these principles are redundant or unnecessary, because other rules and guidelines have already been stated publicly. However, we think the principles above have several important uses. First, they may cover problems and issues not explicitly covered by existing rules or guidelines. Second, they can be helpful in interpreting or justifying existing rules and guidelines. Third, they apply to new and emerging disciplines or practices that have not yet established ethical codes.

Institutional Ethics

While most theories of ethics focus on ethical conduct at the level of the individual (Pellegrino 1992), it is also important to address ethical problems, issues, and choices that occur at the institutional level. Because institutional actions can have important impacts on society, and institutional polices can affect the behavior of individuals, institutions have legal and ethical responsibilities (De George 1995). Research institutions, such as universities, have ethical and legal obligations and policies that can either foster or hinder integrity in research (Shamoo and Davis 1989, Shamoo and Dunigan 2000, Berger and Gert 1997). Thus, it is important for institutions to develop policies on research misconduct, data management, conflicts of interest, intellectual property, human subjects research, animal research, radiation safety, biohazards, research compliance, sexual harassment, tenure and promotion, and faculty–student relationships. One of the most important actions that an institution can take to promote research integrity is to support education in the ethical conduct of research. But if institutions do not take responsibility for promoting an ethical research environment, then programs designed to educate individual researchers in ethical conduct will have only a marginal impact.

ETHICS, EDUCATION, AND LEADERSHIP

Before concluding this chapter, we would like to make a few remarks about the importance of leadership in ethical conduct and ethical decision making. If ethical conduct is important in research, then all of the stakeholders in the research, including individual scientists as well as various organizations, have an obligation to promote ethical conduct and ethical decision making (Swazey and Bird 1997, Resnik 1998a, Panel on Scientific Responsibility 1992). Although it is important to promulgate and enforce standards of conduct in research, promoting ethical conduct requires much more than investigating and adjudicating claims of misconduct. Ethics is not police work. By far the most effective way to promote ethical conduct in research is to teach students at all levels about ethics and integrity in research (Swazey and Bird 1997, Weil 1993, Swazey 1993, Bird 1993). Education in research ethics can help students develop moral sensitivity (an awareness of ethical issues and concerns), moral reasoning (the ability to make moral decisions), and moral commitment (the willingness do to the right thing even at some personal cost; Pimple 1995). Although courses, seminars, workshops, and lectures on research ethics can be an effective way of teaching ethics in research, empirical research suggests that role modeling plays a very important role in learning ethical conduct. That is, all of us, including scientists and other professionals, learn professional norms and virtues, in part, by example (Kuhn 1970, Aristotle ca. 330 BC [1984], Kopelman 1999).

Scientists who set ethical examples for their students and colleagues exhibit moral or ethical leadership. Ethical leadership promotes ethical conduct by setting an example and a general tone or attitude in an organization. Organizational leaders can promote an ethical corporate culture or unethical corporate culture, depending on the example they set. If members of an organization (e.g., students, researchers, employees) can see that ethics is important to the leaders of the organization and that the leaders take ethical issues seriously, then members will also value ethical conduct and take ethics seriously (Fraedrich 1991). However, if leaders do not emphasize ethics, or if they engage in unethical practices, such as dishonesty, deception, negligence, and law breaking, then members of their organization will follow their example.

Today, many large corporations have adopted ethics statements that emphasize the importance of ethical leadership (Murphy 1998). Although all researchers should teach ethics by example, it is especially important for researchers who have important leadership or management positions, in academia and private industry, to lead by example and affirm their commitment to ethics in research. Individuals as well as institutions have a responsibility to promote ethics by developing policies and procedures and developing effective leadership (Berger and Gert 1997). Thus, department chairs, laboratory and center directors, section heads, vice presidents, deans, and presidents should all lead by example. By doing so, they can affect the behavior of students, colleagues, and employees and promote an ethical culture. Good leaders inspire learning, creativity, and a sense of duty to society and our civilization.

Some of the characteristics of leadership are ethics, vision, initiative, and realism (Koestenbaum 1991, Gardner 1995). Ethics is by far the most important quality of excellent leadership. Many leaders who lacked ethics, such as Hitler, Genghis Khan, Stalin, and Pol Pot, have wreaked havoc on our civilization. Virtuous or ethical leaders, such as Gandhi, Roosevelt, Martin Luther King, and Mother Teresa, have brought much good to society. Ethical leadership does not imply perfection; even ethical leaders make mistakes. But ethical leaders respond to mistakes by admitting them, learning from them, and taking steps to amend them, not by denying them or covering them up.

The four characteristics of leadership are as follows:

1. Ethics: Ethical leadership requires a whole host of virtues, including honesty, integrity, truthfulness, courage, humility, compassion, fairness, and a willingness to serve others or make sacrifices for the greater good.
2. Vision: More than 100 years ago, George Bernard Shaw said: "You see things; and you say 'why?' But I dream things that never were; and say, 'why not?'" Leaders think in big pictures. They are able to see a general pattern and put it in perspective. This perspective helps frame general solutions. In research, we take specific data sets and try to generalize them to solve a larger problem. Researchers usually are trained to be visionary in their area of research.
3. Initiative: Leaders are creative and courageous, and they take risks. They come up with new ideas and challenge dogmas and traditions. Leaders also accept the consequences of their decisions and initiatives and do not shy from being held accountable.
4. Realism: Leaders have a good sense of what they can and cannot accomplish; although they have vision, they do not indulge in illusions. Being grounded in reality—relying on facts and data—is also a part of being a good scientist. Scientists understand that their credibility will be eroded if they draw conclusions that are not supported by the evidence.

Many researchers have vision, initiative, and realism. This is not surprising, given that science education emphasizes these three characteristics. However, science education should also emphasize the first quality—ethics. Placing more of an emphasis on ethics in science education will be good for science and good for society.

This concludes our first chapter. Although we may not specifically address elsewhere in this book many of the topics addressed in this chapter, we expect that students and teachers will be able to apply this foundational material in the following chapters in understanding and applying discussions of research ethics and in analyzing and discussing the case studies we have included in each chapter.

QUESTIONS FOR DISCUSSION

1. Do you think that most scientists and science students are ethical?
2. When, how, and why are scientists tempted to violate ethical standards in research?

3. What situations in science present the most difficult ethical problems and dilemmas?

4. Do you think researchers should adhere to the same ethical standards that apply to other professions, such as medicine or law? Why or why not?

5. Do you think researchers have ethical duties and responsibilities "over and above" the ethical obligations of ordinary people?

6. Can you think of any principles to add to our guidelines for ethical research conduct? What would they be and how would they be justified? Do you think our list contains some principles that should be omitted or reworded?

7. We have emphasized practical reasoning in our approach to moral decision making. Can you think of any other methods for decision making that may be useful (or that people may sometimes use)? Is reasoning the best method? Why or why not?

8. Do you think that moral theories and principles have some bearing on practical choices and decisions? Why or why not?

2

Collection, Analysis, and Management of Data

Proper management of research conduct is essential to achieving reliable results and maintaining the quality, objectivity, and integrity of research data. The different steps of research should be monitored carefully, and research design should include built-in safeguards to ensure the quality and integrity of research data. This chapter addresses ethical conduct in different steps of the research process: hypothesis formation, research design, literature review, data collection, data analysis, data interpretation, publication, and data storage. This chapter also discusses methods that can help assure the quality, objectivity, and integrity of research data, such as good research practices (GRPs), standard operating procedures (SOPs), peer review, and data audit.

Scientific research is the systematic attempt to describe, explain, and understand the world. While all three main branches of science—physical science, biological science, and social science—study different aspects of the natural world, they share some common methods and procedures. These methods and procedures are designed to achieve the goals of science by helping researchers to acquire accurate knowledge and information. Researchers' compliance with the scientific methods and procedures will minimize falsehoods and biases and maximize truth and objectivity (Cheny 1993). One pillar of the scientific method is the idea that researchers should subject their theories and hypotheses to rigorous tests (Popper 1959). A test is an attempt to gather empirical evidence (or data) that tends to either confirm or disconfirm a theory or hypothesis. Ideas that cannot be tested, such as metaphysical theories or ideological claims, are not scientific hypotheses or theories. Some (but not all) tests involve experiments. In an experiment, a researcher attempts to control the conditions of a test in order to understand statistical or causal relationships between variables or parameters. For an experiment to be rigorous, a researcher must describe it in enough detail that other researchers can obtain the same results by replicating the experimental conditions (Kirk 1995).

Repeatability is important in experimentation because it confirms that others can carry out the methods and procedures used and attain the same data. Repeatability, or lack thereof, provides substance for public debate and inquiry. Private intuitions, hunches, faith, introspection, or insight can play an important role in generating new ideas to test, but they do not constitute rigorous proof. Therefore, all test results in science, whether from controlled experiments, field observations, surveys, epidemiological studies, computer models, or meta-analyses, should be open to public scrutiny and debate. Peer review is one of science's most important methods because it promotes the public scrutiny of hypotheses, theories, and test results. Peer review also plays an important preliminary gatekeeping role, ensuring that interpretations of data are self-consistent and consistent with existing literature. In this manner, peer review can contribute to the quality and integrity of published research. Once a hypothesis or theory becomes well established, it may be said to be a "fact," and it is no longer subjected to rigorous tests. For example, the idea that the Sun is the center of the solar system is now accepted as a fact, but it was a hypothesis during the time of Copernicus (1542 [1995]). Well-established generalizations, such as Newton's laws of motion or the ideal gas laws, are known as laws of nature (Popper 1959, Hempel 1965, Giere 1991, Resnik 1998a).

Research investigators work in different ways to attain new knowledge and have many different motives for conducting research. Most researchers have a deep desire and curiosity to understand the world, to make new discoveries, and to pursue truth. Others want to make an important contribution to the world by improving the human condition or protecting the natural environment. Researchers may also have goals that are less altruistic or noble. Some seek fame, glory, and prestige, and almost all researchers also have strong economic motivations. For most researchers, science is a career and a way to make a living. For example, the U.S. research enterprise consists of more than 2.8 million individuals with master or doctoral degrees, including about 900,000 professionals directly engaged in research (NSF 1997). Therefore, the scientific enterprise is no different from any other business sector of our society, and its performance reflects the values, motives, interests and shortcomings of our culture (Longino 1990). The failure to understand the selfishness, greed, and bias that is as inherent in science as it is in the other social sectors could lead to unrealistic expectations of the research enterprise and impractical rules and policies.

STEPS IN SCIENTIFIC RESEARCH (OR SCIENTIFIC METHOD): RESEARCH PLANNING AND DESIGN OF THE PROTOCOL

To develop new knowledge, one must follow numerous steps in planning the research project and designing the protocols. (A protocol is a set of rules, methods, and procedures used to obtain the objectives of a research project.) Each event in the chain of planning and design of the protocols is necessary to ensure that quality, integrity, and objectivity of the data and final results. Each scientist, whether consciously or unconsciously, follows something like the chain of events described below. In the twentieth century, these events became more formalized and rigid, especially in large projects. Although we present these steps in linear order, some of them may occur concurrently, and researchers sometimes return to earlier steps when revising the project and protocol. The following steps outline the processes that usually comprise a research project (see figure 1).

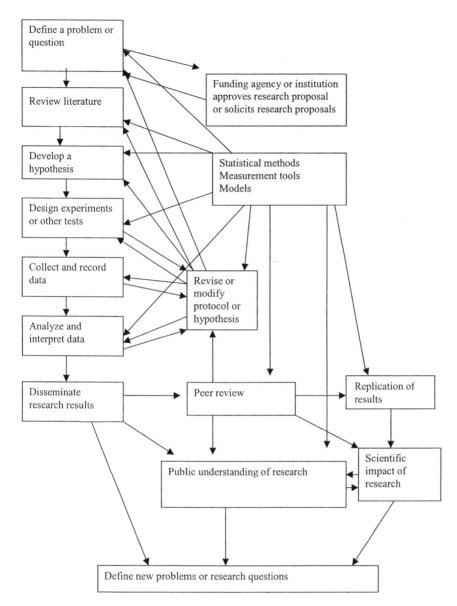

Figure 1. A flow diagram for the research process.

State Objectives of the Research Project

The objectives of a research project are the questions that researchers are attempting to answer or the problems they are attempting to solve (Grinnell 1992). For example, if a research project is addressing the toxicity of a particular drug in laboratory mice, then one of its objectives may be to "test toxicity of certain drug in laboratory mice." The questions answered may be "what is the toxicity of the drug?" The knowledge obtained from answering questions such as this could satisfy the needs of society for improving the health and education of its citizens.

Develop Specific Aims for the Project

Specific aims list the particular goals of the project that need to be achieved in order to attain its overall objective(s). The aims may help meet the objectives of the project either wholly or in part. For example, to test toxicity of a certain drug in animals, one must design specific aims to test for lethal doses, toxic doses, and side effects, and one must describe the species and gender of animals, duration of testing, and types of measurements (such as blood pathology, temperature, biopsies, etc.).

Propose Hypotheses(s)

Hypotheses are statements that are designed to answer research questions (Grinnell 1992). One way to test a hypothesis is to put it in the form of a conditional statement, for example, "If A occurs, then B will occur." The antecedent (A) in the conditional specifies the test conditions; the consequent (B) states predicted results (Giere 1991). Suppose we want to know whether a drug is toxic. The hypothesis could be "drug A is toxic in species S." To test this statement, we can develop a conditional statement that makes predictions about specific results that should occur if the hypothesis is true. For example, the conditional could be "if a drug is suspected to inhibit cancer growth in species S, then we should be able to find the dose where the cancer in the animals used will show stoppage of growth within a month of receiving the dose." If a researcher conducts a test with the dose suspected of stopping tumor growth, but the results are negative, then they tend to disconfirm or disprove the hypothesis. But if a large number of animals show stoppage or reduction in the size of the tumor, then this result confirms the hypothesis. In this example, the test conditions specify the procedure used for administering the drug to the species, and the outcome (or result) is what happens to the animals. Very often, test conditions include unstated or implied assumptions used in conducting research. For example, the type of syringe used to administer the drug, the diet, and overall health of the population may be unstated test conditions. Sometimes researchers may modify a hypothesis based on negative results, unexpected findings, or difficulties in satisfying the test conditions. However, any modifications to the hypothesis should be clearly stated in the project. In other words, the description of the project and protocol must reflect the realities of what has happened—good, bad, or unexpected—to preserve the integrity, objectivity, and quality of the data.

Conduct a Literature Search

The literature search step can be the first step in the overall project. This is an important step for the investigator because it can save the investigator a great deal of time and money by eliminating a flawed objective or a hypothesis. It can also help researchers to learn whether their projects may make an original or worthwhile contribution or whether they merely repeat previous work or would result in knowledge that has little value. A literature search can also help researchers learn about previously used methods, procedures, and experimental designs and can place the project's experimental design and protocol within the known realities of the subject matter. Finally, a thorough literature search can allow researchers to give proper credit to others who have already worked in the area. Failing to acknowledge other relevant work is arrogant and self-serving, and is a type of plagiarism or serious bias if one knowingly or unknowingly claims to be the originator of someone else's idea (Resnik 1998b, Shamoo 1992).

Design Experiments or Tests

As mentioned above, each step is important in the chain of research events to ensure the integrity, objectivity, and quality of the data and results. Each project usually consists of more than one experimental protocol. The design of experiments (and other tests, such as surveys) is one of these crucial steps in preserving the integrity, quality, and objectivity of the research project. It is easy to employ experimental designs that tend to bias the data and results. For example, in the toxicity study mentioned above, using unhealthy or overcrowded mice could affect the data. Because no amount of statistical analysis or interpretation can overcome a design flaw, data that result from a flawed design are virtually useless, and using them can be unethical (Resnik 2000, Irving and Shamoo 1993). Obtaining useless data wastes time, money, and effort, and it can also involve the unnecessary use of human or animal subjects. Indeed, sound experimental design is one of the key ethical principles of human subjects research (Levine 1988, Irving and Shamoo 1993).

Biased designs frequently occur when industries sponsor research projects aimed at promoting their economic interests (Crossen 1994, Porter 1993). For example, researchers at a drug company may be tempted to design a study that would fail to collect adequate data on a side effect of a drug. Because scientists have an obligation to be objective in designing of experiments, the design of an experiment should not only remove bias but test for it. Some forms of bias involve intentional deception (or research misconduct), such as "cooking" the data (the practice of designing an experiment to produce a desired outcome and not subjecting a hypothesis to a rigorous test). Other types of bias are unintentional—scientists, like all human beings, are susceptible to self-deception (Broad and Wade 1982 [1993]). Since it is not always possible to see the biases in one's own work, it is important to solicit critical feedback from colleagues when designing experiments.

Identify and Describe in Detail the Methods That Will Be Used in the Project

In this step, researchers identify and describe methods to be used in the project based on their own methods and previous research, existing literature, laboratory manuals, and other sources. Researchers should follow appropriate standards in applying methods and should keep records of what methods they use and how they use them. During initial tests, researchers should use and identify standard (or well-established) methods, but they can modify these methods to suit new experimental applications or testing procedures. It is important for researchers to note changes they make and state the reasons for them. Furthermore, researchers should not make changes in the middle of an individual test or experiment, because this will bias or corrupt the data. All accidental changes, such as dropping a test tube, should be noted in the laboratory notebook. If researchers perform tests or experiments to produce data for statistical analysis, the procedures should be carried out in the same exact manner each time. Researchers should pick and choose among experiments or tests not to achieve a desired result, but only if they recognize a variable inherent in the protocol that was not first recognized in earlier stages of the project. For example, in testing a new drug in humans, researchers may realize that an unanticipated side effect should be recorded and could therefore change the protocol and design a new experiment that measures this side effect. However, researchers should record these decisions and discuss them in detail at the same time and place where the experiments are recorded, derived, or manipulated.

Collect and Record Data

Proper documentation of the experimental methods, described above, and recording of data are crucial to ensuring accountability in research and keeping a proper paper trail for management and other, future interested parties to authenticate the data. Thorough documentation is also useful for future analysis, verification, and replication by others, or investigations of misconduct, error, or other problems (Shamoo 1989, 1991a,b). Detailed and accurate record keeping is also essential for preserving ownership of intellectual property, such as copyrights and patents. Although this may sound strict to some, we believe that research records can be viewed as quasi-legal documents analogous to medical records, business inventories, or investment accounts.

Raw (or original) data are the records of direct or indirect observations of a test or experiment. Some observations involve the unaided senses, while others involve instruments or devices (Grinnell 1992). For example, when conducting an experiment on rodent maze-learning behavior, the raw data may be the records of the observations made with one's eyes (e.g., the rat completed the maze at a specific time). When testing a metal for electrical conductivity, the raw data would be a record of the output of an ammeter. Raw data, therefore, are those data drawn directly from the experiment or test: data recorded on a laboratory notebook from direct observations, recorder charts, field notes, machine tapes, computer printouts or disks, slides, photographs, and the like.

Researchers record the raw data in a data notebook or its equivalent, such as a computer disk, computer printout, instrument output, and such. The data notebook (or other document) is crucial to future review and to test the integrity and quality of the research output. A laboratory data notebook should be bound and the pages numbered consecutively. Loose-leaf notebooks are hazardous and may tempt a beginning researcher or technician to tear off pages with mistakes. All entries in the laboratory notebook should be made legibly with permanent, nonerasable ink. Ideally, entries should also be signed (or initialed) and dated. Researchers should draw a line through a mistaken entry, without making it completely illegible, and should not use correction fluid. Mistakes that can be traced can be valuable in assessing the progress of the project or observing new, unintended findings. All additive information directly relevant to the raw data, such as derived data, tables, calculations, or graphs, should be either done directly in the laboratory notebook or taped thoroughly on an adjacent page in the notebook. If this is not feasible, files can be used; providing clear identification of the data and the page where the data were derived from is essential (Macrina 2000, NAS 1994). Although many researchers take data with them when they change jobs, we strongly recommend that research institutions keep copies of all raw data while allowing individuals to have copies of data. Some universities follow the example of private industry and treat research data as the property of the institution. Keeping the data within the institution is important so that future interested parties can check the original data against derived data, graphs, or published results.

There are no excuses for not keeping accurate and informative records of methods and data. In the modern age, a large number of principal investigators are far removed in their research operation from these two steps. Therefore, investigators need to exert quality control and insist on proper documentation to assure that the integrity of the data is preserved. Moreover, the existence of an accurate paper trail may provide invaluable data for future discoveries. Some investigators may design detailed standard operating procedures (SOPs) to monitor the research protocol. Other investigators or supervisors may even add test steps (i.e., sample tests not known to the one carrying out the experiments) to ensure quality control and integrity of the process.

Raw data are usually manipulated (or processed) through many stages, depending on the type of research, before they are presented as graphs, charts, or tables or in a publishable form. As data are processed, the risk of introducing (intentional or unintentional) biases, adjustments, or errors increases (Grinnell 1992, Shamoo 1989, 1991a,b). Thus, it is important to introduce quality assurance steps to maintain the quality, objectivity, and integrity of derived data—data obtained, calculated, or derived from the raw data. Derived data appear in many forms. The most commonly known are quantitative and qualitative data such as recorder charts, instrument output such as a spectrum (e.g., optical density vs. length or vs. wavelength), scanning charts, recorder outputs representing variety of parameters, graphs, and many other forms.

In additon to raw and derived data, the data also include samples that are needed to carry out experiments, such as biological samples of bacteria, virus, vectors, certain specialty compounds, and many others. SOPs such as instrument manuals, computer software, and the like are not data but are an adjunct to the research protocol. However, they are needed to correctly carry out the proposed experiments and thus replicate the results.

Analyze the Data

The analysis of data in modern science involves the application of various statistical techniques, such as correlation, regression, analysis of variance (ANOVA), chi-square tests, and so on. These techniques provide a way of drawing inductive inferences from data and distinguishing the signal (the phenomenon of interest) from the noise (statistical fluctuations) present in the data. A responsible researcher will make every attempt to draw an unbiased inference from a data set or to focus on a true signal instead of on the noise. Different disciplines use different statistical techniques, and statistical practices vary a great deal across different disciplines. Most fields have norms or accepted practices for data analysis, and it is prudent for researchers to follow the accepted norms (Resnik 2000). These norms are usually based on two factors: (1) the nature of the variables used (i.e., quantitative, comparative, or qualitative), and (2) assumptions about the population from which the data are drawn (i.e., random distribution, independence, sample size, etc.). There is nothing inherently unethical in the use of unconventional norms. It is important, however, to be forthright in stating clearly the method of analysis, why it is being used, and how it differs from others. It is unethical to deceive or camouflage a new, as yet unaccepted method of analysis or to fail to disclose some important information relevant to the data analysis (Resnik 2000).

Given the complexities of data analysis, it is easy to introduce biases or other errors in the analysis and to misrepresent the data (Bailar 1986). The failure to provide an honest and accurate analysis of the data can have as significant an impact on research results as recording data improperly. Moreover, research indicates that statistical errors are fairly common in science (DeMets 1999). Thus, this step is crucial to ensuring the objectivity, integrity, and quality of research. Some common problem areas in data analysis are excluding outliers, filling in missing data, editing data, analyzing existing records for trends and patterns (or data mining), developing graphical representations of the data, and establishing the statistical and practical significance of the data. While none of these areas of data analysis are inherently deceptive, biased, or unethical, researchers must make sure that they follow good statistical practices and honestly describe their statistical methods and assumptions to avoid errors in data analysis (American Statistical Association 1999). Intentionally misrepresenting the data can be regarded as a type of misconduct (Resnik 2000).

Manipulate the Data

When data are published in a journal article, report, or web page, they are rarely published in raw form and are usually highly processed. Thus, the decision of how to present derived data, which portion, why, how, and to whom, are all important scientific aspects of data manipulation. For example, a researcher may select a set of tables, figures, or spectral analysis, and not others. All of the data (presented in a publication or a report) are part of the supporting documentation of the published material. It is important to keep an adequate and an accurate paper trail of data manipulation for future review and potential use (Shamoo 1989). This information is valuable not only to ensure the integrity of the process but also for the additional use of the data. For example, data from several sources may provide a new finding, or a new investigator may find a whole new way to interpret the data missed by the original investigator.

Researchers should also develop the habit of stamping laboratory note-books and other data indicating the owner of the copyright, who actually is the principle investigator (with dates), and perhaps a signature of a witness. Industry researchers already use such practices to help in future claims regarding issues of intellectual properties, such as copyrights and patents (discussed elsewhere in this text).

There are no set standards of how and where the data should be stored. Most researchers keep their data practically until they retire, or until they no longer have a sufficient space to store them. Recently, the U.S. Public Health Service (PHS) adopted the same storage time requirement for research data as for the financial records: three years from the time of last report filed to the federal agency. There is no adequate justification for this short period of time, because publication of these data may take several years beyond the time of the last expenditure report. It is our view that data should be stored for seven years after the last expenditure report (Shamoo and Teaf 1990). In the event the federal agency is auditing and inquiring about the data, the time is automatically extended to the needed length of time. If the federal agency is investigating certain data, the agency has the right to obtain these data if they are available regardless when they were obtained in the first place. Universities as yet have no provisions for storing data in centralized or any other facilities. Furthermore, granting agencies have not provided the means to store data for future generations. We recommend that research institutions develop computerized data archives and that they require those researchers not working with human subjects to deposit data in these archives on an annual basis. (Researchers have an obligation to destroy some data pertaining to human subjects research if they contain an identifying trail, as discussed in chapter 9.) Like any business keeping a centralized inventory of its stock, a research institution should keep a centralized inventory of its research.

Although it is important to store data, storage introduces problems space allocation and the use of technology. Some projects, such as tissue collections, insect collections, patient records, and outputs from radio telescopes, generate rooms full of data. Furthermore, some data are stored in formats that are becoming obsolete, such as old computer diskettes or audiotapes. Most institutions may have trouble finding room for data storage, maintaining obsolete technologies, or transferring data to new media. Thus, while data storage is important, specific ethical dilemmas concerning the storage of data must be approached with an eye to other important values and concerns in research (Resnik 1998a). The federal government can and should provide funding to develop resources for data storage, such as databanks or archives.

Interpret the Data

If all researchers interpreted the data in the same way, science would be a dry and dull profession. But this is not the case. Many important and heated debates in science, such as research on firearm violence, studies of intelligence tests, and studies of global warming, concern the interpretation of data. Sometimes an important discovery or advance in science occurs as the result of a new interpretation of existing data. Of course, challenging a standard interpretation of the data is risky: those who challenge the existing paradigm either go down in flames or win the Nobel Prize. Most challenges to the existing paradigm turn out to be wrong. But those few times that the new interpretation is correct can change and advance our knowledge in a revolutionary fashion. For example, Peter Mitchell won the Nobel Prize for his chemiosmotic theory. He advanced the notion that a proton gradient across the membrane is the driving force to synthesize adenosine triphosphate (ATP) from adenosine diphosphate (ADP) and inorganic phosphate (P_i). The chemiosmotic theory was originally considered heresy because it contradicted the long-held phosphorylated intermediate theory for the synthesis of ATP.

The path of a trailblazer is full of hazards. Most researchers resist new ideas and stick to generally accepted standards, despite their image as being open-minded and liberal. Although revolutions do occur in science, most research conforms to the model of "normal" science—science that falls within accepted standards, traditions, and procedures (Kuhn 1970). It is often the case that researchers who have new interpretations are scoffed at before their ideas are accepted. For example, the idea of continental drift was viewed as ludicrous, as was the idea that a bacterium could cause ulcers. However, if researchers can find new ways of interpreting data, they should be encouraged. And their new interpretations will be more readily accepted (or at least considered) if they properly acknowledge the existing paradigm (Resnik 1994).

Even within the existing paradigm, the interpretation of the same data can take very different pathways, none of which are likely to be unethical. As stressed above, there is an important distinction between misconduct and error, and disagreement. Just because one disagrees with an interpretation does not mean that the research is erroneous or dishonest. Researchers may, at times, become so obsessed with their view that their scientific approach can become biased, and this may, in rare instances, contribute to deviations that could lead to scientific misconduct. It is especially important, therefore, for those researchers with new interpretations to be even more careful in documenting and leaving a thorough paper trail of their data, so that other researchers will be able to understand their interpretations and not dismiss them as resulting from fraud or error. Ensuring the integrity of research data does not mean straitjacketing the investigator's creativity and latitude in introducing new ideas and interpretation. However, prudence suggests all interpretations of data should be consistent with the existing knowledge. If the interpretation of new data is inconsistent with existing knowledge, an honest discussion of the differences is in order.

Put the Results into a Publishable Format

Putting results into a publishable format, such as a paper or conference presentation, is an important part of the research project, because this is how results are disseminated to the wider community of researchers. Research papers should provide readers with an honest, accurate, and thorough description of all the steps of the research project. Researchers should accurately report data and the contributions of other contributors. They should also disclose sources of funding or outside support as well as any potential conflicts of interest (other chapters cover these issues in more depth).

Most journals require authors to divide their papers into specific sections, such as abstract, introduction, materials and methods, results, discussion, and conclusion. The abstract is a short summary of the paper that reports its key findings. Because computer database programs for literature searches usually search for words found in abstracts, it is important for authors to write an accurate and useful abstract. In the introduction section, researchers usually review previous research in the area of the project, describe its aims and objectives, and discuss its importance. In the materials and methods section, authors describe the design of the tests or experiments as well as materials, methods, statistical techniques, and procedures used. In the results section, authors report processed and sometimes raw data as well as the results of the analysis of the data. In the discussion section, the authors may address a number of different issues relating to the research, such as placing the new data within the existing data in the literature; how and why they differ; potential biases, flaws, or shortcomings; difficulties in conducting the research; significance of the research and its relation to other studies; and areas for further research and exploration. The conclusion section summarizes all aspects of the research.

All papers and presentations should be clearly written. If the authors have some help from an editor or writer in preparing their publication, they should acknowledge this contribution. Note that some researchers in business, the military, or other settings may be required to not publish their results (discussed in chapter 4).

Publish the Results

We discuss aspects of publication of results in more detail in chapter 4 on publication and peer review. For now, we simply note that researchers have an obligation to disseminate work for the obvious reason that science cannot advance unless researchers report and share results. Dissemination can include publication in peer-reviewed journals, publication in monographs or other books, and publication on web pages, as well as presentations at professional meetings. The important ethical consideration is that research should be disseminated to colleagues and the public for scrutiny and review. Indeed, researchers who receive grants from the government or private funding agencies are usually required to specify a plan for disseminating their research in the grant proposal and to report to the agency about publications that result from the grant (Grinnell 1992). On the other hand, researchers who work for business and industry often sign agreements to not publish results or to withhold publication until they obtain approval from management (Blumenthal 1997, Gibbs 1996). For instance, researchers working for the tobacco industry did not publish their work on nicotine's addictive properties for many years (Resnik 1998b). We will explore these issues in a later chapter as well.

Replicate the Results

Once the results are published, it is important for other researchers to be able to replicate the results. Although scientists do not frequently repeat each other's tests or experiments, due to an emphasis on original research, it is important that research be repeatable in principle. Repeatability is the primary assurance of the integrity of research data. Moreover, repeated confirmation of results by others lends greater credence that the data are usable, especially those data that can have an impact on the well-being of millions of people. The ability of other investigators to replicate the experiments by following the method in the published report is crucial to the advancement of science. It is important that the published work give sufficient details for others to replicate it. If there is not sufficient journal space to state the experimental details, several other means should be attempted to publish and provide the experimental details, such as mini-print appendixes, archives, and an invitation to the reader to ask for the full report from the investigator.

Share Data and Results

As noted above, openness is a key principle in research ethics. Scientists should share data and results (1) to promote the advancement of knowledge by making information publicly known; (2) to allow criticism and feedback as well as replication; (3) to build and maintain a culture of trust, cooperation, and collaboration among researchers; (4) to build support from the public by demonstrating openness and trustworthiness. The ideal of openness is considered by many people, including many researchers, to be a fundamental part of research and scholarship. The real world of research does not usually conform to this ideal, however. Although researchers share data within the same team of collaborators working on a common project, they rarely share data with noncollaborators and often do not welcome requests to share data from other researchers in the field, much less people from outside the research community. The resistance to data sharing is especially high among researchers who have concerns about intellectual property, such as potential patents or trade secrets. For several years, the National Institutes of Health has encouraged researchers to share data, reagents, cell lines, and other research materials and has released some guidelines in this regard (Wadman 1999). Although there are no hard data on the prevalence of data sharing or the resistance to data sharing, there are many anecdotal reports of refusals to share data (Munthe and Welin 1996, Harris 1999).

While the progress of science thrives on sharing information and data and as soon as possible, it makes sense to allow researchers who work for private industry to refuse to share data or results in order to protect a company's proprietary and confidential information. This exception to the principle of openness can be justified on the ground that private money is an important part of scientific funding and that businesses need to protect information in order to obtain a return on their R&D investments (Resnik 1998b). However, this argument does not apply to publicly funded research, which should be shared as soon as possible. If public funds pay for research, then that research should be available to the public. Indeed, last year the U.S. Congress adopted a bill requiring federal granting agencies to ensure that all data produced under a federal grant be available to the public through the Freedom of Information Act (Frankel 1999). Scientists raised many objections to this new policy, arguing that it could subject them to harassment from people who want to interfere with their work, could undermine intellectual property claims, or could make it difficult to protect confidential data related to human subjects research (Macilwain 1999). We think these are all good reasons to withhold data. However, we agree with the general idea of making publicly funded research available to the public. Thus, we would argue that researchers have an obligation to share their data with the public provided that (1) they have secured intellectual property rights, such as credit for a discovery or patent rights, and (2) they have removed personal information that could be used to identify human subjects. Although it is important for researchers to be free from harassment from industry representatives, political activists, or other parties, we do not think that researchers who receive public funds can be completely shielded from this threat. It is difficult to know in advance whether any particular request for data would be harassment of researchers. Without having this knowledge in advance, any policy short of answering all requests for data would be arbitrary and possibly biased.

Corrupting Influences in the Current Research Environment

Although following the steps of the scientific method discussed above can ensure and assure the objectivity, quality, and integrity of research data, a number of different psychological, social, economic, political, and institutional influences can undermine or corrupt the research process. The scientific method is an ideal that may be difficult to achieve in practice. The following influences and trends can interfere with and undermine research results and their application.

Pressure to Produce Results

Researchers who receive government funds face enormous financial and institutional pressures to produce results in order to obtain new funding, to continue funding, or to publish papers. The phrase "publish or perish" accurately describes the life of the academic researcher. Researchers employed by private industry face similar pressures to produce results that provide useful information, although they may not face any pressure to publish. Because researchers in private industry who do not produce results can lose their jobs or their sources of funding, the phrase "produce or perish" is more apt. When the research plan is not going well or is taking longer than expected, researchers can be tempted to compromise the integrity of the research process in order to obtain results, which may result in bias, error, sloppiness, or even fraud (Woolf 1986, Broad and Wade 1982 [1993], National Academy of Science 1992,

Resnik 1998b, Shamoo 1989). These pressures often fall most severely on junior researchers and graduate students, who may be under pressure to produce results for senior colleagues in order to advance their own careers or retain their jobs (Browing 1995).

Careerism

Research is no longer an avocation or hobby; it is a career. Career advancement usually results from many different types of achievements, such as publications, grants, intellectual property, special appointments, awards, and recognition. While the desire for a career in research can inspire dedication and hard work, it can also lead researchers to violate standards of ethics and integrity to achieve various goals along the path of career advancement (National Academy of Science 1992, 1994).

Conflicts of Interest

Conflicts of interest, financial or otherwise, can undermine trustworthiness and objective judgment, which are required in virtually all steps of the scientific method, especially study design, data interpretation, and publication (Krimsky 1996, Shamoo 1989, 1992). These are discussed in more depth in chapter 7.

Intellectual Property Interests

Researchers in the private or public sector frequently seek intellectual property rights, such as patents or copyrights (Krimsky 1996a, b). To secure these rights, researchers may be tempted to violate standards of ethics and integrity. Some but not all attempts to secure intellectual property create conflicts of interest.

Complexity

Research projects often involve many different collaborators, institutions, disciplines, research sites, and sources of funding. It may be very difficult for any one person to understand or control an entire research project. This complexity can lead to problems in monitoring data, revising hypotheses or study aims, initiating tests or experiments, and so on. Complexity can also lead to communication problems among different members of the research team, and between the team and institutions, sponsoring organizations, and government agencies (Grinnell 1992).

Remoteness

The principal investigator or the manager of the project sometimes is far removed physically from the project itself and its various collaborators. More important, often the investigator relies on less knowledgeable individuals to carry out daily monitoring and discussions. This remoteness results in the investigator being mentally removed from the day-to-day operations of obtaining research data. Remoteness also results in poor supervision of those directly involved in data acquisition, analysis, and manipulation. According to several

studies, poor supervision of subordinates is one of the chief causes of misconduct, error, and bias in research (National Academy of Science 1992). Because
principal investigators may be so far removed from the day to day research operations, trust is a key component of ethical conduct: PIs and managers must
be able to trust subordinates and vice versa (Whitbeck 1995).

Self-deception

Although self-criticism and skepticism play an important role in research
planning and execution and are part of the ethos of science, scientists, like
other people, succumb to self-deception (Broad and Wade 1982 [1993]).
There are many different types of self-deception, including observer bias
(where one sees what one wants to see), that can infect data collection, research design, and data analysis (Resnik 1998b). The steps of the scientific
method are designed to counteract self-deception, but nothing can change the
fact that research is conducted by human beings who often believe what they
want to believe.

Political and Sociocultural Biases and Pressures

Many research projects address issues that are clouded with political and social
controversy. Researchers on different sides of a controversial topic, such as
gun control, global warming, tissue engineering, consumer safety, environmental management, homosexuality, or human intelligence, may have different stakes in the results of research. These pressures can undermine objective
judgment and decision making in all phases of research as well as for society
and public policy (Crossen 1994, Longino 1990, Resnik 1998b, Shrader-
Frechette 1994).

THE IMPORTANCE OF GOOD RESEARCH PRACTICES

To deal with corrupting influences and assure the quality, objectivity, and integrity of research data, it is important to promote ethical attitudes and good
research practices (GRPs) among the participants in the enterprise (such as
the principal investigator, technician, supervisor, and management) toward
research integrity. An ethical attitude embodies a positive orientation toward
ethics, an awareness of ethical issues, and a commitment to ethics in research. A person with an ethical attitude wants to do the right things for the
right reasons. GRPs (described below) are rules that researchers can follow
to help ensure the quality, objectivity, and integrity of data (Glick and
Shamoo 1993, 1994, Shamoo 1989, 1991b, Shamoo and Davis 1989). People in positions of leadership in research can play a key role in developing a
culture in which ethical attitudes and GRPs prevail. If principal investigators, managers, corporations, and government agencies demonstrate and
tolerate unethical attitudes and poor research practices, then unethical attitudes and poor research practices will prevail. The research culture (attitudes and behaviors) sets the tone for the importance of quality, objectivity,
and integrity of data and results.

GRP AIMS

The following are aims of GRPs (Shamoo 1991b):

Cardinal Rules

1. Published data are verifiable: a paper trail exists documenting the origin of the data.
2. Published data are reproducible: other investigators are able to reproduce the data by following the published procedures.

Commonsense Rule

The conclusions drawn from the published research data should be consistent with the data.

PROCEDURES TO ACHIEVE GRP OBJECTIVES AND AIMS

The aims of GRPs can be achieved by numerous methods. The investigator should be more concerned with making a sincere effort to accomplish these aims rather than with following any proposed specific procedure. All proposed procedures should serve the GRP aims and not hinder them. Therefore any proposed procedure that may result in a contrary outcome should be either modified or discarded.

Quality Control and Quality Assurance

Industries have used quality control and quality assurance processes for years (Shamoo 1991a,b). These concepts are based on common sense and good business practices. Quality control is concerned with developing rules and procedures designed to ensure that products and services during production are of high quality and conform to original specifications. Quality assurance is concerned with reviewing (or testing) the quality of products and services after they have been produced or used (Shamoo 1991a,b).

Unfortunately, these concepts are foreign to researchers, especially to those in academic institutions, but this should not be the case. One reason why many in academic research loath the concepts of quality control and quality assurance is that these ideas are associated with increased bureaucracy and red tape. But we believe that these concepts can be adapted to the research environment without increasing red tape and bureaucracy and without interfering with the creative process (Shamoo 1989).

The following rules can help establish quality control in research:

1. All equipment used should have been calibrated within the time frame recommended by the manufacturer.
2. All equipment should have its standard operating procedure available.
3. All materials consumed during research experiments should be properly labeled with all of the essential information, such as date of man-

ufacture, expiration date, concentration, pH, storage conditions (e.g.,
refrigeration, freezer, room temperature, etc.).

4. Documentation of procedures used to carry out the research protocol is in its proper place, such as lab notebooks, computer software,
   or automated instruments.
5. All research data should be promptly recorded, dated, and signed in a
   permanent manner.
6. Except for some types of human subjects research, all research data
   and records should be retained for a specified period of time (we recommend seven years).

The following rules, which pertain to actions performed after research is
conducted, can help promote quality assurance:

1. Require researchers to keep original data at the institution.
2. Develop centralized data archives that can be used to audit or review
   data.
3. Examine research for potential conflicts of interest and disclose those
   conflicts to the appropriate parties (see chapter 7 on conflicts of interest).
4. Audit or peer review data every three years. The audit or peer review
   should be conducted by the research chief or director, an outside researcher within the research institution, or a researcher from outside
   the research institution.
5. File the results of data audit or peer review with the research institution and the agency sponsoring the research.
6. Verify in peer review/data audit all of the data, from the published
   data all the way to the original raw data.

The Potential Value of GRP and Peer Review/Data Audit

Implementing the rules listed above can help promote good research practices
(Shamoo 1989, Glick and Shamoo, 1994) and can also help protect the human
and financial investment in research (Shamoo and Davis 1990). Peer review/
data audit has some special advantages:

Reduction of Errors   Human errors are a part of any human function, and the
human factor has a large influence on the quality of data produced. Peer re-
view/data audit can uncover errors both before and after those errors have
contributed to large problems. Modern methods of online data processing
certainly have reduced errors but have also contributed to the increased volume of data that requires human judgment, either before or after online data
processing. Thus, the possibility of error in data analysis remains a significant
factor (Resnik 2000).

Reduction of Irregularities   Data audit can uncover both unintentional and intentional errors. Instituting peer review/data auditing itself may discourage
such irregularities, especially those that are intentional. The amount of data to
be fully audited can vary, depending on the preliminary analysis. A strong sys-

tem of quality assurance can promote cost-effectiveness by ensuring accurate and efficient processing of data as well as reducing the cost of the peer review/data audit.

Reduction of Fraud and Potential for Fraud   The existence of a systematic way to examine independently the data, or at least part of the data—or the thought that the data may be examined—may help reduce fraud and the potential for fraud. But peer review/data audit is by no means a foolproof method to eliminate fraud. If a researcher or an organization is intent on deception, there is as much potential for success as for fraudulent financial transactions. Peer reviewers/data auditors should therefore strive to reduce the ability of a person or an organization to succeed in fraud. But at the same time, peer reviewers/data auditors should be aware of their limitations—the system is not perfect.

Protection for the Public, Government, Industry, and the Individual Investigator   All segments of society benefit from the peer review/data audit because it increases the likelihood of actually achieving worthwhile products. The greatest benefit of peer review/data audit falls to the public, which is the ultimate consumer of all goods and services of industry and government. After all, it is people who must suffer the consequences of poorly tested pharmaceuticals or poorly designed cars. Industry can protect itself from overzealous or dishonest employees as well as unintentional errors. The company's reputation as well as its actual services or products would be enhanced by peer review/data audit. Also, individual investigators can be protected from false accusations, rumors, and gossip.

Improvement of Products and Services   Data audit/peer review not only can eliminate error but also can improve the overall quality of a product or service. Toxicological research, for example, is conducted by some in the chemical industry for certain products covered by a regulatory law. Furthermore, management utilizes these research data for the purpose of protecting the consumers and employees from these potentially toxic substances.

There are broad and general benefits to the consumers of the products and services. Industries such as pharmaceutical, chemical, petrochemical, and pesticide manufacturers, are examples of who may use and benefit from these procedures. As a matter of fact, in the area of some toxic substances, there are specific federal regulations. The National Toxicology Program (NTP) uses project management systems and quality assurance (QA) system to monitor and evaluate the toxicological studies performed by the industry.

Establishment and Improvement of Future Research and Development Standards   The study and application of peer review/data audit are in their infancy. Peer review/data audit standards which individuals and organizations involved in research data production should adhere to and abide by have yet to be well established. One of the primary objectives of applying peer review/data audit in organizations would be to establish such standards, first by borrowing from the experience of finance and molding it to the world of research. Another objective would be to consistently review and revise these standards as needed.

Improvement of Risk Assessment   Risk assessment is an important tool that helps policy makers determine regulations regarding such issues as nuclear safety, carcinogens, and pesticides. One of the critical factors involved in risk assessment is the use of the historical database collected from past research. Thus, the accuracy and reliability of these data become crucial for risk assessment. Peer review/data audit, by ensuring the accuracy and reliability of these data, can become an important partner in public health and safety.

Reduction of Liability   Reduction of legal liability is not an immediate or an obvious purpose of peer review/data audit, but it can be a side effect of that process. In the long run, peer review/data audit may contribute to a greater reliability of and confidence in the data in various segments such as markets, courts, government, and insurance companies. For example, the increased confidence in the data could provide an incentive for insurance companies to reduce liability. Peer review/data audit could also strengthen the hand of industry in defending itself against unfair charges.

This concludes our discussion of GRPs. Subsequent chapters address topics that have direct or indirect connections to GRPs, peer review/data audit, and other topics discussed here.

QUESTIONS FOR DISCUSSION

1. What are your thoughts about scientific research? In your opinion, what is the most crucial part of research?
2. How would you list the steps in carrying out of research? Are there some steps you could skip and why?
3. How would you introduce quality assurance and integrity into your steps for carrying out research?
4. Can you give an example of how data can be "modified" to suit inappropriate goals in steps of research?
5. Give an example of an experimental design that would bias the data.
6. When would you be justified in refusing to share data?
7. How many of these GRPs do people follow (or fail to follow) in your research environment? Why?
8. Can scientific research incorporate quality control and quality assurance methods? Would this stifle creativity, or increase workload?
9. How do you ensure that peer review/data audit is workable, and how you would modify it to accomplish its purpose in your research environment? Can you suggest a whole new system to ensure the quality and integrity of research data?
10. How is a lab notebook like (or not like) a medical record?

CASES FOR DISCUSSION

Case 1

A medical student has a summer job with a faculty mentor at a research university. The student is bright, hard working, and industrious and hopes to publish a paper at the end of the summer. He is the son of a colleague of the mentor at a distant university. The student is working on a cancer cell line that requires three weeks to grow in order to test for the development of a specific antibody. His project plan is to identify the antibody by the end of the summer. The student has written a short paper describing his work.

The mentor went over the raw data and found that some of the data were written on pieces of yellow pads without clearly identifying from which experiment the data came. She also noticed that some of the experiments shown in the paper's table were repeated several times without an explanation as to why. The mentor was not happy about the data or the paper, but she likes the student and does not want to discourage him from a potential career in research.

- What is the primary responsibility of the mentor?
- Should the mentor write a short paper and send it for publication?
- Should the student write a short paper and send it for publication?
- If you were the mentor, what would you do?
- Should the mentor or her representative have paid more attention to the student's work during the course of the summer? Should the student been taught some quality control and/or GRP during the summer?

Case 2

A graduate student at a research university finished her dissertation and graduated with honors. Her mentor gave the continuation of the project to a new graduate student. As usual, the mentor gave the entire laboratory notebook to the new graduate student, who had to repeat the isolation of the newly discovered chemical entity with high-pressure liquid chromatography (HPLC) in order to follow up the chemical and physical characterization of the new compound.

The new graduate student found that if he follows the exact method described in the laboratory notebooks and published by the previous student, he obtains the new chemical entity not at the same HPLC location as published, but rather slightly shifted to the left, and there was a different peak at the location stated. However, the new student discovered that if the ionic strength is doubled, he could find the same chemical at the same location in accordance with the previous student's dissertation. The new student discussed with the mentor how he should proceed. The mentor replied, "Why make a fuss about it? Just proceed with your slightly different method and we can move on."

- What are the responsibilities of the new student? Should the new student refuse to accommodate the mentor's request?

- Should the new student have read more thoroughly the relevant laboratory notebooks prior to starting the experiment? Should there have been a paper trail of the error in the laboratory notebook? Do you think the error was intentional, and does it matter?
- If the laboratory notebook does not reveal the error, is it then misconduct? Does it indicate that a better recording of the data would have been helpful?
- Should the mentor have had training and education in responsible conduct of research (RCR)? If the mentor has had the necessary training in RCR, what actions would you suggest?
- Can you propose a reasonable resolution to the problem?

Case 3

A new postdoctoral fellow in a genetic research laboratory must sequence a 4 kDa fragment. After the sequence, he is to prepare a 200-base unit to use as a potential regulator of a DNA-related enzyme. It is suspected that the 4 kDa fragment contains the 200-base unit. The sequence of the 200-base unit is already known in the literature, but not as part of the 4 kDa fragment, and not as a potential regulator. The fact that the 200-base unit is known is what gave the mentor the idea that it may have a functional role.

The new postdoctoral fellow tried for three months to sequence the 4 kDa fragment, without success, and so simply proceeded to synthesize the 200-base unit without locating it within the fragment. After two years of research, the 4 kDa fragment appeared to have an important regulatory role in an important discovery, but at this time the mentor learned that the post-doc never sequenced the original 4 kDa fragment. The mentor could never find a "good" record of the attempts to sequence the 4 kDa fragment.

- What impression do you gather about how this mentor runs the laboratory?
- Should there be records of sequence attempts of the 4 kDa fragment?
- How should the mentor proceed?
- If you were the new post-doc, what steps you will take to ensure proper records of your work?

Case 4

A graduate student prepared for her thesis a table that shows a toxic substance inhibits an enzyme's activity by about 20%. She has done only six experiments. The mentor looked at the data and found that one of the data showed a stimulation of 20% and that this point is the one that skewed the results to a low level of inhibition with a large standard of deviation. The mentor further determined with the student that the outlier is outside the mean by 2.1 times the standard derivation and that it is reasonable not to include it with the rest of the data. This would make the inhibition about 30% and thus make the potential paper more in line with other research results and hence more "respectable." The mentor instructed the student to do so.

- Should the student simply proceed with the mentor's instructions?
- Should the mentor have been more specific as what to do with the outlier? In what way?
- Can you propose a resolution? Should the outlier be mentioned in the paper?
- How should this laboratory handle similar issues in the future? Should each laboratory have an agreed upon standard operating procedure (SOP) for such a statistical issue?

Case 5

A medical school has just established a primate research center and has been conducting experiments on HIV vaccines in chimpanzees. A local animal rights group has been monitoring this research and has protested the center from the beginning. As a result, researchers are very wary of sharing data with anyone outside the institution, because they fear harassment by this group.

- Should these concerns justify secrecy of the data?
- What would be your resolution for a similar problem?

Case 6

A pharmaceutical company conducts 10 different phase I studies on a new drug to establish its safety in healthy individuals. Five of these studies had a P value less than 0.05, indicating significant results; five had a P value greater than 0.05, indicating nonsignificant results. As it so happens, undesirable side effects were observed in four of the studies with the nonsignificant results. None of the studies with significant results had a significant proportion of side effects. The researchers report these results to the FDA and in a publication, but they do not mention the side effects that occurred in the studies with the higher P values.

- Is there an ethical responsibility to report all of the data? Does it make a difference in reporting if the subjects were not human (i.e., animals)?
- What are the responsibilities of the researchers in this company, to themselves, and to society?
- Should there be a federal mandate to report all side effects?
- How could the GRP help in this case? Would a quality assurance program be helpful?

Case 7

A graduate student is planning to write a thesis on the affects of exercise in managing diabetes in dogs. He is planning to do a trial with dogs with diabetes, control matched with respect to age, breed, sex, and other factors. One group will receive no extra exercise; another group will receive 30 minutes of exercise a day; and another group will receive two 30 minute periods of exercise per day. He will measure blood sugar levels in all of these dogs, as well as the quantities of drugs used to control diabetes.

The graduate student is also conducting a literature review on the subject as a background to his research. In conducting this review, he searches various computer databases, such as the Science Citation Index and MEDLINE, for the past five years. He gathers many abstracts and papers. For much of the research, he only reads abstracts and does not read the full papers. Also, he does not include some of the important work on diabetes in dogs that took place more than five years ago.

- Should the graduate student read articles, not just abstracts?
- If he cites an article in a publication or in his thesis, should he read the full article?
- If he cites a book, should he read the full book or only the part that he uses?
- Should the graduate student include articles published more than five years ago?

Case 8

Two physicians in a department of emergency medicine reviewed the medical records of all patients admitted for diabetic crisis to the hospital in the last five years. They correlated several different variables, such as length of hospital stay, survival, cost of care, rehospitalization, age, race, family history, and so forth. If they found any statistically significant trends (P values of 0.5 or less), they planned to publish those results, and they planned to ask a statistician to help them determine if any of their correlations are significant.

- Do you see any potential methodological or ethical problems with this study design?
- Does it conform to the rules described in this chapter?
- Would it be unethical for the researchers to publish their results if they do not make it clear in the paper that they have mined the data for significant trends?
- Would you be more confident in their research if they had a hypothesis prior to conducting the study?

3

Collaboration in Research: Authorship, Resource Sharing, and Mentoring

> Collaboration is a cornerstone of modern science, but it also raises a variety of ethical problems and dilemmas. This chapter explores a variety of issues related to scientific collaboration, including authorship and credit allocation in science; the sharing of data, results, tools, reagents, equipment, and resources; and mentoring responsibilities. The chapter discusses some of the moral dimensions of collaboration, such as trust, accountability, and collegiality. It also considers some reasons why collaborations sometimes fail in research and addresses polices designed to promote collaboration, including policies on authorship, and to promote effective mentoring.

Contemporary research requires a great deal of collaboration among scientists. Although many people still retain the image of the isolated researcher toiling away in the laboratory, modern science is a highly social activity. Archimedes, Galileo, Newton, Harvey, Lavoisier, and Mendel managed to do a great deal of work without collaborating significantly, but today's scientists often must work with many different colleagues. Researchers share data, databases, ideas, equipment, computers, methods, reagents, cell lines, research sites, personnel, and many other technical and human resources. Collaboration takes place within a single institution and among several institutions; it occurs within a particular discipline and among many disciplines; it takes place within the academic realm, within the private sector, or between the academy and industry; and it happens at local, national, and international levels. Collaborators may include graduate students, postdoctoral students, junior and senior researchers, basic scientists, and clinical researchers. Some research projects, such as the Human Genome Project, involve thousands of researchers from dozens of disciplines working in many different countries (Grinnell 1992, Macrina 2000).

Successful collaboration cannot occur without a high level of cooperation, trust, collegiality, fairness, and accountability. Cooperation is essential to collaboration because researchers cannot collaborate if they are not willing to engage in activities that require a great deal of cooperation, such as sharing data and resources or coordinating activities, experiments, and tests. Trust is important in collaboration because researchers need to trust that their collaborators will keep the agreements, will share resources, will disclose important information, will not lie, and so on (Whitbeck 1998). Many different factors can undermine trustworthiness, including selfishness, incompetence, negligence, unfairness, careerism, and conflicts of interest.

Collegiality, one of sociologist Robert Merton's (1973) four norms of science, is important in maintaining a social environment that promotes cooperation and trust: researchers who treat one another as colleagues are more likely to trust one another and to cooperate. The norm of collegiality requires researchers to treat each other with the respect accorded to a friend or ally in pursuit of a common goal. Colleagues not only help one another but also provide constructive criticism. Behaviors that can undermine collegiality include harassment (sexual or otherwise); racial, ethnic, or sexual discrimination; verbal abuse; personal grudges; theft; and jealousy.

Fairness is important in collaboration because collaborators want to ensure that they receive a fair share of the rewards of research, such as authorship or intellectual property rights, and that they are not unfairly burdened with some of the more tedious or unpleasant aspects of research (Resnik 1998a,b). Although research is a cooperative activity, researchers still retain their individual interests, and they expect that those interests will be treated fairly. Plagiarism and undeserved authorship are extreme violations of fairness. Fairness is also very important in other issues relating to collaboration, such as personnel decisions.

Last but not least, accountability is important in collaboration because when many people work together, it is especially important to know who can be held accountable for the successes or the failures of a project (Rennie et al., 1997). Modern research involves a division of cognitive (or intellectual) labor: different people do different jobs in research, such as design experiments, gather data, analyze data, write papers, and so on (Kitcher 1993). Many research projects encompass research techniques, methods, and disciplines so different from each other that no one person can be responsible for or even knowledgeable about all the different aspects of the project. For example, the study of a new DNA vaccine may involve enzyme kinetics, x-ray crystallography, reverse transcriptase, electron micrographs, recombinant DNA, polymerase chain reactions, clinical trials, pharmacology, microbiology, immunology, and statistical analysis.

Because so many people are doing different jobs, it is often hard to keep track of all of these different laborers, the standards governing their work, and the products of their labor. Leading a research team can be in some ways like managing a small organization. Like any organization, problems relating to communication and supervision can occur in scientific research. Indeed, many of the problems related to misconduct in science often boil down to poor communication and supervision (Panel on Scientific Responsibility, 1992, LaFollette 1992, Broad and Wade 1982 [1993]).

In any research project, different people need to be held accountable for different parts of the project as well as the whole project itself. Accountability is often confused with responsibility, but we distinguish between these two concepts (Davis 1995a). People are accountable for an action if they have the obligation to give an account of the action. People are responsible for an action if they deserve to be praised or blamed for the action. A person may be held accountable even if they are not responsible; for instance, if a 14-year-old boy throws a rock through a window, he is responsible for throwing the rock, but his parents may be held accountable for his actions. In a large research

project with many collaborators, different people may be held accountable for
the project as a whole or its various parts. A person who was not responsible
for some aspect of the project, such as recording data, may still be held accountable for the project as a whole. Clearly, accountability and responsibility are both important in research, but it is also important to keep these notions distinct.

With this brief background of collaboration in research, we now describe
some ethical problems and issues relating to collaborative research. The topic
of collaboration also arises in other chapters, for example, in intellectual property issues and interactions between universities and private industry.

AUTHORSHIP AND PLAGIARISM

Authorship is perhaps the most important reward in research. Many key decisions relating to a person's career advancement in academia, such as hiring,
promotion, or tenure decisions, are based on that person's publication record.
Publication is also important in obtaining grants and contracts, fellowships,
and special awards. The phrases "publish or perish" and "authorship is a meal
ticket" reflect the grim realities of academic life (LaFollette 1992). Publication
is important to a lesser extent in the private sector in that private corporations
may not care whether their employees publish, and they may even discourage
publication. However, one's publication record may still be important in obtaining employment in the private sector.

Over the latter half of the twentieth century, the number of authors on scientific papers has steadily increased (LaFollette 1992, McLellin 1995). In biomedical research, the average number of authors per paper increased from 1.7
in 1960 to 3.1 in 1990 (Drenth 1996). It is not at all uncommon for a paper
published in biomedicine to have five or more authors, and multiple authorship in now the norm (Rennie et al. 1997). The average number of authors for
all fields rose from 1.67 in 1960 to 2.58 in 1980 (Broad 1981). In the 1980s,
the average number of authors per article in medical research rose to 4.5
(LaFollette 1992). In physics, papers may have 50–500 authors. In the life sciences, 37 papers were published in 1994 that had over 100 authors, compared
with almost none with 100 authors in the 1980s (Regaldo 1995). This rise in
the number of authors has been accompanied by a rise in disputes about authorship (Wilcox 1998).

There are several explanations for these trends. One is that collaboration in
science has increased: more people are working together on the same project,
so there are more authors. Collaboration is on the rise because research problems have become more complex, demanding, and interdisciplinary. However,
there is another reason why authorship has increased: the pressure to publish
has increased. Universities, corporations, and granting agencies continue to
stress the quantity of publications in making their funding and personnel decisions. Many believe that this emphasis on quantity has also undermined the
quality of published work (Chubin and Hackett 1990) but that is another issue
altogether.

Researchers have used a variety of ethically questionable strategies to increase the quantity of their own publications:

- Gift authorship, in which a person is listed as an author as a personal or professional favor: Some researchers have even developed reciprocal arrangements for listing each other as coauthors (LaFollette 1992).
- Honorary authorship, in which a person is listed as an author as a sign of respect or gratitude: Some laboratory directors have insisted that they be listed as an author on every publication that their lab produces (Jones 2000).
- Prestige authorship, in which a person with a high degree of prestige or notoriety is listed as an author in order to give the publication more visibility or impact (LaFollette 1992).
- Ghost authorship, in which a ghostwriter is used to write a manuscript: The ghostwriter may not be involved in planning or conducting research. In extreme cases, even the researchers are ghosts. Pharmaceutical companies have asked physicians to be listed as authors on papers in order to give the papers prestige or status. These "authors" have been involved in no aspects of planning or conducting the research or writing up the results. They are authors in name only (Jones 2000, Flanagin et al. 1998).
- Publishing papers using the standard of the "least publishable unit" (LPU) (Broad 1981). This practices involves publishing different pieces of a study in different journals at different times in order to maximize the number of publications produced from a study. Why publish only one paper from a project if you can publish 10? Although this practice may not involve improper allocations of credit, it nevertheless creates problems of accountability, fairness, and trust and also wastes human resources (Huth 1986a).

Conversely, researchers also may unfairly deny people credit where credit is due. There are several reasons why one might prevent someone else from receiving credit for intellectual or other contributions. First, the quest for priority has been and always will be a key aspect of research: scientists want to be the first to discover a new phenomenon or propose a new theory (Merton 1973). Many bitter battles in science have been fought over issues of priority, including the international incident over the discovery of the HIV virus involving Robert Gallo and Luc Montagnier (Cohen 1994). A researcher may be tempted to not list someone as an author or acknowledge that person's contribution in order to achieve an edge in the contest for priority. Second, concerns about priority and credit play a key role in intellectual property rights, such as patents. To solidify their intellectual property claims, researchers may attempt to deny authorship as well as inventorship to people who have contributed to a new discovery or invention. Although we focus on authorship in this chapter, much of our discussion also applies to questions about inventions and patents. Just as a person may be listed as a coauthor on a publication, they may also be listed as a co-inventor on a patent application (Dreyfuss 2000).

Third, although multiple authorship is becoming the norm, researchers may want to hold the number of authors to a minimum to prevent authorship from being diluted. For instance, many journals cite papers with more than three authors as "[first author's name] et al." If a paper has three authors, the second and third authors may have a strong interest in not allowing someone to be added as a fourth author, in order keep their names visible.

Extreme examples of failing to give credit include the following:

- Plagiarism: Plagiarism, according to standard definition, is wrongfully representing someone else's ideas, words, paintings, or other expressions as one's own. Plagiarism has been and continues to be a key issue in misconduct cases investigated by the federal government (Steneck 1999). There are many different forms of plagiarism, not all of which are as extreme as copying a paper word for word (LaFollette 1992, Goode 1993).
- Failure to grant authorship or even an acknowledgment, despite a person's genuine contributions to a project (discussed above).
- Failure to acknowledge, disclose, or obtain permission to use material from one's previous publications: This practice, sometimes called "self-plagiarism," can occur when a person recycles previously published material in papers that purport to be original (LaFollette 1992).
- Irresponsible review of the literature, or "citation amnesia": One very important way to give a person credit is to recognize his or her contribution to a body of research or scholarship when reviewing or discussing the literature. For many, citation is almost as important as authorship. Those who fail to cite important contributors present the reader with inaccurate and biased information and unfairly deny others the rewards of research and scholarship (Resnik 1998a, LaFollette 1992).

CRITERIA FOR AUTHORSHIP

In light of these problems related to credit allocation in science, it is imperative that researchers discuss issues related to authorship and establish standards for authorship in research. In the past, many journals have used as the standard for authorship whether the person has made a "significant contribution" to the project through planning, conceptualization, or research design; collecting or analyzing data; or writing and editing the manuscript (LaFollette 1992). But we believe that this popular approach is vague and may not promote accountability, because it would allow a person to be listed as an author as a result of planning a project, even though this person might not know how the project was actually implemented. Likewise, a person may become involved in the project at the very end and not have an important role in designing the study.

Our basic ethical principle is that authorship and accountability should go hand in hand: people should be listed as an author on a paper only if they can defend the paper or its results (Rennie et al. 1997, Resnik 1997). They need not be responsible for every aspect of the paper, but they must be accountable for the paper as a whole. When it comes to the order of authors, another important issue, we follow a similar principle: the order of authors should reflect the order of accountability. The person most accountable for the research should come first; the person least accountable should come last.

Thus, to decide whether someone should be listed as an author, one must decide whether they can be held accountable for the whole project. People may contribute to a project in important ways without being considered an author. Important contributors can be recognized in an acknowledgments section of a publication. Indeed, many scholars are recommending that the research community take additional steps to make contributors accountable in research. For instance, some have proposed that papers list authors as well as contributors and spell out the different roles and responsibilities of the authors and contributors in a project (Resnik 1997, Rennie et al. 1997).

To make sense of authorship issues, it is important to describe the different roles and responsibilities in research, because these will determine who should or should not be listed as an author or as a contributor, as well as the order of the listing. Although research roles vary considerably across disciplines and even among different projects within the same discipline, people may contribute to a project in basic ways, based on our discussion of the process of research:

1. Defining problems
2. Proposing hypotheses
3. Summarizing the background literature
4. Designing experiments
5. Developing the methodology
6. Collecting and recording data
7. Providing data
8. Managing data
9. Analyzing data
10. Interpreting results
11. Assisting in technical aspects of research
12. Assisting in logistical aspects of research
13. Applying for a grant/obtaining funding
14. Drafting and editing manuscripts

The same person may be involved in many of these different aspects of research, although different people may perform different roles. For instance, in academic research, the principal investigator (PI) is usually a professor who proposes the hypothesis, designs the experiments, develops the methodology, writes the grant proposal, and writes the manuscript. However, she or he may use undergraduate, graduate, or postdoctoral students to collect and record data, review the literature, or edit the manuscript. These students may also provide assistance in other aspects of research as well. Lab assistants may provide assistance with technical aspects the experiments and are not usually listed as authors. However, some have argued that in some instances lab assistants could be listed as authors if they make an important contribution in addition to their technical expertise (Resnik 1997). Statisticians may help analyze data and interpret results. Other senior colleagues, such as the laboratory director, may also help the PI by providing data from their research or by helping with experimental design, methodology, or grant writing. The laboratory director is usually a senior researcher who may or may not be the PI. He or she may supervise many different projects and many different PIs.

In an academic setting, the PI is supposed to be in charge of the research, although other lines of authority and responsibility may not be clearly defined (Rose and Fischer 1995). In private industry, the lines of authority and responsibility are usually more clearly defined, because private industry works on a business model rather than an academic model (Bowie 1994). The laboratory director is in charge of many different projects and many different investigators, who may be assisted by technicians or other scientists. The laboratory director reports to the company's upper level managers. Decisions about which projects to pursue are based on market considerations, not on intellectual considerations. In the military, lines of authority and responsibility are delineated even more strictly, and decisions about funding are based on strategic considerations (Dickson 1988).

Clearly, all of these different roles are ways of contributing to research. Thus, anyone who performs one of these roles deserves to be listed as a contributor. But who should be listed as an author? One would think that, given his or her high level of accountability and responsibility for the research, the PI should be listed as an author, perhaps even as the first author. But suppose the PI has nothing more to do with the project than securing funding. Does this qualify him or her for authorship? Who else should be listed? Students? Technicians? Statisticians? What about the lab director? And how should we deal with research projects that are conducted by groups? Should researchers recognize corporate or institutional authorship? Many different organizations, including the International Committee of Medical Journal Editors (ICMJE) (1997), an organization with over 400 members, have wrestled with these issues.

To help address these questions, we propose the following guidelines on authorship, which are intended to promote accountability, trust, and fairness:

1. To qualify as an author, each person must be held accountable for the whole paper. This does not mean that each member is responsible for every part of the paper (accountability and responsibility are slightly different), since different people may perform different tasks, but each person should be prepared to explain the paper and defend it in public. If the paper contains an error or is found to be fraudulent, each author may be held accountable for this problem, even if only one author actually made the error or committed the fraud. Many authors have stressed the importance of this requirement (International Committee 1997, Huth 1986b, Rennie et al, 1997, Resnik 1997, LaFollette 1992).

2. To qualify to be the first author, the individual must have participated in all of the following: (a) conception or design, analysis and interpretation of data, or both; (b) drafting the article for critically important intellectual content; and (c) final approval of the version to be published.

3. To qualify as a coauthor, the individual must have participated in two or more of the following: (a) conception or design, or analysis and interpretation of data; b) drafting or editing portion(s) or revision(s) of the article; and (c) providing the intellectual proposals for funding agencies for the project.

4. For corporate authorship, at least one person should be listed as an author. Institutions, committees, associations, task forces, and so on, author a growing number of publications. Although these types of collaborations are vital to research, they can raise serious problems with accountability if they do not identify one or more people who can defend the whole paper. If a publication lists only a corporate entity as an author, then reviewers, readers, and the lay public have no idea who to hold accountable or responsible for the project.

5. The authorship order should be based on the importance of the individual's contribution to the paper. Some writers (e.g., Diguisto 1994) have proposed quantitative methods for determining authorship order, but we do not find these methods especially useful, because judgments about importance are, in large part, value judgments and cannot be quantified easily (American Psychological Association 1992).

6. In general, all articles that result from a graduate student's thesis project should list the student as first author. We include this recommendation to avoid some of the problems of exploitation of subordinates that unfortunately occur in research, and which we discuss in more depth below under the topic of mentoring.

7. To the extent possible, papers should clearly state the contributions of different authors and should acknowledge all contributors. This policy encourages both accountability and responsibility in that it provides readers with some idea of who is most responsible for different aspects of the paper (*Nature* 1999). Some writers have argued that it is time to do away with the outmoded category of "author" and replace it with a different system of credit allocation that simply details how different people have contributed to the project (Resnik 1997, Rennie et al. 1997). We are sympathetic to the proposal but also recognize the difficulty of overcoming long-standing traditions and institutional personnel policies that place a heavy emphasis on authorship.

8. Many of these guidelines also apply to the concept of inventorship. Inventors, like authors, receive credit for their work and can be held accountable. It is also important to promote trust and fairness when collaborations result in an invention (Dreyfuss 2000).

SHARING RESOURCES

In addition to authorship, another important issue in collaborative research is how or whether to share resources, such as preliminary data, final data, ideas, results, reagents, cell lines, tissue samples, genetically engineered animals, equipment and tools, computers, methods, administrative or technical staff, and research sites (Marshall 1997a–c). This issue arises in collaborative research because the very idea of collaboration involves sharing and working together. But tensions arise because there are often reasons to share and not share resources.

There are several reasons why researchers have ethical obligations to share resources:

1. Sharing resources promotes efficiency. Research proceeds at a more rapid and efficient pace when scientists pool their resources instead of hoarding them—many hands lighten the load (National Academy of Sciences 1994, Resnik 1998a, Munthe and Welin 1996).
2. Sharing resources promotes objectivity and progress. Openness, or the sharing of data, results, and ideas, is a key part of the scientific method itself in that it promotes constructive criticism, peer review, and replication of results (NAS 1994, Resnik 1998a; Munthe and Welin 1996). This argument applies most strongly to the sharing of final data or results, but it also applies, to a lesser extent, to the sharing of preliminary data.
3. Sharing resources promotes collegiality and trust. When people refuse to share resources, they promote a climate of secrecy and selfishness that can lead to contempt and distrust. Sharing resources, on the other hand, creates a climate of openness and cooperation that encourages collegiality and trust (Resnik 1998a).
4. Sharing resources promotes fairness and equity. The idea here is fairly simple: research resources are more likely to be distributed fairly or equitably when researchers share resources than when they hoard them. When hoarding prevails, the most powerful, prestigious, and well-financed groups will be able to acquire the most resources. If research groups with less power are to have an opportunity to contribute to science, then they need access to resources acquired or used by larger groups.
5. Sharing resources, especially data, is sometimes required by law or by specific policies. According to a recently approved amendment to the U.S. Freedom of Information Act, researchers who use federal funds to obtain data must allow the public to have access to the data (Kaiser 1999). However, researchers maintain that this requirement does not apply to preliminary data or confidential data about patients obtained in clinical trials. The National Institutes of Health (NIH) also have specific resources sharing policies (NIH 1998). With respect to resources, many important scientific resources, such as national parks, national forests, national libraries, national observatories, public data-

bases, and some pieces of equipment (e.g., the Hubble telescope), are public property and must be shared. No one owns some resources, such as the oceans, the atmosphere, and Antarctica.

These are all very strong arguments for sharing data and resources, and we advocate sharing as a general rule in science. However, there are also some reasons not to share data or resources:

1. The need to protect preliminary work from criticism: Many researchers hesitate to share preliminary data, ideas, or results because their work is not yet ready for public scrutiny (Resnik 1998a). Charles Darwin, for example, worked on his theory of evolution by natural selection for over two decades before publishing the *Origin of Species* in 1859. During this time prior to publication, Darwin gathered more evidence for his theory and developed his arguments. He knew that his theory would be subjected to tremendous criticism upon publication, and it was.

2. The need to protect claims related to discovery and priority: Many researchers refuse to share preliminary ideas, methods, or preliminary data in order to prevent competitors from winning the race for priority. In science, those who publish first are usually credited with the important discovery (Merton 1973). As long as the quest for priority continues to be part of the scientific ethos, researchers will hesitate to share resources with competitors in order to avoid being "beaten to the punch."

3. The need to protect intellectual property: Researchers often have intellectual property interests, such as possible or pending patents, that can be threatened by premature disclosure or publication (Gibbs 1996, Marshall 1997a–c, 2000a). According to the U.S. patent laws, which we discuss more fully in chapter 6, one cannot patent an invention if it fails the test of novelty. One way of showing that an invention is not novel is to prove that it has already been invented or that it has been disclosed previously in some form (Foster and Shook 1993).

4. The need to protect institutional or local investments: If a university spends its own resources on developing research equipment, such as a telescope or wind tunnel, then it may decide to give priority to researchers from within the institution for use of the equipment. Likewise, if a state invests in a piece of equipment, it may give priority to researchers from within the state.

5. The need to protect confidential information related to peer review or human subjects research. We discuss these important reasons for refusing to share data in other chapters.

6. The need to protect confidential information in private research, military research, or forensic research: Private companies often impose stringent confidentiality conditions on researchers. Business has several ways of controlling private data and resources, including trade secrecy, patenting practices, and contracts requiring prior review of

research (Bowie 1994). Industry sponsorship of research raises many different concerns about secrecy and openness, which we examine in more depth later. The military also has an elaborate system for protecting classified information for the purposes of national security. People who work for the military are given access to information on a "need to know" basis; a person may be given clearance (or access) only to specific items of information. Information itself is classified according to different degrees, ranging from "top secret" to "highly classified," and so on. We do not discuss military research in great depth in this book—see Resnik (1998b) and Nelkin (1972) for further discussion on the topic. Those who conduct forensic research related to criminal investigations, such as pathologists, forensic anthropologists, and forensic psychiatrists, also have legal and ethical obligations to maintain confidentiality.

7. The need to protect confidential information related to personnel or student records: This is a fairly obvious reason for keeping some aspects of research confidential.

Ethical dilemmas often arise regarding the sharing of data and resources. We do not attempt to solve these dilemmas here; we believe that they are best addressed by considering information, options, and values case by case. We offer the reader the following rules of thumb (see also our method for ethical decision-making discussed in chapter 1):

1. Researchers working on the same project *must* share data and resources. This may seem rather obvious to some, but sometimes researchers working on the same project do not share resources. We use the strong verb "must" here because accountability, trust, and collegiality will break down if researchers on the same project refuse to share information.

2. Researchers *must* share relevant information with committees and organizations in charge of overseeing research, such as institutional review boards, animal care and use committees, biological safety committees, radiation safety committees, data monitoring boards, the U.S. Food and Drug Administration, and conflict of interest committees. Once again, this seems rather obvious, but we mention it here because sometimes researchers do not report adverse events in human experimentation (Shamoo 2001), deaths in animal research, biological hazards, conflicts of interest, and so forth. These committees and organizations have important responsibilities to promote health, safety, animal welfare, and human rights, but they cannot meet their obligations if they do not have the information they need.

3. Researchers should also share data and resources with colleagues, in descending order of importance: (a) colleagues in the same laboratory, (b) colleagues in the same institution, (c) colleagues in the same discipline, (d) other colleagues conducting research or other scholarly activities, and (e) the general public, including reporters, indus-

try representatives, and citizen advocates. This last group covered is highly diverse. Although we believe that researchers have a strong obligation to educate and inform the public, the public often includes people who will disrupt or misinterpret research. Scientists need to be careful when sharing ideas, data, or results with the public.

MENTORING

Mentoring is a very important part of scientific education and training. Although mentors provide students with knowledge and information as well as wisdom and advice, mentors also teach their students by example. Most people have different mentors at different times for different reasons. A mentor could be a family member, a pastor, a coach, a friend, a teacher, a business leader, a policeman, or anyone a student knows and admires. In science, a mentor is usually a senior researcher who supervises a number of different graduate students. Usually students' graduate advisors or thesis advisors are also their mentors, but many research students obtain mentoring from senior researchers who have no formal advising responsibilities (Weil and Arzbaecher 1997). Many students consider more than one person their mentor, but unfortunately, some students have no one whom they would consider a mentor. Students who benefit from mentoring include graduate and undergraduate students, postdoctoral students, and even junior level professors. The mentor-student relationship is the social foundation of research (Panel on Scientific Responsibility 1992, National Academy of Sciences 1997, NIH 2000).

Mentors interact with their students in many ways. Some of the most important activities include the following:

1. Teaching students how to do research: Mentors help students learn the techniques, methods, and traditions of research. They show students how to design experiments, conduct experiments, collect and record data, analyze data, and write up results.
2. Critiquing and supporting students' research and teaching: Mentors read lab notebooks, research protocols, and manuscripts (Macrina 2000) and scrutinize research design and data analysis. They may attend classes that the students teach, read students' evaluations of teaching, or provide feedback on teaching style and technique. Although it is very important for mentors to criticize students, they also need to offer support and encouragement, and they need to carefully tread the line between constructive and destructive criticism.
3. Promoting their students' careers: Mentors help students to enter the job market. They help students find jobs and submit job applications, they write letters of recommendation, and they help students prepare for job interviews (Macrina 2000).
4. Helping students understand the legal, social, and financial aspects of research: Mentors teach their students about research rules and regulations, such as animal care and use regulations, human experimen-

tation regulations, and biological and radiation safety regulations. They also help students understand the social structure of the research environment, including relationships with colleagues, students, administrators, funding agencies, and the public. They help students understand the funding of research and help them write grant applications and obtain scholarships and fellowships.

5. Teaching students about research ethics: Mentors play an important role in teaching students about the ethical aspects of research (Macrina 2000, Weil and Arzbaecher 1997, Swazey and Bird 1997, Panel on Scientific Responsibility 1992). Such teaching may involve didactic lectures, workshops, and seminars as well as informal discussions. Most important, mentors need to provide students with a good example of how to behave ethically in research, because students learn a great deal of ethics by example.

6. Involvement in their students' personal lives: Mentors may also become involved in their students' personal lives if, for example, a student is having difficulties with family or friends or is having psychological, medical, or legal problems. A student's mentor may help the student in these difficult circumstances.

The list above shows that mentors perform many important duties for their students. Mentors are more than mere teachers: they are also advisors, counselors, and friends. Because students often work for mentors as teaching and research assistants, mentors also serve as employers and supervisors. These different roles may sometimes conflict. For instance, a mentor may give a student so much work to do that the student does not have adequate time for her own research. In this case, the mentor's role of employer/supervisor conflicts with the role of teacher. Or a mentor may believe that it is in the student's best interests to transfer to a different university to work with someone who has more expertise in that student's chosen area of research, but yet may hesitate to convey this advice to him if the mentor needs him as a research or teaching assistant.

To understand the ethical dimensions of the mentor–student relationship, it is important to realize that mentors have more power, experience, knowledge, and expertise than do their students (Macrina 2000, Weil and Arzbaecher 1997). Students also depend on their mentors for education, training, advice, and employment. Mentors may also depend on students for assistance in teaching or research, but students are far more dependent on mentors than vice versa. Given their minimal power, experience, knowledge, and expertise and the high degree of dependency, students are highly vulnerable. It is very easy for mentors to manipulate, control, or exploit their students, because students often may be unable to prevent or avoid such abuses of power. Thus, the mentor–student relationship resembles other professional relationships where one party is highly vulnerable, such as the doctor–patient relationship and the lawyer–client relationship. These relationships are sometimes called fiduciary relationships because the vulnerable party must trust the powerful party to provide knowledge, advice, skill, or expertise and the powerful party has ethical duties toward the vulnerable party, such as beneficence, nonmaleficence, confidentiality, respect, and justice (Bayles 1988).

Although it should be fairly obvious that mentors have a variety of ethical duties to their students, ethical problems can still arise in this relationship. Unfortunately, various forms of exploitation are fairly common in mentoring. Mentors sometimes do not protect their students from harm or treat them fairly. For instance, mentors often do not give students proper credit for their work. They may fail to give students acknowledgments in papers or include them as coauthors (Banoub-Baddour and Gien 1991). They may fail to list students as first authors when students make the most important contribution to the research. In some of the more egregious cases, mentors have stolen ideas from their students without giving them any credit at all (Marshall 1999c, 2000a, Dreyfuss 2000). One well-known case of this type of exploitation involved the famous scientist Robert Millikan and his student Harvey Fletcher. Millikan was conducting experiments to measure the minimum electrostatic charge, the charge of an electron. In his experiments, he dropped charged water droplets through charged plates. By comparing the rate of fall of the droplets without charged plates to their rate of fall through the plates, Millikan would be able to determine the electrostatic force on the droplets and therefore the minimum charges. His experiment was not working well, and Fletcher suggested that Millikan use oil droplets instead of water droplets. Millikan took this advice and ended up winning the Nobel Prize in 1923 for the discovery. However, Millikan did not acknowledge Fletcher's contribution in his papers on these experiments (Holton 1978).

Mentors may also overwork their students by assigning them too many experiments to run, too many papers to grade, too many undergraduate students to tutor, and so on. If students are assigned too much work, they will not have enough time for their own education and research. In recent years, graduate students have formed unions to deal with poor working conditions. Postdoctoral students often face especially demanding and exploitative working conditions. They are usually nontenured researchers who are paid through "soft money," that is, money from research grants. Postdoctoral students get paid much less than do regular faculty members even though they have doctoral degrees and they do just as much research or teaching. They also do not receive the usual benefits package, and they have little job security (Barinaga 2000). Although some postdoctoral students enjoy their work, others feel mistreated or exploited. Given their vulnerability, it is very hard for these students to complain about working conditions or about their mentors, because they face the real threat of retaliation. For example, the mentor could refuse to work with the student any longer, recommend that the student be expelled from the program, write an angry letter about the student to colleagues, and so on.

Other examples of ways in which mentors may abuse their students include the following:

- Giving students misinformation or poor advice
- Intimidating or harassing students

- Discriminating against students or showing favoritism
- Failing to help students advance their careers
- Not recognizing when students are having psychological troubles that require counseling

Given the importance of the mentor–student relationship for scientific research, and the kinds of problems that routinely arise, many universities and professional organizations have developed programs and policies aimed at improving mentoring (NIH 2000, National Academy of Sciences 1997). Some of these policies include the following:

1. Rewarding mentors for effective mentoring: Most universities do not emphasize or even consider "mentoring skills" when they review faculty for hiring and promotion, but this needs to change if we want to improve mentoring (Djerassi 1999).
2. Providing mentors with enough time for mentoring: Professors who do not have adequate time for mentoring will do a poor job of mentoring. Professors who have heavy mentoring responsibilities should be released from other administrative or teaching obligations.
3. Developing clear rules concerning workloads, teaching duties, research opportunities, authorship, time commitments, and intellectual property: Many of the problems that occur in mentoring are due to poor communication. Communication can be improved by clearly defining expectations and obligations (Macrina 2000).
4. Establishing procedures and channels for evaluating mentoring and for allowing students and mentors to voices their grievances.
5. Ensuring that students who "blow the whistle" on mentors are protected: We discuss this recommendation in chapter 5 on scientific misconduct.
6. Promoting a psychologically safe work environment: Students and mentors both need to have an environment that is free from sexual, religious, ethnic, and other forms of harassment (Panel on Scientific Responsibility 1992). Sexual harassment is unethical and can also be illegal. Although most researchers agree on the need to protect students and others from sexual harassment, there are disputes about the definition of sexual harassment as well as the proper response to sexual harassment (Swisher 1995). For further discussion, see Resnik 1998b.
7. Promoting a nondiscriminatory work environment: Racial, ethnic, sexual, religious, and other types of discrimination are also unethical and often illegal. Women have for many years labored under the yoke of sex discrimination, although the culture of science has improved the position of women in the latter part of the twentieth century. Racial and ethnic discrimination continue to be a problem in science as more minorities enter the workplace (Johnson 1993, Manning 1998). Although African Americans have historically been the most frequent victims of discrimination, Asian Americans also experience discrimination (Lawler 2000). Scientists should be judged by the

quality of their research, education, and character, not by the color of their skin, their national origin, their religious views, or their gender. Effective mentoring cannot take place when discrimination infects and affects the laboratory (for further discussion, see Resnik 1998b).

8. Promoting a diverse workforce in research: Because mentors serve as role models as well as advisors and friends, one could argue that it is important to promote diversity in science in order to enhance mentoring and education. Science students have different gender, racial, ethnic, and religious characteristics. The scientific workforce should reflect this diversity so that students can benefit from having role models with whom they can identify (Mervis 1999, Holden 2000). An excellent way to promote the effective mentoring of women in science is to hire and promote more women scientists (Etkowitz et al 1994, National Science Foundation 1999), which will also encourage more women to enter science. This same "diversity" argument also applies to racial and ethnic diversity, which raises the question of affirmative action in science: should hiring and promotion of scientists be decided based on racial or ethnic features of a person? This is a complex legal, moral, and political question that we do not explore in depth here. We favor a weak form of affirmative action that increases the diversity of the workforce without compromising quality. Racial, ethnic, and gender considerations should come into play only when different candidates for the same position (job, place in the class, or fellowship) are otherwise equally qualified. Affirmative action should not be used to promote incompetence or tokenism.

RECOMMENDATIONS FOR RESEARCH COLLABORATION

Overall we recommend that collaborators discuss important research issues before and during their collaborative work:

1. Authorship: Who will be an author? Who will be a second author?
2. Research roles and responsibilities: Who will be responsible for different aspects of the research, such as conception and design, collecting data, analyzing data, and so forth? Who are the various personnel working on the project?
3. Extent of the collaboration: How much of a commitment of time, effort, and money is involved in the collaboration?
4. Intellectual property: If the project involves potential patents or other property rights, how will these be shared or assigned?
5. Funding: How will the project be funded? Who will apply for funding?
6. Conflicts of interest: Are there any financial or other interests affecting the research that collaborators should know about?
7. Resource sharing: How will data and other resources be managed and shared?

8. Dissemination of results: How and where will the research be published or disseminated? Is there a plan for discussing research results with the media or the public?
9. Deadlines: Are there any institutional, funding, or other deadlines relevant to the project?
10. Regulations: What regulations (if any) pertain to the project?

Some of these issues have been discussed in this chapter; others are discussed in the chapters that follow.

QUESTIONS FOR DISCUSSION

1. How would you describe the current state of collaboration in research?
2. Why is collaboration important for research?
3. Can you think of any examples, from your own experience or from the experiences of colleagues, where collaboration was lacking?
4. Have you been an author or a coauthor of a research paper? What was your experience, and why did you deserve to be an author/coauthor?
5. What is wrong, if anything, with the "least publishable unit"?
6. Can you think of a situation where granting honorary authorship is justified?
7. Is ghost authorship ever justified?
8. How would you react if someone you do not know wants a sample of research material or data?
9. Can you describe how you are being mentored? Are there modifications you could suggest?
10. What are the qualities (or virtues) of a good mentor?

CASES FOR DISCUSSION

Case 1

A postdoctoral fellow got into a severe conflict with her mentor. Her mentor provided her salary from his grant resources, and she was working in one of his primary projects. She found another job and took all three laboratory notebooks with her when she left. The mentor was very angry when he found out. He asked her to return the lab notebooks immediately or she would be accused of theft. He claimed the lab notebooks belonged to him and to the university, but he invited her to copy the books for her use. She returned the notebooks after making copies.

Two years later, the mentor learned that she had published a paper without mentioning his name anywhere, but that his grant was acknowledged. What should the mentor do?

Case 2

A graduate student worked for a year with an advisor on replicating a new small protein. He spent part of the year developing the methodology before conducting the replications. However, the graduate student did not like his advisor and moved to a different advisor within the same department, who happened to be the director of the graduate program in that department. The student's new research program was in a different area from the previous work.

A year later, the student learned that a subsequent student of his former mentor had used his method for replicating the protein in subsequent research, and that they were writing a paper without listing him as a coauthor. He protested but was told that the new graduate student had to do the whole thing all over again and that they were not using his data. The student argued that the new technique used to collect the data was a novel technique developed by him and not available in the open literature. The student's former advisor, after meeting with everyone including the director, reluctantly agreed to publish at a later date a small technical paper on the technique naming the student as coauthor. The first paper will still appear, much sooner, and without his name. The student agreed, under protest, but he knew his life would be difficult if he insisted on a different outcome.

- What would you have done under these circumstances?
- Should the first advisor have done what she did?
- What should the new student have done, and what should he do now? The director?

Case 3

A graduate student was studying at a university where his faculty mentor is also a full-time employee of the affiliated hospital. He and his mentor discovered a major environmental airborne toxin, and the media covered the story. The mentor then died suddenly of a heart attack. They had a manuscript already written and about to be submitted for publication in a prestigious journal.

The chair of the department, who worked in a closely related area, became the new student's mentor. She took the manuscript and put her name as the senior author (last) and eliminated the name of the deceased. She had no involvement in the project prior to the death of the former mentor. The paper was published after minor revision.

- What should the student do?
- What should the mentor do?

Case 4

The physics department at a university consists of twelve men and no women. The chancellor of the university has said that the department needs to make a superior effort to hire well-qualified women and has promised the department extra money for a new employee's salary, travel, and other benefits if she is a well-qualified woman.

The department posts two new job openings, both at the assistant professor level, and receives 100 applications; only five are from women. The top seven male candidates have a better educational background and publication record than do the three female applicants who are qualified for the job. The department chair has said that they must hire a woman. They plan to hire the best woman they can get as well as the best man. Is this policy discriminatory? Is it fair?

Case 5

Dr. Barnes has been telling dirty jokes in his anatomy and physiology class for as long as anyone can remember. He is a very friendly, outgoing teacher, gets excellent evaluations on his teaching, and has won several teaching awards. Dr. Barnes has three teaching assistants who help with various aspects of the course.

During one of the labs for the course, one of teaching assistants, Heather, overhears two female students complaining about his jokes. They find his jokes both rude and offensive. Heather talks to the two students. She says that she also found his jokes rude and offensive at first, but that she got used to them and they don't bother her anymore. They say that they do not want to get used to his jokes and that they are planning to talk to the Dean of Students. What should Heather do?

Case 6

Dr. Gribnick is testing HIV vaccines on rhesus monkeys. In his experiment, he vaccinates an experimental group of monkeys and then exposes them to the simian version of HIV (SIV). He also exposes an unvaccinated control group of monkeys to SIV. In these experiments, a dozen monkeys have developed the simian version of AIDS, and several have died. The NIH funds his research.

Yesterday, he received a letter requesting data from his research under the Freedom of Information Act. An animal rights group made the request. He is very concerned that the group will try to disrupt his research and possibly destroy his lab, if it has access to his data.

- Should Dr. Gribnick turn over the data as requested?
- Does this outside group have a right to see his data?

Case 7

Dr. Watson and Dr. Gramm are developing a genetic test for adult-onset (type II) diabetes. Their assay tests for several thousand mutations that are strongly predictive of type II diabetes. Of those patients who test positive for these mutations, 60% will develop type II diabetes. Watson and Gramm hope that their test will be used on children and adolescents to provide information that may be helpful in preventing type II diabetes or managing its effects. If people learn early that they have these mutations, then they may be able to undertake a diet and exercise program to prevent this disease or prevent some of its devastating consequences, such as loss of limbs or blindness.

Watson and Gramm plan to patent the test when their work is complete. They have been collaborating with several researchers at other institutions, sharing data, reagents, methods, and so on. They recently received a request for some preliminary data from several colleagues, including their collaborators as well as other colleagues in the field.

- Should they share their data?
- Would it make any difference if a private corporation funded their research?

Case 8

Dr. Thomas published a review article on recent developments in mitochondrial genetics. In the article, he mentioned his own work prominently but failed to mention the work of several other researchers who have made key contributions to the field. Dr. Thomas is clearly one of the most important researchers in the field, and he has done some important work. But he also has some long-running feuds with some of the other prominent researchers in the field, based in part on fundamental disagreements about the role of the mitochondrial DNA in human evolution. In his review article, in several instances he cited his own work instead of giving proper credit to colleagues who had published their articles before his. Is this plagiarism? Is it unethical?

4

Publication and Peer Review

This chapter provides a historical overview of scientific publication and peer review and describes the current practices of scientific journals and granting agencies. It also examines a number of different ethical issues and concerns that arise in publication and peer review, such as quality control, confidentiality, fairness, bias, electronic publication, wasteful publication, duplicate publication, publishing controversial research, and editorial independence. The chapter also addresses the ethical responsibilities of reviewers and concludes with a discussion of the relationship between researchers and the media.

A BRIEF HISTORY OF SCIENTIFIC PUBLICATION AND PEER REVIEW

Throughout history, advances in communication technologies have helped to accelerate the progress of science (Lucky 2000). Written language was the first important innovation in communication that helped promote the growth of science. The Egyptians used hieroglyphics as early as 3000 BC, and by 1700 BC the Phoenicians had developed an alphabet that became the basis of the Roman alphabet. With the invention of writing, human beings were able to record their observations and events as well as their ideas. The Egyptians and Babylonians, for example, made detailed observations of the movements of constellations, planets, and the moon in the night sky, as well as the position of the sun in daytime. Ancient Greek and Roman scientists communicated mostly through direct conversations and occasionally through letters. Philosopher-scientists, such as Pythagoras, Hippocrates, Plato, Aristotle, Euclid, Hero, Ptolemy, and Archimedes, discussed their ideas with students and colleagues in their respective schools, academies, and lyceums. Although these scientists also published some influential books, such as Euclid's *Elements*, Plato's *Republic*, and Ptolemy's *Almagest*, books were very rare because they had to be copied by hand on papyrus rolls.

Egypt, especially the city of Alexandria, was the cultural province of Greece and later Rome. The Roman Empire built the largest network of roads and bridges in the world, which increased commercial and scientific communication between the Far East and Middle East and the West. From about 40 BC to 640 AD, most of the world's recorded scientific knowledge rested in the great library of Alexandria. Invading forces burned the library three times, in 269 AD, 415 AD, and 640 AD. Each time the library burned, scholars rushed to save books from being lost forever—to people in the modern, developed world the idea of there being only a single copy of a book that, if lost, is lost forever is almost inconceivable (Ronan 1982).

Aside from the development of written language, the invention of the printing press during the 1400s by the German goldsmith Johannes Guttenberg was the single most important event in the history of scientific communication. The Chinese had developed paper in the second century AD. By the ninth century, they had printed books using block print and woodcuttings. These inventions were brought to the Western world through trade with Arabic/Islamic countries. Gutenberg added to these established printing technologies and key innovation, moveable type, which allowed the printer to quickly change the letters of the printing template. In 1450 Gutenberg established a printing shop and began to print the first works using his press, which included sacred texts, such as the Bible (1454) and prayer books, grammar books, and bureaucratic documents. The selection of books soon expanded to include guidebooks, maps, how-to books, calendars, and currency exchange tables. In 1543 two influential and widely distributed scientific works also appeared in print, Vesalius' *The Fabric of the Human Body* and Copernicus' *The Revolutions of the Heavenly Bodies*. During the sixteenth century many important scientific and technical books, often originally written in Latin or Greek, were translated into vernacular and printed (Burke 1995).

The printing press increased the rapidity and quantity of scientific communication like no other invention before or since (Lucky 2000). It also helped transform Europe from a medieval to a modern culture and worldview and thus helped stimulate the Scientific Revolution (see chapter 12). The printing press helped transform Europe from a society based on oral tradition and memory to a literate society based on permanent, shared records and writing. People learned to read and developed a passion for books and learning. The Catholic Church lost control of the interpretation of the Bible when this work was translated into the vernacular, and people began fashioning their own interpretations of what they read, an event that helped spur the Protestant Reformation. Martin Luther printed copies of his *95 Criticisms of the Church* (1517) and nailed them to a bulletin board in his own church in Wittenberg, Germany. As others printed copies, Luther's complaints about indulgences, corruption, and paganism spread all over Europe in less than a month (Burke 1995).

By the 1600s, scientific books were common items in libraries throughout the world. But because it took several years to research, write, and publish a book, more rapid communication was needed as well. Scientists continued to correspond with letters, of course. Indeed, the letters of Descartes, Galileo, Newton, Boyle, and Harvey are considered to be key documents in the history of science. An important step toward more rapid and more public communication took place in 1665, when the world's first two scientific journals, *The Philosophical Transactions of the Royal Society of London* and the *Journal des Scavans*, were first published. The first scientific association, the Royal Society of London, was a private corporation formed in 1662 to support scientific research and the exchange of ideas. Its journal is still published today. The world's second scientific society, the Academy of Sciences of Paris, was formed in 1666 as an organization sponsored by the French government. By the 1800s, many other scientific associations and scientific journals had arisen (Meadows 1992).

The advantage of scientific journals is that they provide rapid communication of ideas, data, and results. Journals can also print a high volume of material. However, journals must face the problem of quality control. The Royal Society addressed this issue in 1752, when it started evaluating and reviewing manuscripts submitted to its journal (Kronic 1990). The Royal Society took this step because its members became concerned about the quality of papers that were published in the journal. Some of the papers published before then had included highly speculative and rambling essays, as well as works of fiction (LaFollette 1992). Soon other journals followed this example, and the peer review system began to take shape.

Other important innovations in communication technologies included the telegraph (1837), the transatlantic telegraph (1858), the telephone (1876), the phonograph (1877), radio (1894), and television (1925–1933). Developments in transportation also enhanced scientific communication, because printed materials still must be transported in order to disseminate them widely. Important developments in transportation included the steam locomotive (1804), transcontinental railways (1869), the automobile (1859–1867), and the airplane (1903) (Williams 1987).

After the printing press, the computer (1946) is arguably the second most important invention relating to scientific communication. Computers allow researchers to collect, store, transmit, process, and analyze information in digital form. Computers are also the key technology in the Internet, which combines computers and other communication technologies, such as telephone lines, cable lines, and satellite transmitters, to form an information network. The Internet allows researchers to publish scientific information instantaneously and distribute it to an unlimited audience via electronic mail, discussion boards, and web pages. The Internet also allows scientists to instantly search scientific databases for articles and information (Lucky 2000). It is like having a library, newspaper, shopping catalogue, magazine, billboard, museum, atlas, theater, and radio station all accessible through a computer terminal (Graham 1999). Although the Internet is a monumental leap forward in the rapidity and quantity of scientific communication, it also poses tremendous problems relating to quality control, because anyone can publish anything on the Internet (Resnik 1998b).

THE CURRENT PEER REVIEW SYSTEM

Although peer review had its origins in scientific publishing in the eighteenth century, it was not institutionalized until the twentieth century, when it began to be used to legitimize specific projects that required the expenditure of large sums of public funds (Burnham 1990). In 1937, the requirement of peer review for awarding grants from the National Cancer Institute (NCI) was made into a public law. Today, all major federal funding agencies, such as the National Institutes of Health (NIH), the National Science Foundation (NSF), the Department of Energy (DOE), the Environmental Protection Agency (EPA), and the National Endowment for the Humanities (NEH), use peer review to make decisions on awarding funding.

Peer review brought together two potentially conflicting concepts—expertise and objectivity (Shamoo 1993). The need for peer review of public funds arose in order to provide a mechanism of quality control and to prevent favoritism, the "old boy network," and fraud in allocating public money. The system was implemented in order to make objective decisions pertaining to the quality of grant proposals. Peer review arose in scientific publication in order to evaluate the quality of manuscripts submitted for publication and to provide a quality control mechanism for science. Another advantage of peer review is that it is less centralized and bureaucratic than other processes one might use to fund research (LaFollette 1994c). Scientists, not politicians or bureaucrats, control peer review. On the other hand, peer review also allows for a certain amount of government oversight, and thus it provides a venue for public participation in the setting of funding priorities (Jasanoff 1990).

There are numerous types of peer review processes developed for variety of purposes. However, there are three sectors of the scientific enterprise that rely heavily on peer review to in decision making: government contracts and grants,

Government Contracts and Grants

Grants are the most important area where peer review is used, not only because government grants provide public money to fund a large portion of research across the country, but more important, because this is the only area of peer review under direct public scrutiny where citizens can raise issues of fairness, equity, justice, and public accountability with the public. In addition to public funding agencies, many private corporations, such as pharmaceutical and biotechnology companies, sponsor research through grants to investigators or institutions.

A contract, on the other hand, is a specific contractual agreement between the investigator and a government or private agency. A contract stipulates the conditions to be met, and both parties must agree to these conditions. A contract may or may not go through peer review. Even when contracts undergo peer review, it is selective and does not conform to the usual "independent" peer review used to evaluate grant proposals. Because contracts do not conform to the standards set by independent peer review, one may question the current practices in granting contracts in science, but we do not explore that issue here. We concentrate here on the "grant-dependent" peer review standards.

Grants in broad terms originate from two funding sources, the private sector and the public sector. The public sector includes agencies of the federal government such as the NIH, NSF, and NEH. The private sector ranges from very small foundations awarding hundreds of dollars to large foundations such as the Howard Hughes Medical Foundation, which awards millions of dollars each year. Private foundations follow whatever review process they deem suitable for their purpose, and many use methods that evaluate proposals on ethnic or religious grounds. There is very little public scrutiny of their decision-making process other than what little is prescribed by the Internal Revenue Service (IRS) for nonprofit status. Although these foundations are philanthropic and public service institutions that contribute to the advancement of knowledge, most are indirectly subsidized by taxpayers because they are classified by the IRS as nonprofit (501C3) organizations, which are tax-exempt. One could argue that these organizations should be held more publicly accountable if they receive tax breaks.

In the peer review process for government agencies, on the other hand, the first step is the selection of peers and definition of "peers." The Government Accounting Office (GAO 1994) report of peer review provides a thorough evaluation of this process. The selection of peer reviewers differs among the NIH, the NSF, and the NEH. Further, the hierarchy of peer review structure and its impact also differ at the three agencies. NIH has an initial peer review at the proposal's study section level (it has over 100 study sections). These study sections belong officially to the Division of Research Grants, which reports directly to the NIH director and not to each institute within NIH. The independence and division from actual program managers at each institute preserve the integrity of the review process. However, in special cases, institutes can construct their own study sections, especially for large program projects and center grants. Study sections usually consist of 18–20 members. Their decisions are not final, because the NIH Advisory Council has the final authority. However, the council usually follows the study section ratings. The executive secretary of each study section is the one who recommends new members for the study section, at the approval of senior administrators. The executive secretary keeps a large list of potential study section members, based on discipline, knowledge, gender, age, and so forth. The executive secretary is usually a career staff member of the NIH with an M.D. or a Ph.D. degree. The NIH uses 6,000 to 7,000 reviewers annually (GAO 1994).

At the NSF, most of the initial peer review occurs by mail, followed by a meeting of a panel of 8–12 members who review the comments made by mail. The panels are headed by NSF program directors, who are NSF career employees with advanced degrees. Each program director has the authority to select panel members and mail reviewers, and keeps a large list of potential reviewers based on discipline, publications, gender, race, age, and knowledge. NSF uses over 60,000 reviewers annually (GAO 1994).

At the NEH there is only one peer review system, which is based on standing panels of about five members, who are selected from a large list based on qualification similar to the criteria used by NIH and NSF. At times, NEH program managers solicit evaluation from external reviewers to supplement the panel's deliberations. Annually, the NEH uses about 1,000 scholars for this review process (GAO 1994).

In evaluating proposals, reviewers at government agencies consider and address a number of different criteria:

1. The scientific or scholarly significance of the proposal
2. The proposed methodology
3. The qualifications of the principle investigator (PI) and other participants

4. Prior research or data that support the proposal
5. The level of institutional support and resources
6. The appropriateness of the budget request
7. Dissemination plans
8. Compliance with federal regulations
9. The proposal's potential social impact

Reviewers take these factors into account and rate proposals based on a relative point scale. The NIH uses comparative merit scores based on the scores of several previous review cycles. These comparative scores are given as percentile scores from lowest (0 percentile) to highest (100 percentile). The NSF allows each program to develop its own scoring method, but each program uses the same scoring method for all proposals it reviews. NSF criteria for scoring are similar to those of NIH, except there is a larger variation in scoring since most scoring is done by mail. For both the NIH and NSF, there is a good relationship between ratings and funding decisions. However, funding decisions are also greatly influenced by the program or project managers. The NSF's program directors have much greater ability to bypass the scores in order to expand opportunities for women, minorities, and geographic areas and to initiate what they think are new and innovative projects. The NEH panels review proposals beforehand, deliberate at their meeting, and then score each proposal. The NEH's criteria for scoring are similar to those of the NIH and the NSF.

Journals

Although the concept of peer review for publication has its origins in the eighteenth century, in the twentieth century peer review evolved into a method for controlling quality of publications as well as providing a stamp of approval by the established peers in a given field. The peer review of manuscripts varies from journal to journal, though the usual procedure has the editor-in-chief (or an associate if it is a large publication) select two reviewers, often experts in the field, to review each manuscript. A few editorial offices of journals that receive a large volume of manuscripts, such as *Science*, *Nature*, and *The New England Journal of Medicine*, screen papers for quality and suitability beforehand to select a small percentage of manuscripts to send to reviewers. Reviewers are given guidelines on reviewing the paper, but in reality reviewers are like jurors in courts: they can ignore the guidelines and base their opinion on whatever they deem to be appropriate. Most reviewers, however, evaluate manuscripts based on the following criteria:

1. Appropriateness of the topic for the journal
2. Originality or significance of the research
3. Strength of the conclusions, results, or interpretations as supported by the data or evidence
4. The validity of the research methods and the research design, given the research goals or aims
5. The quality of the writing

Reviewers may recommend that a manuscript be

- Accepted as is
- Accepted with minor revisions
- Accepted with major revision
- Rejected, but encouraged to resubmit with revisions
- Rejected, not encouraged to resubmit

Usually, if both reviewers highly recommend the acceptance or the rejection of the manuscript, the editor-in-chief follows that recommendation. However, when the reviewers are lukewarm in acceptance or rejection of the manuscript, or if the reviewers conflict in opinion, the editor usually has some latitude in making the decision. Some editors may simply accept or reject a paper, whereas others may send it to a third reviewer for deciding between two conflicting opinions. Of course, editors may also decide, in some rare cases, that the reviewers are completely mistaken and they may accept a paper that reviewers have rejected, or vice versa (LaFollette 1992).

Promotion and Tenure

In public and private academic and research institutions, personnel decisions such as appointment, promotion, and tenure are based on committee recommendations. The criteria followed in making these personnel decisions vary considerably among community colleges, small colleges, local universities, research universities, industrial research organizations, and government laboratories. Although small colleges and community colleges emphasize a person's contributions to teaching, advising, or their service to the institution, most of the other institutions place a greater emphasis a person's research record, that is, the quantity and quality of publications and presentations, and the person's success in obtaining contracts or grants. The committee members as well as relevant administrators are in essence conducting an internal peer review of the candidate's past performance and potential contributions. The committees also solicit reviews of publications and contracts/grants from established researchers/scholars from outside the institution. The input of internal and external peer reviewers is crucial to the personnel decisions. If the committee recommends a candidate for tenure, for example, then other administrators and committees will usually follow this recommendation. Because most institutions emphasize research over teaching, advising, and service, individuals who are seeking tenure or promotion often face difficult choices in balancing their commitments in these different areas.

In our discussion of mentoring in chapter 3, we noted that one way to improve mentoring is to ensure that researchers are adequately rewarded for high-quality mentoring. We recommend that mentoring play a key role in personnel decisions. Many commentators have also noted that the pressure to publish contributes to a variety of ethical problems in science, such as plagiarism, fraud, undeserved authorship, and careless errors (Panel on Scientific Responsibility 1992). To address these pressures to publish, it is important to consider ways of reforming the tenure and promotion system. One key assumption that needs to be examined is the idea that, for publication, "more is better." The emphasis on the quantity of publications, as opposed to quality, is a key factor in the pressure to publish. To address this issue, some universities have decided to only review a select number of publications and to focus on the quality of the candidate's work.

PROBLEMS WITH PEER REVIEW

The idea of peer review makes a great deal of sense. Indeed, peer review is regarded by many philosophers of science as a key pillar of the scientific method because it promotes objectivity and repeatability (Kitcher 1993). Science can be "self-correcting" because scientists review and criticize research methods, designs, and conclusions and repeat experiments and tests. Indeed, it is hard to imagine how science could make progress without something like a peer review system (Abby et al. 1994). However, the peer review system has come under severe criticism in recent years.

Bias and Lack of Reliability

Numerous scholars have provided evidence that peer reviewers have significant bias and low agreement of opinions on the same proposal or potential publication (Cole and Cole 1981, Cole et al. 1978, Chubin and Hackett 1990, Bower 1991, Roy 1993, Shamoo 1993, 1994, Fletcher and Fletcher 1997, Oxman et al. 1991). Some of the biases that can affect peer review include theoretical, conceptual, and methodological disagreements; professional rivalries; institutional biases; and personal feuds (Hull 1988, Godlee 2000). There is considerable evidence that the peer review process may not catch even simple mistakes and that it is certainly not effective at detecting plagiarism and fraud (LaFollette 1992, Peters and Ceci 1982, Goodman 1994). From our own experience, we have come across many published papers that still have obvious and nontrivial mistakes.

Because editors and review panels may reject papers or research proposals based on one negative review, biases can profoundly affect the peer review process. Most scientific journals assign only two or three reviewers to a given paper. Although a peer review panel includes many reviewers, usually only a few people are assigned as primary reviewers for a given proposal. Other panel members will not read the proposal very closely and will not be asked to make extensive comments. It may only take on a single biased primary reviewer to eliminate a grant proposal.

This problem is especially pronounced in the realm of controversial research (Chalmers et al. 1990, Godlee 2000; Barber 1961). Controversial research does not fit neatly into well-established research traditions, norms, or paradigms. It is what the famous historian of science Thomas Kuhn (1970) dubs "revolutionary science" (in contrast with "normal science"). Research can be controversial for a number of reasons: it may be highly creative or innovative; it may challenge previously held theories; or it may be interdisciplinary. Interdisciplinary work provides an additional challenge for reviewers because reviewers may come from different disciplines, and no single reviewer may have all the education or training required to evaluate an interdisciplinary project.

Because reviewers often are established researchers with theoretical and professional commitments, they may be very resistant to new, original, or highly innovative ideas. Historians of science have understood this phenomenon for many years. For example, Kuhn (1962) notes that quantum mechanics was not fully accepted until the old generation of Newtonian physicists died off. Although research carried out within specific disciplinary parameters (i.e., "normal" science) plays a very important role in the overall progress of science, the most important advances in science occur through controversial or "revolutionary" science (Kuhn 1962, Shamoo 1994). History provides us with many examples of important theories that were resisted and ridiculed by established researchers, such as Gregor Mendel's laws of inheritance, Barbara McLintock's gene jumping hypothesis, Peter Mitchell's chemiosmostic theory, and Alfred Wegener's continental drift hypothesis.

The debate over cold fusion in many ways fits this model, although it is too soon to tell whether cold fusion researchers will ultimately be vindicated (Fleischmann 2000). Critics of cold fusion have lambasted this research as either fraudulent or sloppy, while proponents have charged that critics are close-minded and dogmatic. As a result of this controversy, it has been difficult to conduct peer-reviewed work on cold fusion, because mainstream physics journals select reviewers with strong biases against cold fusion. This has not stopped this research program from going forward, however. Cold fusion researchers have established their own journals and societies in response to these rebukes from the "hot" fusion community.

To provide objective and reliable assessments of controversial research, journal editors and review panel leaders should be willing to do what it takes to "open the doors" to new and novel work. If they close these doors, then they are exerting a form of censorship that is not especially helpful to science or to society. What it takes to open the door to controversial research may vary from case to case, but we suggest that editors and review panel leaders should always try to understand controversial research within its context. For instance, if an editor recognizes that a paper is likely to be controversial, then he or she should not automatically reject the paper based on one negative review; before rejecting it, he or she should seek other reviews and give the paper a sympathetic reading.

The issue of publishing controversial research reveals an important flaw in the idea of quality control: if a journal tries to be sure that all articles meet specified standards related to quality, then it may not publish some controversial (but good and important) studies. On the other hand, one way to ensure that controversial ideas are not ignored is to publish a larger quantity of articles with less control over quality. Thus, the scientific community faces a dilemma of quality versus quantity. One partial solution to this dilemma is to increase the number of journals as well as the number of ways to disseminate information, to allow outlets for controversial studies. The advent of Internet publishing has increased the quantity of published material without a proportional increase in the cost of publication, which allows researchers to publish more data and results. It will still be difficult to get controversial work published in the top, peer-reviewed journals, but controversial work can still be published in mid- to lower-range journals, on web pages, and so forth (Bingham 2000).

Fairness in Journal Review

As discussed above, the decisions of individual reviewers, editors, and panel leaders control the outcomes of peer review. A great deal often depends on who is selected to review an article or proposal and on how the reviewers' assessments are interpreted. The system is designed in such a way that it is very easy for someone to affect the outcome in order help someone they know and like or to hinder someone they either don't know or like. For example, an editor's biased choice of reviewers can have an impact on the review outcome.

Many factors can give unfair advantages (or disadvantages) to the authors of manuscripts. Factors such as the author's name and institutional affiliation affect the judgments of editors and reviewers, who are more likely to give favorable reviews to well-respected authors from prestigious institutions than to unknown authors from less prestigious institutions (LaFollette 1992, Garfunkel et al. 1994). Most scientific journals currently use a single-blind system, where authors do not know the identity of reviewers, but reviewers know the identity of the authors. One way that journals have attempted to deal with this problem is to use a double-blind peer review system, where reviewers do not know the identity of authors.

There has been some debate about the strengths and weaknesses of blinded peer review. Several studies have shown that often the reviewers can still identify authors even when they are not given the authors' names or institutional affiliations (Rooyen et al. 1998). The effects of blinding on the quality of peer review are not clear. While some studies have shown that masking the identities of authors improves peer review (McNutt et al. 1990, Blank 1991), other studies indicate that masking the identities of authors does not improve the quality of peer review (Rooyen et al. 1998; Justice et al. 1998). Laband and Piette (1994) examined 1051 full articles published in 1984 in 28 economic journals. They then compared the citations of these articles in the following five years, 1985–1989. They found that papers from journals using masked peer review were cited more often than were papers from journals using unmasked review. These results suggest that the quality of published papers after masked reviews are better on the average than that of papers published after unmasked reviews. On the other hand, the results may be due to the fact that the journals that use masked review are better than or more prestigious than journals that use unmasked review. Even if the evidence does not show that masking the identities of authors improves the quality of peer review, one can still argue that this practice is important in promoting fairness and integrity of peer review.

Some writers have argued that unblinded review would best promote integrity, fairness, and responsibility in peer review, because the current system allows reviewers to hide behind the mask of peer review (DeBakey 1990). If their identities could be discovered or were made public, reviewers would be more likely to be responsible and careful. Recently, anonymous peer review has been challenged in courts. One the other hand, one can argue if reviewer identities are not anonymous, then they may be less likely to be critical or un-biased, because they may fear repercussions from authors (LaFollette 1992).

Fairness in Grant Review

When it comes to grant review, there is evidence that people who know mem-bers of the review panels and who know how the process works are much more likely to have their grants approved than are people who lack this inside information (Shamoo 1993).

Other studies have shown that the peer review system may give favorable treatment to researchers from large or more prestigious institutions, that it may disfavor researchers from certain geographic areas, and that men get higher grant awards than do women (Marshall 1997d, Agnew 1999a). Thus, something like an "old boys' network" exists in peer review (Chubin and Hackett 1990, Glantz and Bero 1994, Godlee 2000, Marshall 1997d, Arm-strong 1997).

One reason why fairness has become such an important issue in peer review is that scientific resources and rewards, such as grants and publications, are scarce. When rewards are scarce, questions about how to distribute rewards fairly are paramount. Not every paper will be published in a top journal, and not every grant will be funded. Indeed, many top journals have acceptance rates of 10% or less (LaFollette 1992). Although NIH funding has increased considerably in recent years (Malakoff and Marshall 1999), the NIH still funds less than 30% of the proposals it receives (Gross et al 1999). Other agencies, such as the NSF, have not kept pace with NIH in recent years and tend to fund an even lower percentage of proposals.

The selection of peers to review papers or proposals can profoundly affect the review process. Glantz and Bero (1994) showed that the professional in-terests of reviewers play a critical role in their level of enthusiasm for a grant proposal, which affects its score. The overall effect of reviewer selection is that it gives an unfair advantage to applicants who know the professional interests of potential reviewers. These applicants are likely to be those people who know the potential reviewers—the "old boys' network."

The requirement of preliminary data can create an unfair disadvantage to beginning investigators or those who lack sufficient funding. Even though no federal agencies officially require preliminary data, the General Accounting Office (GAO) report on peer review (1994) includes testimony from investi-gators who said that preliminary data are an essential component of a new grant application. Even more troubling for the new investigator is where to obtain funding for his or her preliminary data. If investigators already have funding for another project, they must funnel some of that funding to obtain preliminary data for a new project. There are very few resources to produce truly preliminary data. Therefore, this policy pushes investigators into "theft" of funding from one project to another, an unethical zone of behavior that could manifest itself elsewhere. The fact that there is little or no funding for preliminary data also encourages investigators to "stretch the truth" on grant applications by overestimating the significance of their preliminary work (LaFollette 1992,Grinnell 1992).

Those who are involved in the peer review process, especially members of advisory councils, can also gain unfair "insider information" relating to how the process works, what types of proposals agencies would like to fund, what it takes to write convincing applications, and so on. In securities trading, financial institutions or individuals can go to jail for using "insider information" for economic gains. In science, those with insider information are not punished but are free to use and gain greater chances for funding for their projects. For example, evidence shows that NIH's members of the study sections and advisory councils (past, present, and nominated) are twice as likely to have their research grant applications funded compared with the rest of the scientific investigators (Shamoo 1993). Evidence also supports the conclusion that members of the advisory councils are more likely to have their proposals funded than are nonmembers despite the fact that their merit scores by the study sections were no different (Shamoo 1993). According to the GAO (1994), 97% of NSF applicants who were successful in obtaining funding had been reviewers in the last five years. One may explain these results by arguing that insiders are more likely to obtain funding because they have better expertise, a better understanding of peer review, or better knowledge of research or methods. While we do not deny this point, we doubt that these factors can completely explain these results. We believe it is likely that funding decisions are often influenced by access to the right people with the relevant insider information.

Failure to Control the Quality of Published Work

There is evidence that peer review often does not improve the quality of published work. Some studies have shown that peer review may not be a very effective gate-keeping mechanism, because most articles rejected by more prestigious journals are eventually published elsewhere (Lock 1991). However, as noted above, this is not entirely bad, because it ensures that controversial research is published. Studies have also shown that peer review is effective at improving the quality of published articles even if does not make articles perfect (Goodman 1994, Callahan et al. 1998).

IMPROVING THE PEER REVIEW SYSTEM

Although the peer review system is far from perfect, it does work very well for the vast majority or papers and grants proposals. Moreover, it is hard to imagine any reasonable alternative to peer review. Without peer review, researchers would have no way to control the quality of articles or funded research or to promote objective, reliable research—there would be no way to separate the wheat from the chaff. From its inception in 1752, peer review was never meant to be infallible. As Knoll (1990) states: "We tend to forget that just because peer review reviews scientific work does not mean that it is itself a scientific process" (p. 1331).

On the other hand, the fact that we have no reasonable alternatives to peer review does not mean that we cannot or should not make an effort to improve the current system. It is important to conduct more research on how the current system works (or fails to work) and to experiment with different peer review practices. To its credit, the NIH is considering ways to reform its system of grant review, such as awarding longer grant periods, reviewing grants retrospectively, inviting public participation in study sections, and finding ways to fund controversial research (Zurer 1993, Marshall 1997d).

Journals have also considered ways to reform the peer review system. One recent innovation by a number of journals is the concept of "target articles with open commentary." In this practice, authors submit an article for publication, which is peer reviewed. If the editors decide to publish the article and they think it will generate interesting discussion, they then solicit or invite commentaries to be published along with the article. They may also use e-mail discussion boards to allow further debate (Bingham 2000). The advantage of this system is that it combines the virtues of quality control (blinded peer review) with the virtues of openness, diversity, and accessibility. We encourage researchers to experiment with other innovations in peer review.

A challenge for journals and granting agencies is to find ways to give a fair review to creative and controversial projects or papers, as discussed above. Because science often makes progress through creative or unconventional leaps, it is important to test innovative or controversial ideas. Because a few of these ideas may bear fruit, editors and granting agencies may be willing to take some risks in order to reap potentially high rewards. Because these controversial projects may use controversial methods, it may be necessary to modify the normal peer review process somewhat to accommodate these proposals. For example, granting agencies could loosen their informal requirements of prior work as well as their demands to produce results within certain deadlines. To ensure that research is still of high quality, agencies could perform more frequent site visits and data audits.

ETHICAL DUTIES IN PEER REVIEW

This section briefly describes some ethical duties of editors, panel directors, reviewers, and other research involved in peer review, and gives a brief rationale for these duties.

Confidentiality

Everyone involved in the peer review process should maintain the confidentiality of materials being reviewed. Papers submitted for publication or grant proposals often contain data, results, ideas, and methods that have not been previously published. This material belongs to those who are submitting the paper or proposal, and it is privileged information. If a reviewer discusses a paper with an outside party, a paper still in the review process, then that outside party could use that information to his or her advantage, for example, to steal the ideas or results. The whole system of peer review would collapse if those who submit papers or proposals could not trust that their work will remain confidential (Godlee 2000, LaFollette 1992). Most granting agencies and journals now require reviewers to agree to treat all materials that they review as confidential, and some even require reviewers to destroy papers or proposals after they complete their review.

Respect for Intellectual Property

The ideas, data, methods, results, and other aspects of a paper or proposal submitted for review should be treated as the intellectual property of the authors or principal investigators (PIs). Those involved in the process should therefore not use any of this property without the explicit permission of the authors or PIs (Godlee 2000). Many scientists can attest to having their ideas stolen during peer review. One common scenario is as follows: researchers submit a paper to a journal. The journal takes a long time to make a decision on the paper and then finally rejects the paper. In the meantime, another research team publishes a paper on the exact same problem using identical methods with almost identical results. Is this sheer coincidence, or theft? Most researchers will not be able to prove that their ideas have been stolen, but they will remain suspicious. However, many researchers are so wary of this problem that they will omit important information from papers in order to prevent others from replicating their work before it is published (Grinnell 1992, LaFollette 1992). It almost goes without saying that the peer review system could not function if authors or PIs could not trust that their work would be protected from theft. Why would anyone submit a paper or proposal if they thought someone else would steal their work?

Disclose or Avoid Conflicts of Interest

If reviewers have a personal, professional, or financial interest that may undermine their ability to give a fair and unbiased review, then they should declare that conflict to the relevant parties, such as editors or panel leaders (Shamoo 1994, Godlee 2000, Resnik 1998b). One very common type of conflict of interest in peer review is where the reviewers have relationships with authors or PIs, who may be current or former students, colleagues at the same institution, or bitter rivals. Although it is important to disclose these conflicts, some should be avoided altogether, such as reviewing the work of a current or former student or a colleague at the same institution. Many granting agencies and journals also now require reviewers to disclose conflicts or interest. We discuss conflicts on interest in depth in chapter 7.

Punctuality

Reviewers should complete their reviews within the stated deadlines, especially for papers submitted for publication. If a reviewer cannot complete the review by the deadline, he or she should not accept the assignment, and may recommend someone else (LaFollette 1992). Scientific research occurs at a very rapid pace. Slow reviews can have adverse effects on the careers of researchers: one research team may be "beaten to punch" by a different research team while they are waiting for their work to be reviewed. In research related to public policy or current events, much of the material in a paper submitted for publication may go out of date if the paper is not published in time. A researcher may fail to get tenure, promotion, or a good rating if he or she has some major papers that have not been reviewed in a timely fashion. Although the length of review varies from journal to journal, most have a decision within six months of submission, and many have a decision in less than three months. With the use of e-mail and electronic submission, review can be even more rapid. Authors should not hesitate to contact editors if they are concerned about the status of a manuscript or its stage in the review process.

Professionalism

Reviewers should conduct careful, thorough, critical, and responsible reviews of papers or proposals. Reviewers should not offer to review a paper or proposal if they lack the expertise to make an informed judgment about its quality. In writing comments, reviewers should avoid insults, personal attacks, and other unprofessional remarks and make every effort to provide authors or PIs with useful comments for improving the manuscript or proposal (LaFollette 1992, Resnik 1998b).

Although these ethical rules may seem obvious, there are not always observed. Unfortunately, many researchers have had to deal with unprofessional reviews. Although senior researchers can develop some understanding of the peer review process and learn to accept harsh and irresponsible criticism, beginning researchers and graduate students may have an especially difficult time dealing with unprofessional reviews of their work. Insults can undermine a person's self-confidence and trust in his or her colleagues. Low-quality reviews are often of little use to the author or PI. Who can learn anything from a review of a manuscript that says: "reject" and does not even offer a reason for rejecting the manuscript? Worse yet are reviews of manuscripts that are so poor that it is clear the reviewer did not understood or even read the manuscript.

OTHER ISSUES IN SCIENTIFIC PUBLICATION

Wasteful and Duplicative Publication

Chapter 3 discusses authorship and mentions the tendency to publish papers according to the least publishable unit (LPU). Many commentators have criticized this practice as wasteful and irresponsible (Huth 2000, Jones 2000). We concur with this assessment and encourage researchers not to divide substantial papers into LPUs. On the other hand, there are sometimes advantages to dividing larger papers into smaller parts, because a large paper may cover too many topics. Authors should consider dividing their papers to improve the quality, focus, and clarity of their arguments and analysis.

The practice of duplicative publication has also been criticized (Huth 2000). For example, some researchers have published the exact same paper in different journals without telling the editors. Others have published papers substantially similar to papers they have published elsewhere (LaFollette 1992). Duplicative publication is unethical because it is wasteful and deceptive: Most journals expect that papers submitted for publication have not already been published, even in a different but substantially similar work. The editors may ask authors to certify that the manuscript is original. Some types of duplicative publication are warranted, however, because they may serve important educational purposes, for example, when papers are published in a different language or for a completely different audience. If an older paper has historical significance, it may be appropriately republished so that the current generation of researchers can become familiar with it. In all of these cases where duplicative publication is appropriate, the editors should clearly reference the original work.

Multiple Submissions

Most journals forbid multiple submissions, and some even require authors to certify that their manuscripts are not under submission elsewhere (LaFollette 1992). There seem to be two reasons for this practice. The first is to save resources: if a journal is going to go to the trouble to review a paper, then it does not want the paper snatched by another journal. The second is to avoid disputes among journals: journal editors do not want to have to negotiate with other journals or authors for the rights to publish papers. On the other hand, the rest of the publishing world does not follow this exclusive submission policy. Law journals, poetry journals, magazines, newspapers, and commercial and academic presses allow multiple submissions. Indeed, one could argue that the peer review process would be improved if journals did not require exclusive submissions, because this would force journals to compete for papers and to improve the quality and punctuality of the review process. Indeed, established researchers who can afford to wait can often choose among competing journals, even if they only submit a paper to one journal at a time. If researchers submit a paper to a journal and decide that they do not want to make changes recommended by the reviewers, then they can submit the paper to another journal.

Editorial Independence

Many journals are sponsored by professional organizations. For example, the American Association for the Advancement of Science sponsors *Science*, the American Medical Association sponsors the *Journal of the American Medical Association* (*JAMA*), and the Federation of American Societies for Experimental Biology sponsors the *FASEB Journal*. Other journals are sponsored by government or paragovernmental organizations, such as the *Proceedings of the National Academy of Sciences of the USA* and the *Journal of the National Cancer Institute*. Some journals are sponsored by private think tanks, such as *The Hastings Center Report* and the *Cato Institute Report*. Other journals are sponsored by religious, political, or business organizations. Some journals are completely independent and have no sponsors.

For those journals that have official sponsors, problems relating to editorial independence sometimes arise. In one recent example, it appears that the American Medical Association fired *JAMA*'s editor, George Lundberg, after he decided to publish a controversial study on sexual practices and perceptions among adolescents (Glass et al. 1999). We strongly support the idea of editorial independence as vital to the peer review process and the progress and integrity of research. On the other hand, we also recognize that private organizations have a right to control the materials they publish. A Jewish organization, for example, has no obligation to publish anti-Semitic writings. One way to settle these conflicts is for organizations that sponsor specific publications to publicly state the editorial goals of those publications. This will allow readers and prospective authors to understand a journal's particular editorial bent and to plan accordingly. If authors realize that their work goes against that stated aims of the journal, they may submit their work elsewhere.

Controversial Research

We have already discussed questions related to reviewing controversial research, but ethical dilemmas can also arise even when the reviewers agree on the merits of a controversial paper. The editors may still have some reservations about publishing the paper even when the reviewers recommend publication as a result of the potential social or political implications of the research. For example, in 1998 *Science* and the *Proceedings of the National Academy of Sciences of the USA* both published papers on human embryonic stems cells. Many people oppose research on embryonic stem cells because it involves the destruction of human embryos, but these journals decided to publish these papers to promote progress in these important new areas of research and to help stimulate public debate on the topic (Miller and Bloom 1998). Other areas of research that have generated a great deal of public debate (and at times acrimony) include cloning, human intelligence, genetic factors in crime, and sexuality. Although we recognize that editors must consider the social or political implications of articles, their primary obligation is to publish new findings and stimulate debate, not to protect society from "harmful" or "dangerous" research. Only a few decades ago Kinsey and his colleagues had difficulty publishing their research on human sexuality because of its controversial nature. Indeed, much of this research was conducted with private money and published with private support.

Electronic Publication

Many journals today, such as *Science, Nature, The New England Journal of Medicine*, and *JAMA*, publish simultaneously in paper and electronic form. Some journals are now entirely in electronic form, and almost all journals publish article abstracts in electronic databases. It is likely that these trends will continue and that one day almost any article will be available in some form through the

Internet and electronic databases and bibliographies. Given their high costs, printed journals may soon become obsolete (Butler 1999a).

Electronic publication offers many important benefits to researchers. It can allow more rapid review and publication. It can increase access to publication for those who do not have access to regular print journals. Researchers can more easily search for specific articles, topics, or authors with a search engine, which can locate in one second work that may have taken a month to find using older methods. Electronic publication also increases the quantity of published material and reduces the cost.

Despite all of these advantages, electronic publication also has some disadvantages, as mentioned above. The chief disadvantage is the problem of quality control: how to separate the wheat from the chaff, to tell the difference between good science, bad science, pseudoscience, and fraudulent science. Before electronic publication, researchers could rely on the reputation of the journal to help them make judgments about the quality of published material, a method still useful today. However, as more and more electronic articles are published outside of well-established journals, it will become much more difficult to rely on journal reputation.

The recent controversy over the NIH's "E-Biomed" proposal illustrates the problem of quality control (Marshall 1999a,b). The proposal would link all electronic biomedical publications in one public web site. Critics worried that E-Biomed would increase the quantity and speed of biomedical publication at the expense of quality control (Relman 1999). Although there are problems with the specific E-Biomed proposals, many researchers still endorse the idea of a central electronic publication index. One way to make this proposal work would be to develop a web site that links together existing peer-reviewed journals but does not bypass the normal mechanisms of peer review (Butler 1999b).

Data Access

Access to data has become an issue in publication in recent years as private companies have sought to protect their proprietary interests in research data while also publishing the data. Researchers are publishing sequence data as they become available from the human, mouse, rice, fruit fly, and other genomes. For research funded through public funds, data are available free of charge. Private companies that publish these data, such as Celera Genomics, are making data available free of charge for academic scientists but for a subscription fee for all for-profit users. Many researchers cried "foul!" when *Science* magazine published Celera's human genome data because of Celera's policy of charging for-profit users a fee (Kennedy 2001). These scientists argued that all published genome data should be deposited in a public and free-access site, such as GenBank. Although we believe in openness in science, we recognize that data also have economic value, and that the best compromise may involve some combination of publication with fees for access or use. Many private companies, such as Celera, are investing heavily in research and are producing important results that benefit science. Companies need some way of obtaining a return on their investments, and a fee for data access to nonacademic researchers seems reasonable. Private companies may also charge fees for data services, such as indexing and analysis.

Science and the Media

Many scientific discoveries and results have a significant bearing on public health and safety, education, the economy, international relations, criminal justice, politics, and the environment. These research findings are newsworthy in two different ways: first, they are events that the public should know about; second, they are events that many people find intrinsically interesting. For many years, scientific discoveries and results have been reported in newspapers and magazines and on radio and television. Science is also discussed in popular fiction and movies. We believe that scientists have a social responsibility to report their findings to the media because these findings are often useful to the public (see further discussion in chapter 12). Research findings can help prevent harm to individuals or to society and can promote general welfare. Reporting discoveries and results in the press can also enhance the public's understanding of science. But some problems can arise when scientists engage the media.

One problem concerns publication in the media prior to peer review, or "press conference" science. The controversy over cold fusion illustrates this problem. Stanley Pons, chairman of the chemistry department at the University of Utah, and Martin Fleischmann, a chemistry professor at Southampton University, announced their results at a press conference on March 23, 1989 in Salt Lake City, Utah. They claimed to have produced nuclear fusion at room temperatures using equipment available in most high school laboratories. Researchers around the world rushed to try to replicate these results, but the Utah press release did not provide adequate information to replicate these results. Pons and Fleischmann made their announcement to ensure that they would not be scooped by other research groups in the race for priority, and to protect their pending patent claims. As mentioned above, other researchers failed to replicate their work, and mainstream physicists came to regard their work as "careless," "irresponsible," or simply "loony." Although cold fusion research continues to this day, and Pons, Fleischmann, and others continue to publish results, the cold fusion community has become isolated from the traditional fusion community.

In retrospect, one wonders whether this press conference actually hindered the cause of cold fusion by calling too much attention to the subject before the work was adequately peer reviewed. If the work had been published in a low-profile physics journal and others with an interest in the subject had reviewed the work in an orderly fashion, then cold fusion research could still have been regarded as controversial but not "irresponsible" or "loony." Fleischmann (2000) considered this option and favored delayed publication in an obscure journal. Thus, this press conference science may have hindered the progress of science. Another problem with this prior publication in the media is that it wasted valuable resources as researchers scrambled to replicate the results with insufficient information. This probably would not have happened if this research had been published in a peer-reviewed journal first.

The whole cold fusion episode also undermined the public's trust in science in that the researchers made extraordinary claims in their press conference that have not been verified. This makes scientists look foolish or incompetent. Other types of press conference science have the potential to do much more damage to science's public image as well as to the public. Premature announcements of research on diseases or new medical treatments can have adverse effects on public health and safety (Altman 1995). For example, if researchers announce in a press release that they have discovered that a blood pressure medication has some serious drug interactions, then patients may stop taking the medication, and some may have a hypertensive crisis as a result. If this claim has not been subjected to peer review and turns out to be false, then the press conference will have resulted in unnecessary harm to patients. On the other hand, if researchers have very good evidence and they feel that it is important for the public to know their results as soon as possible, then they may choose not to wait for their work to go through the peer review process, because a delay of several months could result in unnecessary loss of life or injury.

To deal with issues relating to prior publication in the media, many journals have adopted policies requiring authors to certify that they have not discussed their work with the media before submitting it for publication (LaFollette 1992). Many journals also forbid authors from prior publication of their works on web pages as condition of acceptance. Many top journals, such as *Science*, *Nature*, *JAMA*, and *The New England Journal of Medicine*, have adopted an embargo policy for science journalists (Marshall 1998). According to this policy, journals allow reporters to have a sneak preview of articles prior to publication on the understanding that the reporters will not disclose the information to the public until the article is published. This policy allows reporters to have early access to newsworthy stories, and it allows journals to ensure that communications with the media do not undermine peer review and that scientists get adequate publicity. Many researchers, such as astronomers and space scientists, actively seek publicity in order to win public support for their work. Although embargo policies often work well, confusion can arise regarding the status of work presented at scientific meetings: if a reporter working on an embargoed story learns about the story at a scientific meeting, would it break the embargo to cover the story at the meeting? A similar confusion can arise with journals' own prior publication policies: does presenting results at a scientific meeting count as prior publication?

Misunderstandings can also result from communications between scientists and the media. Consider a scientist discussing with a journalist her research on the beneficial effects of moderate alcohol consumption. Communication problems between the scientist and the journalist can arise in several ways. Even if the journalist writes a perfect science news story, communication problems can arise between journalist and the public. For example, our science journalist may title a story on the research "Moderate Alcohol Consumption Protects Against Heart Disease," and members of the public may read the headline (and possibly the first paragraph) and conclude that the best way to avoid heart disease is to drink more alcohol. Although this example may seem a bit contrived, the issues are real and important: how should scientists discuss their work with the media? How can they communicate openly and freely while helping people to make informed, rational choices? To avoid these communication problems, scientists may "prepackage" their results for public consumption. They may boil down their research to specific key points and attempt to simplify complex findings for a general audience. However, preparing research for public consumption has its own problems: when does simplification become oversimplification? When does useful communication become paternalistic communication? These problems occur in all areas of public scientific communication but are most acute in public health communication, because researchers are attempting to develop guidelines and educational materials that will be used by the public to make decisions about diet, exercise, lifestyle, sexual practices, child rearing, and so on. To explore these issues in depth see Friedman et al. (1999) and Resnik (2001c).

QUESTIONS FOR DISCUSSION

1. What is the premise of peer review (i.e., what are the reasons behind it? What is the goal?)? Can you change the premise and why?
2. What suggestions would you make to improve the current manuscript review process for journal publication?
3. What is your personal experience or your colleagues' or mentor's experience with peer review?
4. How would you promote ethical practices among your colleagues regarding peer review?
5. Do you think researchers should disseminate their findings in the media? How and why?

CASES FOR DISCUSSION

Case 1

A very busy researcher is also a member of an NIH study section. He received 25 proposals to review in four weeks. He is the primary or secondary reviewer for 10 proposals. The primary and secondary reviewers are supposed to prepare a report about each proposal. Also, all reviewers are supposed to read all of the proposals.

The researcher delayed reading the material until the night before the meeting. He read thoroughly five of the ten proposals where he was the primary/secondary reviewer and prepared reports. Lacking in time, he skimmed the other five proposals and wrote reports laden with generalized statements of praise or criticism. He never read the other 15 proposals.

- What should he do?
- What would you have done?

Case 2

The same busy researcher received the same 25 grant proposals to review in four weeks. He gave 10 of them (five for which he was primary/secondary reviewer and five others) to his most senior postdoctoral fellow to read and comment on. During the study section deliberation four weeks later, the chairman of the study section realized that the researcher had never read those five proposals, because he was not able to discuss them.

- What should the reviewer do?
- What should the reviewer have done?
- What should the chairman of the Study section do?

Case 3

A member of an NIH study section hands over a proposal to her postdoctoral fellow to read, to learn how to write a good grant proposal. The postdoctoral fellow then copied the proposal so that he could read it at his leisure and underline the important points. He also found a number of good references that he could use. The researcher found out what her postdoctoral fellow did and admonished him.

- What should the researcher do?
- What should the postdoctoral fellow do?

Case 4

A senior scientist at a major eastern medical school was also a member of the grant review board for a large medical foundation. He was also a member of an NIH study section. During foundation review deliberations of a grant proposal from a relatively junior scientist, he stated, *"We just turned down his NIH research proposal, which was basically on the same topic."* However, the outside reviewers recommended this proposal be funded by the foundation. Prior to the senior scientist's comments, the discussions were moving in favor of funding. After his comments, the entire discussion became negative, and the proposal ultimately was not funded.

- What should the senior scientist have done?
- What should the junior scientist do if she hears what happened?
- What should the chairman of the review group at the foundation have done?

Case 5

An associate professor in a university is also on the editorial board of a major journal in her field. She receives a paper to review in her field. While reading the manuscript, she recognizes that the paper's researcher is on the path to discovering an important peptide that the professor's close friend is also pursuing. She calls her close friend and discusses her friend's project and how he is progressing with it. She never mentions that she is reviewing the submitted paper. But at the end of their conversation, she informs her friend, "If I were you, I would hurry up and submit the work quickly before someone else beats you to it." She repeats the same sentence twice and adds, "I would recommend that you send it as a short communication so that it can be published shortly." The associate professor then mails her review paper three months later. She recommends acceptance with major modifications and few additional experiments.

- What should the associate professor have done?
- What should her close friend have done?
- What should the author of the submitted paper do if he hears about it?

Case 6

An assistant professor receives from her chairman a manuscript to review informally. The chairman is the associate editor of the journal where the paper was submitted. The assistant professor prepares a thorough review and recommends publication. The chairman receives reviews from two editorial board members he selected. Both reviewers recommend rejection. The chairman tears up the informal review and rejects the paper.

- What should the chairman have done?
- What should the author do if he hears about it?
- What should the assistant professor do if she hears about what happened to her review?

Case 7

An editor of a journal receives a controversial paper in the field questioning the existing paradigm. The editor knows that if he sends the manuscript to two experts on his editorial board, they will most likely reject it. He sends them the manuscript for review anyway, and he also sends it to an outside third reviewer who is neutral on the subject. To his surprise, one of the two editorial board members recommended acceptance, while the other recommended rejection. The outside third reviewer also recommended acceptance. The editor decided to accept the paper but he felt obligated to call the reviewer who recommended the paper to be rejected and inform him of his decision. The purpose of the call was to keep editorial board members happy and content. The editorial board member informed the editor that if he accepts this piece of garbage, she would resign from the board.

- What should the editor have done? And do?
- What should the two editorial board members have done?
- What should the author do if she hears about it?

Case 8

An editor of a major ethics journal receives a paper dealing with a controversial topic on the use of human subjects in research. The paper deals with surveying the open literature for questionable ethical practices toward a vulnerable population. The editor mails the article to several reviewers, among them two researchers whose own work was part of the survey. These two reviewers are not members of the editorial board, and so they were being used as ad hoc reviewers. The instruction to reviewers carries with it clearly the notation that this is a privileged communication.

The two ad hoc reviewers copy the manuscript and mail it to about a dozen researchers whose work is mentioned in the paper. After three months, the paper is accepted based on the other reviewers' comments, because the two ad hoc reviewers never mailed back their reviews. The author receives the page proofs, makes a few corrections, and mails it back to the production office. A few weeks later, the editor calls the author to inform him that the paper will not be published because of a threat of a libel lawsuit from "some researchers" cited in the paper. She tells the author that the publisher does not have the resources to fight a law suit.

- What should the editor do or have done?
- What should the ad hoc reviewers have done?
- What should the author do?

Case 9

A university's promotion and tenure committee is deliberating on the promotion of an assistant professor to an associate professor with tenure. This is a crucial step in a faculty member's career. The assistant professor's package before the committee contains six strong letters of recommendation (three from inside and three from outside the university), a strong curriculum vita that includes 30 papers in peer-reviewed journals, an R01 grant for $1 million for five years, and a good but not exemplary teaching record. The letter from the chair of the department is supportive but not glowing. The department chair's concerns are legitimate in that this faculty member is not a "good" citizen and is hard to manage. He resists any additional duties that are not related to research. The department chair wants the committee to turn him down so she will be off the hook. She took additional informal steps to stop his promotion, including talking to the chair of the committee and two of its members about her concerns.

- What should the department head do or have done?
- What should the chair and members of the promotion and tenure committee have done and do?
- What should the faculty member do if his promotion is turned down? If he hears about why?

Case 10

An associate professor at a large research university in the midwest receives a package from a committee chair at an East Coast university, asking him to evaluate the promotion of an assistant professor within four weeks. The associate professor has a grant deadline coming up in a month and has a heavy teaching load. He does not want to say no to the chair, who is an important figure in his field. Moreover, he does not have first-hand knowledge of the candidate for promotion. He will probably have time to read one or two papers from the candidate's 40 publications, but no more.

Near the end of the four weeks, the associate professor writes a letter that neither recommends nor rejects the promotion, and in this way he protects himself from all sides. The chair is an experienced person and realizes that this associate professor did not do an adequate job. But he does not want to alienate a colleague by not using the evaluation.

- What should the chairman do?
- What should the evaluator have done?

Case 11

A faculty member is also a reviewer for a major journal. Her graduate student is having difficulty setting up a unique and novel method to test for low-temperature electron tunneling in a specific metal. Development of the method must be done before the student proceeds with work on his project. The faculty member receives a paper from the journal to review that lays out the method in detail. She gives the paper to the student to read.

- Should the students read the paper?
- If the student reads the paper, should he then use the method?
- Who are the parties involved and why?
- Is there a responsible way to deal with this issue?

Case 12

Three authors submit a paper on superconductivity to a prestigious journal. They become irritated when the journal does not make a decision after six months. Finally, after nine months, the journal decides to reject their manuscript. The journal does not provide them with any substantial comments and says that there was a delay in getting a review back from the second reviewer. The editor recommends that they try to publish their paper elsewhere.

The next month, a paper comes out in a different journal that is suspiciously similar to their paper. That research used the same methods and techniques and its data appear to be almost identical to the data in their study. The paper uses several sentences in the discussion section that bare a strong resemblance to sentences from their paper. It also draws similar conclusions.

- What might have happened in this case?
- Can you find fault with the conduct of the editor or reviewer(s)?
- What should the authors do now?

5

Scientific Misconduct

In the 1980s and 1990s, well-publicized examples of scientific misconduct increased public concerns and stimulated responses from government, universities, and other research institutions. The result has been the formulation of policies and procedures that are designed to investigate, adjudicate, and prevent scientific misconduct. Some aspects of these deliberations are controversial, including even basic agreement on the definition of misconduct and appropriate forms of disciplinary action. Nevertheless, there is now a functioning system in place designed to deal with misconduct allegations, and efforts to prevent misconduct are increasing. This chapter discusses the definition of scientific misconduct as well as policies and procedures for reporting, investigating, and adjudicating misconduct.

Although breaches of scientific integrity have been part of our culture for many years, a book by two science journalists, William Broad and Nicholas Wade, *Betrayers of the Truth: Fraud and Deceit in the Halls of Science* (1982, [1993]), played an important role in focusing public attention on research misconduct. The authors recounted both historical and current cases of scientific fraud and criticized the scientific community for its indifference to the problem.

The book challenged scientific icons. According to the evidence presented by the authors, Galileo made the data for falling objects better than they really were; Newton made his experimental results fit his theories better by fudging his predictions on the velocity of sound, the procession of equinoxes, and gravitational forces; Dalton cleaned up his data on the ratios of chemical reactions, which remain hard to duplicate; Mendel manipulated the heredity ratios on his experiment with peas; Millikan selectively reported oil drop data on his calculation of electronic charges; and even Pasteur was guilty of announcing his anthrax vaccine before he completed his experiments (Broad and Wade 1982 [1993], Geison 1978 [1995], Shamoo and Annau 1989).

Among the most famous historical examples of misconduct is the story of the "Piltdown Man." In 1908, skull bones were found in Piltdown, a town not far from London. The bones were presented by a brilliant young curator as being thousands of years old and belonging to a person who had the characteristics of both monkey and man. It was sensational scientific news: here was the "missing link" to prove that man had evolved directly from apes. Forty-five years later, however, some scholars concluded that the curator had pieced together contemporary skull bones from the two different species and had aged them chemically (Barbash 1996). At the time of the discovery, the curator's colleagues had accepted his findings without critical appraisal, largely because "the researchers [had] shaped reality to their heart's desire, protecting their theories, their careers, their reputations, all of which they lugged into the pit with them" (Blinderman 1986 p. 235).

A host of contemporary cases complement these historical examples. Some of them have been widely publicized by the media, while others have appeared only as footnotes (Broad and Wade 1982 [1993], Shamoo and Annau 1989):

- In the early 1970s, the fabrication of animal testing data by Industrial Biotech Corporation (IBT) sparked the legislation for the Good Laboratory Practices (GLP) regulations enforced by the U.S. Food and Drug Administration (Marshal 1983).
- In his 1950s studies of IQ and inheritance, Cyril Burt created nonexistent twin subjects and phony coauthors and fabricated data to support his theory that IQ is inherited (Shamoo and Annau 1989).
- In 1974 John Summerlin, in his studies of host-graft disease, painted the coats of mice black in order to indicate successfully grafted skin transplants (Broad and Wade 1982 [1993]).
- In 1981, doctoral candidate Mark Spector published a series of papers on enzymes involved in cancer initiation. He fabricated data by intentionally placing radioactive phosphorus onto thin-layer chromatography sheets, thus falsely indicating that it was a reaction by-product (Fox 1981, Wade 1981, Lock 1993).
- Between 1980 and 1983, Dr. Steven Breuning of the University of Pittsburgh published 24 papers funded by a National Institute of Mental Health (NIMH) grant to study powerful neuroleptic antipsychotic drugs for the treatment of retarded patients. The principal investigator was Dr. Robert L. Sprague, Director of the Institute of Child Behavior and Development. Dr. Breuning's results questioned the use of neuroleptics in retarded children and led to a change in their clinical management nationally (Garfield, 1990). In a renewal application for a four-year extension to the grant, Dr. Breuning submitted additional new data. Dr. Sprague questioned these data and informed NIMH of his concerns. According to Dr. Sprague, NIMH's first response was slow and accusatory. Ultimately, Dr. Sprague's frustration with NIMH spilled over to the media and led to congressional hearings. Meanwhile, Dr. Breuning remained active and funded. Finally, an NIMH panel in 1987 found that Dr. Breuning had committed scientific misconduct by reporting nonexistent patients, fabricating data, and including falsified results in a grant application. The panel recommended barring Dr. Breuning from receiving any grants from the U.S. Public Health Service, including NIMH, and referred him for criminal prosecution. Dr. Breuning was convicted in 1988—the first scientist to receive such action—was sentenced to 60 days of imprisonment and 5 years of probation, and was ordered to pay $11,352 in restitution to the University of Pittsburgh. During this process, Dr. Sprague lost all funding for his grants and was investigated by the NIMH. He was ultimately cleared of wrongdoing (Shamoo and Annau 1989, Monson 1991, Sprague 1991, 1993 Wilcox, 1992).
- In a highly publicized case in 1981, Dr. John Darsee, a postdoctoral fellow at the Harvard laboratory of Dr. Braunwald, was accused of

using fraudulent data in the assessment of drug therapy to protect is-chemic myocardium (Wade 1981, Lock 1993). Stewart and Feder (1991), dubbed "fraud busters" by the media, published a paper in *Nature* showing that Dr. Darsee's publications contained excessively fa-vorable language, fabricated experimental data, and fudged control data.

- In another well-known case, Dr. Robert Slutzky, a Harvard cardiolo-gist who was being considered for promotion in 1985, listed 137 pub-lications on his curriculum vita, of which 12 were found to be clearly fraudulent and 48 were questionable (Engler et al. 1987).
- In 1986, postdoctoral fellow Thereza Imanishi-Kari was the lead au-thor of an MIT team of five who published a now famous paper in the journal *Cell* (Weaver et al. 1986). Among the authors was the 1975 Nobel Prize winner in Medicine, David Baltimore. The paper showed that foreign genes had stimulated the production of large amounts of antibody by the genes in normal mice, which was considered to be a remarkable achievement. However, Margot O'Toole, a postdoctoral colleague, was not able to reproduce a key part of the experiment. She also discovered that the published data did not fully match the data in the laboratory notebook. A series of charges and countercharges once again attracted the "fraud busters" Stewart and Feder. A widely dis-tributed 1987 paper detailed analysis of their notes and their 1991 paper in *Nature* led to an investigation by the National Institutes of Health (NIH). Congressional hearings were held that featured angry exchanges between the congressional committee chair and David Bal-timore, who spoke in defense of Imanishi-Kari's work. The NIH in-vestigations concluded that fraud had indeed been committed. How-ever, after nearly nine years of controversy, the appeals board of the Department of Health and Human Services dropped the charges (Weaver et al. 1986, Friedly 1996a, Kevles 1996, Baltimore 1991, Eisen 1991, Hamilton 1991, Imanishi-Kari 1991, Kuznik 1991, Stew-art and Feder 1991).
- In 1984 Robert Gallo and his colleague Mikulas Popovic published in *Science* the first paper that identified the HIV virus, based on research that was done at the National Cancer Institute. Luc Montagnier of the Pasteur Institute, with whom Gallo had previously collaborated, ac-cused Gallo of stealing the HIV virus. The major question in the case was whether the virus given by Montagnier to Gallo in the early 1980s had contaminated Gallo's virus line or whether Gallo had perpetuated the same virus and claimed it to be his own discovery. Claims, coun-terclaims, and the loss of primary data made it impossible to prove the origin of the virus line (Cohen 1991, Culliton 1990). After failing to resolve the issues despite years of investigation, the Department of Health and Human Services dropped the case in 1993. A significant factor in the inability to resolve the case was the failure to regularly keep laboratory notebooks (Culliton 1990, p. 202).
- In 1996 one of the students in the laboratory of Dr. Francis Collins,

head of the Human Genome project was discovered to have fabricated data on the genetics of leukemia (Marshall 1996).

- In 1996, Dr. Michail Washbaugh, a biochemist at the Johns Hopkins University, was accused by a graduate student and later found guilty of placing unverified data on a graph in an NIH grant proposal (Forkenflick 1996).
- In 1996, the U.S. Office of Research Integrity found Dr. James Abbes of the University of Wisconsin guilty of publishing previously reported data on Alzheimer patients (Friedly 1996b).
- In 1997, a German panel of expert investigators discovered that two biomedical researchers published 37 papers containing falsifications and/or data manipulation (Koenig 1997).
- From 1996 to 1998, a series of reports appeared that exposed a decades-long abuse of schizophrenics involving the introduction of chemicals into patients to induce symptoms of the illness. Additionally, patients were left in the community for months without medication, sometimes suffering psychosis and delusions during washout/relapse experiments (Shamoo and Keay 1996, Shamoo 1997c,d, Shamoo et al. 1997, Shamoo and O'Sullivan 1998).
- In 1997, after a seven-year court battle, Carolyn Phinney, Ph.D., won a $1.67 million jury judgment against the University of Michigan. Dr. Phinney had accused her supervisor of stealing her data. The court's award was both for retaliation and for personal damages related to the use of her data without her permission (New York Times News Service 1997).
- Other recent examples of scientific misconduct include allegations and revelations of poor record keeping, bias, and fraud in the Federal Bureau of Investigation's (FBI) forensic research laboratories (Watson 2000, Associated Press 2001); data fabrication in crucial tests of the Strategic Defense Initiative (Weiner 1994); and data falsification in large, multicenter clinical trials of treatments for breast cancer (Resnik 1996b).

THE COLD FUSION CONTROVERSY

One of the most celebrated cases of continuous claims and counterclaims of scientific misconduct occurred in the "cold fusion" debacle. (Even though the original authors did not coin the term "cold fusion," we use this term here because it clearly conveys the topic and the controversy.) The main question in this debate remains whether "cold fusion" is a real phenomenon or an artifact of poorly understood experimental procedures. The issue of whether there was scientific misconduct by the original authors and their supporters or by their detractors still remains unresolved. In this short description, we are not taking sides on the controversy, but the discussion is worthwhile in terms of how norms of scientific research and discourse have been violated repeatedly by many on both sides of the argument. More important, this saga has cast a shadow on how not to conduct research. The best article for the general reader on the subject was published in 1994 by David Goodstein of the California Institute of Technology, which has been republished with a commentary by the author in a series of eight articles on the topic (Goodstein 1994).

In 1989 Martin Fleischmann and Stanley Pons of the University of Utah reported that they observed a greater production of energy (in the form of excess heat) from an electrolytic cell at room temperature than would be produced through electrical or chemical reactions. The electrolytic cell consisted of a solution of lithium deuteroxide (LiOD) in heavy water (deuterium is D_2O) and two palladium (Pd) electrodes. Known physical laws could not explain this key observation, according to the authors. Fleischmann and Pons also claimed to have observed neutrons, the normal by-product of nuclear reaction (for details, see Chubb 2000, Beudette 2000).

The well-known reactions of deuterium are that two deuterium atoms combine, to form a helium isotope (^{3}He atom) + a neutron + 3.3 million electron volts (MeV) or (with equal probability) to form a tritium (^{3}H) atom + a proton + 4.0 MeV. There is, however, a theoretical probability of 10^{-6} that two deuterium atoms would combine to form an ^{4}He helium atom + gamma rays + 24 MeV. This is highly unlikely because the nuclei of two deuterium atoms are highly positively charged and will repel each other as they come close together in order to merge and form the helium atom. Therefore, what all physicists have known for years is that you need a very high temperature, on the order of 10^8 degrees Kelvin (i.e., hot fusion), to fuse two deuterium atoms to form an ^{4}He atom. What is even more remarkable about Fleischmann and Pons's result is that gamma rays were not emitted but heat was. In a similar experiment, Steven Jones of Brigham Young University announced (almost simultaneously) that with a similar apparatus he had observed neutrons but no excess heat. Fleischmann and Pons, due to pressures from university administrators, announced their findings at a news conference, as did Jones. The U.S. Department of Energy (DOE) funded Jones's research on the subject. Prior to the news conference, Pons had submitted a grant application to the DOE. The development of cold fusion as a source of energy would have profound implications for our civilization, because it would offer an inexhaustible and clean source of energy.

As one can imagine, this case drew a great deal of attention from the media. Headlines ran across the globe. Scientists were interviewed regardless of whether they did such experiments or not. Also, hundreds of scientists all across the world tried to repeat the experiment. Claims were made daily and weekly concerning the reproducibility of the experiment. However, more often claims were made that the experiments were not reproducible. Those who could not reproduce the experiments often described the work of Fleischmann and Pons and of Jones as unethical, and sloppy.

Unfortunately, in this case the process of scientific research failed in many ways. Many different parties on all sides of this dispute violated ethical norms. These transgressors included university administrators who attempted to lay claim to research findings and potential funds through newspapers and headlines; researchers who cut corners to prove their points and gain recognition and priority; researchers who were quick to denounce their peers and insinuate misconduct; journalists who assumed the worst; journalists who beamed with naive credulity; journal editors who became censors for one side or another; reviewers who divulged confidential information; federal grant administrators who decided funding based on public perceptions; researchers who failed to cite accurately the work of others; and universities that violated academic freedom. The parties demonstrated a lack of civility, respect for individuals, respect for society, and respect for science.

The obvious violations of ethical norms began when the University of Utah announced the findings of Fleischmann and Pons at a news conference. The announcement was made presumably to protect intellectual property for the university and the inventors, so these parties may have had a conflict of interest. Fleischmann and Pons contributed to these violations through their enthusiasm at the news conference. Moreover, the inventors were not immediately forthcoming with details. The original article submitted for publication by Fleischmann and Pons was leaked and distributed all across the world. Thus, the editors of the journal as well as countless individuals violated ethical norms of confidentiality in peer review. This case illustrates the need for better methods to differentiate scientific misconduct from errors and honest disagreement. It also illustrates ethical problems with disseminating scientific results in the media before they have been reviewed by peers for quality and consistency (Resnik 1996c, 1998a).

All of these cases raise many questions. What exactly is meant by misconduct? What is the range of its manifestations? Are some kinds of misconduct worse than others? What are the factors that lead someone to be involved in misconduct? How often does it occur? What has been done thus far to prevent it? What is the process by which misconduct is being identified and dealt with? How is innocence or guilt determined? How effective are the current efforts to manage misconduct and to prevent it? How are whistleblowers being protected and is the process adequate? What yet remains to be done?

Before proceeding to these topics, we need to understand exactly how misconduct is defined. However, because the term has been defined by the agency whose responsibility it is to regulate it, we first turn to a discussion of the structure and function of the Office of Research Integrity (ORI).

CREATION OF THE OFFICE OF RESEARCH INTEGRITY

In the late 1970s and early 1980s newspaper reports of high-profile cases of scientific misconduct and a series of congressional hearings spurred the National Institutes of Health (NIH) to deal seriously with the issue of scientific misconduct (Pascal 1999, 2000). The pressure was intensified by the poor treatment of whistleblowers and by the inadequate responses of research institutions to instances of scientific misconduct.

In 1989, the Department of Health and Human Services (DHHS), in compliance with the 1985 Health Research Extension Act, established the Office of Scientific Integrity (OSI) within the NIH Director's office, and the Office of Scientific Integrity Review (OSIR) within the Office of the Assistant Secretary for Health. Almost immediately, the presence of OSI within the NIH was criticized because of potential conflicts of interest: the NIH, the chief provider of funds for research, was now also responsible for the investigation and punishment of scientific misconduct. As a result of the criticism, reorganization took place in 1992, 1993, and again in 1995, resulting in the establishment of the ORI within the Office of the Assistant Secretary for Health to replace both OSI and OSIR (ORI 1996, 1999).

The responsibilities of the ORI are very broad, including everything from the promotion of responsible conduct and the formulation of policy, to the oversight and/or investigation of both the intramural programs of the U.S. Public Health Service (PHS) and also the larger group of extramural programs. These responsibilities in part are as follows:

1. Ensure that all institutions receiving PHS funds have a mechanism in place for dealing with scientific misconduct and that the mechanism includes the protection of whistleblowers.
2. Oversee and review all scientific misconduct investigations conducted by institutions receiving PHS funds and impose administrative action on those who are found guilty.
3. Conduct all scientific misconduct investigations within the PHS intramural programs, such as those at the NIH campus in Bethesda, Maryland. Also, conduct investigations at extramural institutions when necessary.
4. Develop regulations and policies to deal with scientific misconduct.
5. Encourage and promote responsible conduct in research in collaboration with institutions, professional organizations, and other federal agencies (ORI 1996) .

DEFINITION OF MISCONDUCT

As a beginning activity, the newly formed OSI defined misconduct in order to establish the range of activities that should be investigated and that deserve sanctions if guilt is determined, which the ORI still uses today. Under current ORI mandates, all institutions receiving PHS funds must use this definition of misconduct.

The OSI defined scientific misconduct as follows: "Fabrication, falsification, plagiarism, or other practices that seriously deviate from those that are commonly accepted within the scientific community for proposing, conducting, or reporting research. It does not include honest error or honest differences in interpretations or judgments of data" (Code 7 Federal Regulation 1989). The terms "fabrication, falsification, and plagiarism" are commonly referred to as FFP. Neither the OSI nor ORI has ever defined the components of this definition. Other organizations have used other definitions of misconduct. The National Science Foundation (NSF) also uses FFP (without defining it) as well as the category "other serious deviations" from accepted practices (Federal Register 1991).

Despite no formal adoption at the time of specific definitions of FFP, research institutions throughout the country have used these terms without major difficulties. However, problems have arisen concerning what is meant by the ORI's "other practices" and the NSF's "serious deviation from accepted practices" (NSF 1991, Goodstein 1992, Buzzelli 1993, Sundro 1993). From the start, the scientific community has been uncomfortable with the broad and open-ended aspects of this definition as a whole, because it does not adequately distinguish misconduct from methodological or factual disagreement (Pascal 2000). Adding to the difficulties is the fact that ORI, in its own approaches to the management of misconduct, uses the narrow FFP definition of scientific misconduct almost exclusively (Pascal 2000).

Not included in the narrow definition (FFP only) are such activities as disputes on authorship, ownership of data, methodology claims, sexual harassment, careless mistakes, poor scientific practices, biased selection or suppression of data, the misuse of privileged information, poor data quality, incompetence, breach of confidentiality, and criminal activities (Pascal 2000). Also, issues involving human subjects and animal use are left to other agencies. Some authors have argued that the exclusion of some of these activities is narrow-minded and simplistic (Parish 1996).

One problem with any definition of misconduct is proving intent, because misconduct is not the same as error, which does not imply intent (Panel on Scientific Responsibility 1992). There have been two high-profile cases in which the ORI ruling of guilt was overturned by the DHHS Appeals Board based on insufficient proof that the researcher must have acted intentionally (Pascal 2000). Schmaus (1990) points out that the intent to deceive is difficult to prove and that sloppiness or carelessness probably occurs much more often than intentional deceit.

Despite the widespread concerns about a more inclusive redefinition of scientific misconduct, such broad definitions may be an opening to abuses by some officials and therefore may ultimately be destructive to science (Goodstein 1992). For example, a National Academy of Science (NAS) report raised concerns about allegations of misconduct "based solely on [the researchers'] use of novel or unorthodox research methods" (NAS 1992, p. 5). Nevertheless, critics of the narrow definition, including the 1995 report of the Commission on Research Integrity (CRI 1995), stress that the narrow definition can miss occasions of serious misconduct.

One aspect of the CRI's activities was concerned with a proposed new definition of misconduct: It would change FFP to MIM—misappropriation, interference, and misrepresentation. The CRI points out that the new terms are expressions of either dishonesty or unfairness. The definition attempts to clarify the role of intent and distinguishes between scientific misconduct and other forms of research-related professional misconduct, including obstruction of investigations of research misconduct and noncompliance with research regulations. Because at the present time it is unlikely that this definition will be generally accepted, we do not discuss it here.

The most recent proposed definition is contained within the proposed new policy on scientific misconduct that came from the highest federal authority on the subject: the Office of Science and Technology Policy (OSTP 1999) at the White House. Based on all available information, Goodman (2000) predicted correctly that this policy would become the core of the federal policy on scientific misconduct. The final policy ruling from OSTP includes a definition—which includes the subdefinitions of FFP—that satisfies institutional demands for the narrow definition of scientific misconduct, which reads as follows:

> Research misconduct is defined as fabrication, falsification, or plagiarism in proposing, performing, or reviewing research, or in reporting research results.
> . . .
> Research, as used herein, includes all basic, applied, and demonstration research in all fields of science, engineering, and mathematics. This includes, but is not limited to, research in economics, education, linguistics, medicine, psychology, social sciences, statistics, and research involving human subjects or animals.
> . . .
> Fabrication is making up data or results and recording or reporting them.
> . . .
> Falsification is manipulating research materials, equipment, or processes, or changing or omitting data or results such that the research is not accurately represented in the research record.
> . . .
> The research record is the record of data or results that embody the facts resulting from scientific inquiry, and includes, but is not limited to, research proposals, laboratory records, both physical and electronic, progress reports, abstracts, theses, oral presentations, internal reports and journal articles.
> . . .
> Plagiarism is the appropriation of another person's ideas, processes, results, or words without giving appropriate credit.
> . . .
> Research misconduct does not include honest error or differences of opinion.
>
> II. Findings of Research Misconduct
>
> A finding of research misconduct requires that:
>   There be a significant departure from accepted practices of the relevant research community; and
>   The misconduct be committed intentionally, or knowingly, or recklessly; and
>   The allegation be proven by a preponderance of evidence.

(OSTP, 2000)

The new federal policy also separates the three phases of handling a potential case of misconduct: "(1) an inquiry—the assessment of whether the allegation has substance and if an investigation is warranted; (2) an investigation—the formal development of a factual record, and the examination of that record leading to dismissal of the case or other appropriate remedies; (3) adjudication—during which recommendations are reviewed and appropriate corrective actions determined."

The final OSTP policy also separates the investigative process from the adjudicative process. Institutions perform the investigations and then take actions that are within their prerogative, such as reprimand, demotion, or termination of employment. The federal agency then reviews the deliberations of the institution and can take additional action if necessary. The accused may then appeal the decision through the agency's appeal procedure. The new policy basically conforms to existing practices. Institutions already have performed the investigative step in over 90% of all cases of misconduct (Pascal 2000). On the other hand, allowing investigations to be conducted solely by the institutions has been criticized because of the reluctance of institutions to reveal their own wrongdoing and the early lack of diligence by institutions in their pursuit of investigations.

Federal agencies are responsible for the implementation of these policies. However, federal agencies refer that implementation to the research institutions receiving federal funding. In most cases, federal agencies will rely on research institutions to manage scientific misconduct policies. The policy reserves the rights of the federal agency in question to proceed with inquiry and investigation under the following circumstances, among others: (1) the institution lacks the ability to handle the case; (2) the institution cannot protect the public interest, such as public health and safety; and (3) the institution is too small to conduct an investigation.

Note that there is an important difference between legal and institutional definitions of "scientific misconduct" discussed above and the concept of scientific misconduct in general. In a very general sense, one could argue that scientific misconduct occurs whenever a scientist deviates from well-established ethical norms in research, administration, peer review, or other settings. To commit "misconduct," in this sense, is to "intentionally violate ethical norms." When the community lacks agreement about ethical standards, an action may be ethically controversial or questionable but not a form of misconduct. The legal and institutional definitions of misconduct discussed above focus on those aspects of research where there is widespread (indeed, nearly unanimous) agreement on the difference between ethical and unethical conduct. If scientists decide that practices other than FFP are clearly unethical, then those practices may one day be classified as "misconduct."

One reason why government agencies focus on a narrower definition of "misconduct" is that they approach the problem from a legalistic rather than from an ethical viewpoint (Resnik 1998a). That is, research misconduct while receiving a government grant or contract is regarded as a type of fraud, which is a legal notion. A person who commits misconduct while conducting research for the government is therefore defrauding the government. On the other hand, there is a different sense of misconduct as behavior that is regarded by most people as unethical, even if it is not also illegal. In this view, conduct ranges from "ethically acceptable" to "ethically questionable" to ("ethically unacceptable misconduct"). Although we believe that the ethical notion of misconduct makes the most sense and is most useful in promoting responsible conduct in research, we can understand why government agencies (and institutions) focus on the legalistic notion.

WHAT IS THE INCIDENCE OF MISCONDUCT?

In their 1982 book, Broad and Wade claimed that there was more misconduct in the research community than it wants to admit (Broad and Wade 1982 [1993]). Furthermore, by the time misconduct is reported, it probably is the culmination of a spectrum of unethical activity of which misconduct is only the end point (LaFollette 1994a, 2000). Therefore, one may surmise that the reported cases of misconduct are but the "tip of the iceberg" (AAAS–ABA 1988). Although scientists, politicians, and the public regard the problem of scientific misconduct as extremely important, the scientific community still lacks solid evidence concerning the incidence of misconduct. Estimates of the misconduct rate, based on surveys that asked researchers whether they know about misconduct that has occurred, range from 3% to 32% (Steneck 2000). A 1987 survey of scientists found that 32% suspected a colleague of plagiarism (Tagney 1987). A 1992 study showed that the reported incidence of fraud affected 0.01–0.1% of all published research (Glick 1992). A 1993 survey of science students and faculty estimated that the percentage of questionable research studies, including fraud, may range from 6% to 12%. The results further showed that 44% of the responding students and 50% of the faculty reported being exposed to two or more types of misconduct or questionable research practices. Finally, 6–9% of faculty and students reported having direct knowledge of plagiarism or data falsification (Swazy et al. 1993).

Another way to estimate misconduct is to extrapolate from confirmed cases of misconduct reported to the government. With 200 confirmed cases in 20 years, this works out to a misconduct rate of 1 out of 100,000 researchers per year (Steneck 2000). However, because both surveys rely on confirmed cases of misconduct they are susceptible to an underreporting bias. Consider estimating the rate of tax fraud, for example. One could mail out surveys and ask people if they have ever committed fraud or know of tax fraud occurring, or one could make some estimate based on tax fraud convictions. Both of these methods, especially the second one, would probably estimate a fraud rate lower than the actual rate of fraud occurring. One may argue that the only way to get a good estimate of the rate of scientific misconduct is to randomly audit research procedures and research data—other methods would introduce underreporting biases.

Regardless of what the exact rate of misconduct turns out to be, misconduct is still a very important concern for researchers, because it undermines trust, trustworthiness, integrity, and accountability in research (Panel on Scientific Responsibility 1992). For example, murder is still regarded as a serious crime worthy public attention even when the murder rate is low. Thus, those who maintain that misconduct is not an issue in science because it is so "rare" do not understand the seriousness of the crime. Moreover, given the growing influence of money in research, misconduct may be more common than people think.

WHAT ARE THE FACTORS THAT LEAD TO MISCONDUCT?

Before discussing how institutions respond to allegations of misconduct, it is worthwhile to consider why scientists sometimes engage in any of the various forms of misconduct. How important to the etiology of misconduct are the pressures to publish and to be funded? To what extent is misconduct due to problems in our institutions as opposed to the personal flaws of our scientists?

The etiology of scientific misconduct is probably as complex as any other form of unacceptable human behavior. The theories of nineteenth-century French philosopher Emile Durkheim and twentieth-century American sociologist Robert K. Merton provide a theoretical framework for its genesis (Zuckerman 1977a,b, Garfield 1987). According to these theories, the values and norms pertaining to the conduct of science ordinarily become internalized during the period of education and are reinforced later with a system of "social control" that includes both rewards and sanctions. Deviant behavior is likely to occur when values break down and an individual's aspirations and goals come into conflict with society's structure and controls.

Although it is tempting to blame misconduct on the occasional "bad apple" (AAAS–ABA 1988, NAS 1992), it probably results from a variety of factors, including the ambitions, interests, biases, and personal flaws of individual scientists; economic and financial pressures to obtain and maintain funding; political and institutional influences; and inadequate education, training, supervision, and oversight at all levels of research (Shamoo 1989, Panel on Scientific Responsibility 1992). Misconduct may be the unintended result (or side effect) of a system of scientific research, education, and funding that overemphasizes career advancement, institutional prestige, money, and a "win at all costs" attitude.

Factors that have been identified as fostering misconduct include the pursuit of fame, money, and reputation; the quest for promotion; pressures to produce; poor training in research methodology; and an increased complexity of the research environment (Shamoo 1989, Shamoo and Annau 1989, NAS 1992). Inappropriate and large collaborative groups may diffuse accountability and thus also contribute to misconduct (Shamoo and Annau 1989, Davis 1990, NAS 1992). Additionally, three common factors are shared between financial misconduct and scientific misconduct: conflict of interest, the complexity of the research, and the remoteness of the laboratory manager from day-to-day operations (Shamoo and Annau 1989).

HOW HAVE SCIENTISTS RESPONDED TO THE ISSUE?

Scientists themselves (and their leadership) seem reluctant to confront the issue of misconduct. Often their response to the problems in data integrity is analogous to the denial and anger that terminally ill patients experience when they are first told about their disease. The stages of reluctance, depression, and acceptance may follow. In the words of the biologist and Nobel Laureate Dr. Peter B. Medawar: "The human mind treats a new idea the way the body treats a strange protein; it rejects it" (cited in Byrne 1988, p. 62).

The failure of the scientific community to manage the problem of scientific misconduct quickly and adequately is apparent from several standpoints. In 1981, then Senator Al Gore held hearings emphasizing that the research enterprise rests on the trust of the American people in the scientific process (cited in LaFollette 1994a). In subsequent hearings, strong concerns were raised about resistance to change and the betrayal of public trust within the scientific community. In response, in 1981 the NIH began to formulate proposed guidelines for the management of misconduct that eventually resulted in the formation of the OSI (LaFollette 1994a). However, because of resistance from the scientific community and foot dragging by the NIH, especially in the formulation of a definition of misconduct, the OSI was not created until 1989.

Other examples of the reluctance to accept the problem of scientific misconduct include the observation that corrections in the literature necessitated by misconduct have been slow in coming (Friedman 1990). Additionally, the scientific community has suggested that the media has overblown the problem with its sensationalistic coverage of the few cases of misconduct (LaFollette 1992). Scientists also contend that the existence of fraud signifies only that science, like other disciplines, has its own share of pathological individuals, and that this says nothing about the integrity of the system (NAS 1992). A recent survey of scientists showed that they would not report 50% of unethical scientific behaviors (by their own definitions) to the responsible person or agency either within the school or outside the school. Instead, they would opt for collegial solutions to the problems of misconduct (Wenger et al. 1999). Finally, the scientific community has resisted calls for random data audits to determine the prevalence of scientific misconduct (Shamoo 1988, 1989, Shamoo and Annau 1987, Loeb and Shamoo 1989, Glick and Shamoo 1991, Glick 1992, Rennie 1989a,b).

THE PROCESS OF DEALING WITH MISCONDUCT

The ORI has formulated general guidelines for the process of dealing with misconduct and requires that each institution receiving PHS funds have specific procedures that ensure compliance with the guidelines. Consequently, there are many similarities and some differences among these documents around the country. The ORI requires that institutions be the primary sites for handling misconduct allegations, and the process described below deals with that issue. We use the procedures currently in use at the University of Maryland, Baltimore to illustrate the process (UMB 1997). (These procedures conform to the ORI's model policy for dealing with scientific misconduct.)

A complaint can be made by anyone connected with the research. The complainant may direct the allegation either to the dean of the appropriate college or to the campus Vice President for Academic Affairs, who is the UMB's responsible official. The vice president consults with the complainant, reviews the allegations, gathers all necessary documentation, and determines whether to initiate the inquiry process within 10 days after receiving the complaint. If so, the vice president appoints an inquiry committee within 30 days after the decision to proceed. In circumstances where additional information is required, the UMB process provides for a preliminary review that takes place prior to the inquiry decision.

The inquiry committee consists of three tenured faculty members without conflict of interest with respect to either the complainant or the accused. It has the authority to meet with individuals, including the accused, who may have information about the case. It may also request information, records, expert opinions, and so forth. The accused may consult legal counsel. The inquiry committee should, if possible, complete its proceedings within 60 days. The purpose of its deliberations is to determine whether misconduct has occurred and whether there is sufficient justification to warrant the formal stage of investigation. If the committee so decides, it does not represent an assumption of guilt. In this way, it is analogous to an indictment by a grand jury. The committee's findings are communicated to the vice president, who consults with legal counsel and decides within 15 days whether to proceed to a formal investigation, terminate the process, or undertake alternative actions such as a correction of the literature that does not require a full investigation. If an investigation is warranted, the vice president appoints an investigation committee within 30 days after the decision to proceed.

The investigation committee at UMB consists of three to five tenured full professors or professors emeritus without conflict of interest in the case. At least one member must not be connected with the entire University of Maryland system. While due process and confidentiality are integral components of all phases of the process, the formal assurances during the investigation are significantly more rigorous. For example, meeting and hearing dates are provided in writing 72 hours in advance, and the proceedings are tape-recorded with copies made available to the accused if so desired.

The investigation should be completed, if possible, within 120 days. The accused again may choose to consult legal counsel. During the course of the investigation, the committee may expand the documentation provided during the inquiry process and may also expand the scope of the investigation beyond the scope of the original allegations. During its final deliberations, the investigation committee applies the standard of "preponderance of evidence." The committee must write a report that details the findings and its recommendations. The committee, if it finds that academic misconduct has been committed, may recommend sanctions. Note that the committee is also obliged to consider the restoration of damaged reputations, retractions, or disclaimers as necessary.

The report of the investigation committee is sent to the vice president. A copy is then sent to the accused, who is provided 15 days to offer written comment. Appropriate portions of the report are also sent to the complainant, who has the same opportunity to respond. The final report, along with any additional required documentation, is sent to the director of the ORI.

Within 30 days after receiving the report of the investigation committee, the vice president, after consulting with legal counsel and other academic personnel, should make a determination as to the finding of misconduct. The vice president informs the president and then submits a report to the ORI that includes the decision and the description of the case and reason for the decision. The process is then complete, except for the possibility of appeal, which is provided for in UMB's procedures.

Simply counting the number of days required to navigate the process just described begins to illustrate its cost in time, dollars, and emotions. Assuming that the timetable is met precisely, and that no hitches occur—never a safe assumption—the process takes almost 10 months from allegation to final institutional action. Add to that an appeal and the deliberations at the ORI, and more than a year has elapsed. The gravity of the process is apparent from beginning to the end. Lives can be affected significantly, especially those of the accused and the complainant. Tens of thousands of dollars can be spent on legal counsel. Hundreds of difficult hours of university personnel time are spent in activities related to judging colleagues. The process is significant from every aspect—including the necessity for its existence.

What have been the actual experiences of research institutions around the country and their interactions with the ORI in the management of scientific misconduct? The ORI compiled and published statistics on their experiences with the management of scientific misconduct (ORI 1999) over a five-year period, 1993–1997. Data compiled from these experiences are presented in tables 5.1–5.4.

These tables show that medical schools and hospitals have experienced the lion's share (79%) of investigations, with the remaining 21% spread approximately equally for research institutes and other organizations (table 5.1). In most instances, 83% of the allegations were handled by the same institutions (table 5.2).

Table 5.3 shows that during 1993–1997, the ORI received 987 allegations of misconduct from institutions around the country. Whistleblowers were the main source of the allegations, and most allegations did not meet the definitions of misconduct. Some of them (140, 14%) involved such issues as non-PHS funded research, sexual harassment, or problems with human subjects that were handled in other agencies or divisions of the institutions. But in most cases (660, 67%), no actions were possible. Only 19% (187) of all allegations went to the inquiry stage or beyond. Of those that reached the inquiry stage, the great majority (150, 80%) were sent on to the investigation stage. Approximately half of those (76) concluded with findings of guilt. Thus, although most allegations of misconduct (81%) do not proceed to the stage of inquiry, approximately 40% of those that do are ultimately resolved with a finding of guilt.

Table 5.4 shows that the great preponderance of misconduct (86%) in-

Table 5.1. Types of Institutional Settings in 140 Investigations

Institutional Setting	Total	%
Medical Schools	95	68
Hospitals	15	11
Research Institutes	14	10
Other	16	11

Adapted from ORI (1999).

Table 5.2. Conduct of 140 Investigations by Institution versus ORI

	Total	%
Institution	117	83
Institution and ORI	11	8
ORI	12	9

Adapted from ORI (1999).

Table 5.3. Disposition of 987 Allegations to ORI from 1993 to 1997

Disposition	Total	%
Inquiry or Investigation	187	19
Referred to Other Agencies	140	14
No Action Possible	660	67

Adapted from ORI (1999).

Table 5.4. Types of Misconduct in 150 Cases

Types of Misconduct	Total	%
Fabrication	18	12
Falsification	64	43
Plagiarism	8	5
Fabrication/Falsification	47	31
Other	13	9

Adapted from ORI (1999).

volved dishonesty in the presentation of data, with falsification observed more often than fabrication. Plagiarism and the "other" category together represented only 14% of the total.

What do these data mean? Is the system working well, or should the definition of misconduct be broader? Are other components of institutions handling too many cases of true scientific misconduct? Do these findings tell us anything about the existence of unacceptable scientific behavior? Are those who submit the allegations excessively zealous? It seems that many questions remain unanswered.

THE COMMISSION ON RESEARCH INTEGRITY

In 1993, the Secretary of the U.S. Department of Health and Human Services (DHHS) created the Commission on Research Integrity (CRI) in response to the continued failure to resolve issues related to scientific misconduct. The function of the CRI was to provide advice to the Secretary of the DHHS on such issues as a new definition of misconduct, improvements in monitoring and institutional compliance processes, and a possible regulation to protect whistleblowers.

In 1995, the CRI issued its report, entitled *Integrity and Misconduct in Research*. As of this writing, the report of the interagency task force to implement the commission's recommendation has not yet been acted upon by the Secretary of the DHHS.

The CRI produced nine major recommendations designed to foster an environment that nurtures research integrity. They suggested that particular institutions and disciplines implement these recommendations with an eye toward their specific research methods, goals, and procedures. The recommendations were wide ranging and advocated adoption of a new federal definition of research, education in research integrity for everyone supported by PHS funds, standards for protection of whistleblowers, increased monitoring of intramural PHS programs, streamlined misconduct management mechanisms, and the promotion of organization codes of ethics in research (CRI 1995).

Most of the recommendations will probably be implemented eventually. Of particular concern, however, are the recommendations calling for more education in research integrity, improvements in the protection of whistleblowers, and the redefinition of misconduct. With respect to education, the assumption is that an awareness of the foundational relationship between research and scientific integrity, an understanding of the current ethical issues, and knowledge of the accepted practices in research are likely to have a sanguine effect.

Previously, the only formal educational step taken had been the 1989 NIH requirement that all research trainees on federal grant awards have an educational experience in ethics in research. This requirement has been met in a variety of formats ranging from half-day seminars to graduate-level courses. Nevertheless, during the 1990s the number of full courses in research ethics around the country increased significantly. A preliminary survey of institutional response to the requirement of training in the responsible conduct of research for NIH trainees indicates that the overwhelming majority of institutions have provided some form of education (Mastroianni and Khan 1999). However, less prevalent was the provision of this training to all researchers as NIH policy has encouraged. Furthermore, late in 1999 the ORI indicated that it would mandate educational experiences in the responsible conduct of research for all persons conducting research with funds from the DHHS (ORI 1999). This requirement took effect in the second half of 2000, and was withdrawn later after objections from a powerful congressman.

The CRI's action regarding whistleblowers was to develop a regulation guaranteeing appropriate standards for the protection of whistleblowers, based on the development of a Bill of Rights for whistleblowers. The CRI helped focus the attention of all institutions receiving DHHS funds on several current regulations that protect whistleblowers and the need for compliance with these already existing regulations (CRI 1995). Among them is the PHS act that requires "undertaking diligent efforts to protect the positions and reputations of those persons who, in good faith, make allegations." The CRI further reminds institutions to comply with the NIH Revitalization Act of 1993, which contains a whistleblower protection statute (see CRI 1995). To reinforce the CRI's stand, the ORI has issued two publications. One provides institutional guidelines for responding to retaliation against whistleblowers (see the web site for ORI or the web site for this book) (ORI 1995). The other, possibly more important, is a Bill of Rights for whistleblowers (ORI 1998). Collectively, these provide reminders of the legal necessity to protect good-faith whistleblowers, discourage retaliation, provide a fair due process, and avoid conflicts of interest.

OTHER APPROACHES TO MISCONDUCT PREVENTION

Thus far, the ORI has emphasized defining, reporting, investigating, and adjudicating misconduct in its approach to the problem of scientific misconduct. However, the ORI has recently moved more in the direction of empirical research and professional education. Although it is important to formulate and enforce specific rules and policies on misconduct, such a legalistic approach has limitations. It is much more effective to encourage good conduct than to attempt to catch and punish criminals. One of the most important ways to prevent misconduct, according to many scholars who have studied research ethics, is to promote education and instruction in ethics and integrity in research (Hollander et al. 1996). Current initiatives emphasize education in research ethics during graduate school, but undergraduate and even high school students can benefit from ethics education. Education can take place through formal courses on research ethics or during informal discussions in the laboratory, small group exercises, brown bag lunches, workshops, or other settings. Role modeling also plays a key role in ethics education: beginning scientists learn about ethics and integrity in research by following the examples set by their teachers, advisors, mentors, and peers. The current generation of scientists has an ethical responsibility to help transmit standards of conduct to the next generation.

In addition to education, the idea of data audit was first introduced in the late 1980s as an approach to the prevention of misconduct (Shamoo and Annau 1987, Shamoo 1988, Loeb and Shamoo 1989, Rennie 1989a,b, Glick and Shamoo 1991, Glick 1992). It was patterned after experience in the financial field, where cooperative experience between auditor and corporate executives is the norm. Auditors have total access to records, and personnel answer questions forthrightly. In the field of science, however, data audit is looked upon with suspicion.

In 1991, Glick and Shamoo published a prototypical example of how data audits can work in the scientific world. Shamoo, an experienced biophysicist, agreed to have his work audited by Glick, a much-audited biotechnology corporate executive as well as an experienced scientist with a scholarly interest in data audit. The audit was to be a retrospective evaluation of a research project that culminated in the publication of a paper in 1983. The ground rules were that Dr. Glick had total access to any records, could ask any question, and could arrive at any conclusion. The audit process involved tracking the data from the published paper back to the original raw data in the laboratory notebooks. At the conclusion of the audit, a report was written providing the details of the audit process and its results (Glick and Shamoo 1991).

Data audits could be funded through the regular funding process. Every grant proposal would contain funds for data audit (Shamoo 1988, Shamoo and Dunigan 2000). Glick (1992, 1993) has argued that a scientifically conducted data audit can become an effective management tool in saving the public not only from poor data but also from unnecessary expenses. He estimated that 10–20% of all research and development data funds result in questionable data because of inappropriate research activities ranging from sloppy work to outright misconduct. If data audit were to result in a 50% reduction of questionable data production, there would be a savings of $5–10 per audit dollar spent. Twenty years into the data audit program, the public save $40–90 per audit dollar (Glick 1992).

Subsequent to the introduction of the proposal for data audits, Grimlund and Doucet (1992) developed detailed scientific statistical auditing techniques for research data based in part on financial auditing methods. The key new element in this technique is the development of stratified sampling for rare events. Two years later Doucet and Grimlund collaborated with others, including one of the authors of this textbook (A.E.S.; Doucet et al. 1994), to apply their statistical technique to existing data in toxicology that had been audited using a 100% random auditing method. They found the stratified method to be faster, more reliable, and more economical than 100% random auditing, because fewer actual data were audited.

Additional activity pertaining to data audits include a 1992 report by the ORI (Price and Hallum 1992) on their use of several data analysis methods to detect scientific misconduct, including statistical auditing and sampling techniques. Similarly, a statistical approach that identified lack of randomness in detecting fabricated data was published by Mosimann et al. (1995). The biotechnology industry appears to use data audit technique widely as a quality assurance method (Glick 1993).

Finally, it may also be important to provide an educational and policy framework pertaining to research practices and arrangements that can tempt, challenge, or corrupt even those researchers who have a strong sense of integrity and ethics. While these initiatives would not deal specifically with misconduct, they would complement efforts to prevent misconduct by helping to create and maintain a research environment that emphasizes honesty, openness, fairness, integrity, responsibility, and other ethical norms (Koppelman 1999). Some of these complementary policies and educational efforts could address the wide variety of ethical issues in science that go beyond mere misconduct, such as issues relating to data storage, data sharing, authorship, publication, conflicts of interests, contractual arrangements, peer review, whistleblowing, human subjects research, animal research, and intellectual property, to name but a few. To be sure, the research community already has policies and procedure relating to most of these issues. We discuss these as well as other ethical issues in the remainder of this book.

QUESTIONS FOR DISCUSSION

1. Based on the current information available about the incidence and significance of misconduct, do you think the press has exaggerated its implications? Does the process currently mandated by the federal government adequately manage the issue? How could it be improved? Do you think more or fewer regulations are needed to manage scientific misconduct?
2. What comments do you have on the causes of scientific misconduct? Which factors do you think are the most important? Do you think that the etiology of scientific misconduct resides primarily within the individual or within the system?
3. Can you give an example of possible scientific misconduct from your own experience or one that you have heard about? How was it dealt with? How should it have been dealt with?
4. How would you evaluate the process (inquiry, investigation, etc.) for the management of misconduct described in the text? Is it fair to the accused? To the accuser? To the university? To the public? Can you think of any changes that would improve the procedures?
5. If you were charged with scientific misconduct, would you hire legal counsel? If so, at what stage in the process?
6. Do you think that it could be possible to fully protect a whistleblower such as Dr. Robert L. Sprague (cf p. 94)? What would be the essential safeguards of an effective policy to protect whistleblowers?
7. Is data audit contrary to the personal liberty of scientists? Is it destructive to the principles of the scientific method? Could data audit stifle creativity and engender distrust? What system you would design to ensure scientific integrity?

CASES FOR DISCUSSION

Case 1

A graduate student was conducting a behavioral study on drug addicts as part of a larger NIH grant that had been obtained by his mentor. The study was to be the core of his Ph.D. thesis. However, the intended sample size of 50 was proving even more difficult to recruit than he had expected. Despite his most diligent efforts and the help of a social worker who had recently joined the grant, he was able to recruit only 44 subjects. The prospects for getting more seemed dim. He was more successful, however, in his rapport with the social worker, and they began living together. Still, he was faced with the practical academic problem of completing his thesis. The conclusions that he could make from the statistical data from his 44 subjects supported his hypotheses. Nevertheless, he was still short on subjects. His solution to the problem was to make up fictional data for the four remaining, nonexisting subjects. The conclusions from the statistical data were basically the same whether he used 50 or 44 subjects, but he presented all 50 for his thesis.

Within a year he had defended his thesis successfully and received his Ph.D. He submitted and had accepted two papers based on his thesis in a refereed journal. He took a job at another college in the area so that his living arrangements could remain the same. A year later, after a nasty fight, he broke off his relationship with the social worker. Unbeknownst to him, she had been aware of the entire fraudulent episode. In anger, she wrote a letter to the ORI. The ORI informed the university and requested a report.

- What responsibility does the social worker have for the actions of the graduate student? Should she be considered a candidate for charges of misconduct?
- Should the graduate student's mentor have known what was going on in the activities of her grant?
- Does the mentor bear any responsibility for her student's actions?
- Can the university and the ORI take action even though the Ph.D. degree has already has been given?
- Assuming a guilty verdict, what do you consider appropriate sanctions in this case?

Case 2

A postdoctoral fellow published a paper on the fluorescence spectrum of a newly discovered compound bound to a fluorescent dye. The spectrum of this bound compound in experimental animals differed substantially from that of the control group. This was considered to be a significant finding and he published his results. Later, one of his colleagues informed the mentor that she had discovered the control animal experiments had never been conducted. She said that the postdoc had relied on her control data from previous studies. Furthermore, the colleague had spoken to the postdoctoral fellow, who had said that he thought that it was acceptable to use historical data, but admitted that he had not mentioned the source of the data in his paper.

- Considering that the postdoctoral fellow says that he thought the use of historical data was acceptable, do you think that his behavior constituted misconduct? Is it viewed as misconduct by the definitions provided by federal government or your definition?

- Is the colleague obligated to tell the fellow of his decision to go to his mentor?
- Should the colleague have considered other alternatives rather than telling the mentor, for example, informing the appropriate university official and/or ORI or insisting that a correction be published?
- What alternatives does the mentor now have, and which one(s) should she seriously consider?
- If you were the university official in charge of the research integrity program, would you be likely to send it to the inquiry stage?

Case 3

A new assistant professor was accused of misconduct by a technician at the university where she had trained. The accusation was that she published a questionable abstract for a national meeting based on research that was supported by an NIH grant. The problem was that the abstract contained data that the technician cannot find in any of the laboratory notebooks. The technician also determined that this data had never been used in any other full-length published paper but had been part of the professor's dissertation. The technician discussed his concerns with the mentor, who in turn called his previous graduate student. Subsequently, the former student said that she was not able to find the data and claimed that it must have been misplaced. The technician made an official complaint both to the ORI and to the university.

- If the grant had been from a non-NIH source, would the university still have jurisdiction over this issue?
- What, if any, is the mentor's responsibility for the action of his former graduate student, either while she was a student or in the preparation of this abstract? Does the mentor have any obligations beyond his call to his former student?
- How do you assess the technician's response, including both the scope of his fact-finding activities and his decision making regarding his complaint?
- Now that the complaint has been made, what do you think should be the response of the assistant professor? The mentor? The ORI? The university?
- How could the situation in this case have been prevented?

Case 4

An assistant professor presented his department chair with a Howard Hughes Foundation grant proposal for her signature prior to sending it off. The dean's signature and those of other university officials were already on the routing form. As usual, like most overworked administrators, the chair checked the budget but did not read the grant. However, unlike many administrators, this chair, after the grant was submitted, took the time to read it. She became suspicious that several figures and tables in the grant application had not been based on valid data. A discussion with the assistant professor did not alleviate her concerns, and she filed a complaint to the university. After the university completed its investigation, the chair's suspicion was borne out: several tables and figures had been altered to fit the overall hypothesis of the grant proposal. The assistant professor finally admitted the falsification.

- In this case, misconduct has already been determined. The question here is whether the misconduct simply involved the actions of a "bad apple" and was unavoidable, or whether the necessity of the university's investigative process could have been prevented, "bad apple" or not. If it was avoidable, how could prevention have occurred? By individuals doing their jobs better within a system that works, or by changing the system? In either alternative, how?
- Should the university have ever investigated this problem, given that the grant proposal is submitted to a private foundation?

Case 5

An associate professor in a large university submitted a major grant proposal to the NIH. During the grant review at the study section, a reviewer noticed that the P-value calculated for the table was based on eight experiments. However, the methods section had stated that the experiments had been conducted four times in duplicate. A preliminary inquiry by the study section staff raised further questions about the authenticity of the data. The executive secretary of the study section felt compelled to write to the university's grant office for clarification, with a copy to the ORI. The university responded by conducting an inquiry. The faculty member admitted that she always uses the number of experiments times the number of replicates to obtain the total number of experiments. The university chose not to proceed to the investigation. Instead, it warned her to stop using such methods. The university informed ORI of its decision.

- What failed, and what preventive remedies you would recommend?
- Discuss the appropriateness of the university's action.
- Now that the case is in the ORI's hands, should it accept the university's decision?

Case 6

A newly appointed assistant professor applied for his first NIH grant. A member of the study section noticed that parts of the proposal looked unusually familiar. The reason was that entire paragraphs in the methods and the perspective/significance sections had been lifted from her own grant proposal that she had submitted last year. Although it was obvious that the new assistant professor had not been a member of last year's review process, the current reviewer knew that the submitter's department chair and former mentor had been a member of that study section. The reviewer called the department chair to find out what had happened. The chair reluctantly told her that he had showed the grant proposal to his then postdoctoral fellow for an opinion because he was too busy to read it thoroughly.

- Did the assistant professor do anything wrong when he agreed to read the grant proposal?
- Besides the assistant professor, does anyone else share responsibility for what happened?
- Was it appropriate for the member of the study section to first call the chair? Did the study section member have other alternatives?
- If the university hears about these events, what should it do?
- Discuss whether this is a personal or a systemic failure.

Case 7

A new graduate student working in a senior professor's laboratory conducted experiments testing the modification of telomerase activity. The student was careful to do triplicate experiments for every variable. She found that the compound had no effect on telomerase activity. The professor himself took over the experiment and conducted the same experiment with slight modifications, but did only duplicate experiments for each variable. The professor found an important inhibition of telomerase.

By this time the student had moved on to other areas of interest, but she was suspicious that the professor may have falsified the data, especially given the fact that the experiments had not been done in triplicate. She made a complaint to the university. The university conducted an inquiry, during which the professor claimed that he had not altered any data. He explained that he had not used the student's data because of lack of confidence in her ability to carry out the procedure. The inquiry concluded that there was insufficient evidence to recommend moving to an investigation.

- Discuss the appropriateness of the student's action. Were there other alternatives she should have considered?
- Should the professor have accepted the student's data without further direct experimentation on his part?
- Do you agree that the case should have proceeded to the stage of inquiry? Should it have gone further?
- At this point, does the university have any obligations to the accused? To the complainant?
- Now that the university has effectively closed the case, could ORI reopen it?

Case 8

A paper was written and submitted for publication as a result of the collaboration of three investigators. One of the authors noticed that the data in a table in the paper that was finally submitted was not the same as those in the penultimate draft. This author then made several inquiries to his coauthors about what had happened but received unsatisfactory answers. He then accused the other two authors of scientific misconduct and informed the university. The university conducted an inquiry, which was not conclusive because no one could trace who actually modified the content. The data in the laboratory notebooks justified the data in the table up to the final draft but not in the submitted paper. The university's inquiry found that it could not place blame on any individual and closed the case.

- Where was the failure among the three authors?
- Was there a need for an inquiry because the paper was not yet published?
- Was the university's response appropriate? Did the university make a sufficient attempt to find out who changed the data? Are there other responses that should have been considered? Should the paper have been withdrawn?

Case 9

An administrative assistant, after leaving her current job to take other employment in the same institution, accused her former boss of falsifying a letter of support from a collaborator. The letter was appended to an NIH grant proposal. The assistant wrote directly to the ORI, which requested that the university initiate the misconduct process. An inquiry found that the professor had actually falsified the letter. However, the collaborator had verbally agreed to write such a letter of support but was unable to do so because of travel commitments. If the researcher had waited until the collaborator had come back, he would have missed the grant submission deadline. Based on the collaborator's confirmation that the agreement of collaboration had already been made, the university found that there was no scientific misconduct.

- Although the professor falsified the letter, the university found that scientific misconduct had not occurred. Do you agree with this action? What are the implications of this action? In what way does the professor's falsification of the letter meet or not meet the definition of misconduct?
- Could the professor have handled his dilemma differently?
- What other options did the assistant have when she discovered the falsification of the letter? Did she make a good choice?

Case 10

A postdoctoral fellow made a complaint to the university that his mentor, an associate professor, had falsified the data in a newly published report. The fellow alleged that patients' reports of ovarian cancer did not represent the actual data. The university convened an inquiry committee, which determined that among the 120 subjects in the study, only 80 reflected actual data. The records of the other 40 subjects contained various types of errors as well as information that did not support the investigator's hypothesis. The inquiry committee concluded that although the investigator showed considerable carelessness, there was no proof of intentional falsification of the data.

- Discuss the university's decision to not find that scientific misconduct had been committed. Do you think there are circumstances where sloppy work should be considered misconduct, regardless of the ability to prove intent?

- Do you think that the university has any responsibility to comment further on the investigator's management of data or to require assurances of appropriate data management in future research?
- The postdoctoral fellow went directly to the university without first discussing the issue with his mentor. Did the fellow have any obligation to contact his mentor first?
- Should the investigator's report be rescinded even though she was not found guilty of misconduct?

6

Intellectual Property

This chapter provides a history of intellectual property and an overview of the U.S. intellectual property system. It discusses patents, copyrights, trademarks, trade secrets, and ownership of research data. It also examines some key pieces of intellectual property legislation, such as the Bayh-Dole Act, and intellectual property cases, such as *Diamond v. Chakrabarty*. And it discusses the moral and political foundations of intellectual property as well as some ethical controversies, such as patents on biological materials.

Note: Nothing in this chapter should be taken as a legal advice. The authors are not attorneys. Engaging an intellectual property attorney is recommended in the event of contemplating issues related to a patents, copyrights, or trademarks.

HISTORY AND OVERVIEW OF INTELLECTUAL PROPERTY

When most people think of their property, they imagine their house, their land, their car, their book collection—something that they can touch, see, feel, hear, smell, or taste. Many of the property rights that people have pertain to tangible objects located in time and space. But people also claim to own things that are not located in any particular time or space, such as a song, a poem, computer software, a play, a formula, or an invention. These kinds of intangible things that we claim to own are known as intellectual property (Foster and Shook 1993). In general, property rights are collections of rights to control some thing, such as a house. Someone who owns a house has a right to sell, rent, modify, paint, use, or tear down the house. People who have intellectual property have rights to control intangible objects that are products of human intellect (Garner 1999). For instance, if you have a copyright on a play, you are granted the right to prevent other people from performing the play without your permission. You also have the right to sell your copyright on the play.

Modern property right laws have their basis in Roman laws, which influenced the development of legal systems in Europe and the United States. Nations recognized property before the advent of the Roman Empire—Jewish laws dating to the time of Moses address property issues, for example—but the Romans developed what was at that time the world's most comprehensive and precise legal system. The U.S. Constitution draws heavily on the property rights theories of the eighteenth-century English philosopher John Locke.

Although the Western world has recognized property for thousands of years, intellectual property is a more recent development. While ancient Greek and Roman authors and inventors were concerned about receiving proper credit for their discoveries, they did not have intellectual property laws. Although the origins of patents are obscure, some of the world's first patents were granted in England in the 1400s when the Monarchy granted privileges, known as Letters Patent, to manufacturers and traders. King Henry VI granted the first known English patent in 1449 to John of Utynam for a method of making stained glass (U.K. Patent Office 2001). During the next 200 years, patents became a routine part of commerce and industry in England, although disputes arose concerning the length of the patent period and the conditions for patenting.

The steam engine (1769) was probably the single most important patent awarded by the British government. This invention helped to provide additional justification for patents and served as a model of science–industry collaboration. James Watt (1736–1819) developed a more efficient version of the steam engine, which had been developed by Thomas Newcomen and Thomas Savery. He was awarded a patent in 1765 titled "A New Method of Lessening the Consumption of Steam and Fuel in Fire Engines." Watt collaborated with the entrepreneurs John Roebuck and Matthew Boulton. Roebuck made two thirds of the initial investment required to develop the steam engine but went bankrupt. Boulton bought Roebuck's share of the patent and helped to market this new product. Watt's steam engine was initially most useful in draining mines but was later used for machinery in factories. Watt and Boulton made a considerable sum from the steam engine, which was the product of scientific ingenuity and private investment and marketing (Burke 1995).

The need for copyright coincides with the development of the printing press in the 1500s. Before the printing press, copying of books and author's writings was rare and most people were illiterate. Books and other documents were copied laboriously by hand in Europe. Because it took so much effort to copy a book, the problem of unauthorized copies did not arise. After the printing press was invented, it was possible to make thousands of copies with relative ease, and literacy increased. The question naturally arose as to who would control the making and selling of these copies, and whether "unauthorized" copies would be allowed. Thus, the idea of a "copyright" was developed in eighteenth-century England as a way of giving authors some control over their works. In 1710, the English Parliament passed a statute granting copyright protection to books and other writings. Prior to this statute, copyrights were protected by common law (U.K. Patent Office 2001).

The first U.S. patent was awarded in 1641 to the Massachusetts Bay Colony for the production of salt. The framers of the U.S. Constitution were aware of the scientific and technical developments that were occurring before their eyes and the need to grant intellectual property rights to authors and inventors to encourage the advancement of science, technology, industry, and the practical arts. The primary author of the Constitution, Thomas Jefferson, was himself an author and inventor. Benjamin Franklin, who helped draft the Constitution and the Declaration of Independence, was both a statesman and a prolific inventor whose inventions included the harmonica and the lightning rod. Given their familiarity with science and technology and their appreciation of the importance of free enterprise and commerce, it should come as no surprise that the founding fathers included a provision about intellectual property rights in the U.S. Constitution. Article 1, Section 8, provides the basis for intellectual property laws in the United States when it states that Congress shall have the power "to promote the progress of science and useful arts, by securing for limited times to authors and inventors the exclusive right to their respective writings and discoveries." (U.S. Constitution 1787). In 1790, Congress enacted the first patent and copyright laws, although the U.S. Patent and Trademark Office was not officially established until 1836. The patent laws have been amended numerous times, including significant revisions in 1952 and 1984, and most recently in 1995 (U.S. Patent and Trade Office 2001). Congress also enacted laws establishing the U.S. Copyright Office. These laws have also been revised several times, with the most significant revision occurring in 1976 (U.S. Copyright Office 2001).

During the 1800s, science–industry and government–industry collaborations continued to bear fruit, led by the German universities and the German dye industry. The modern chemical industry began when German companies developed private laboratories for making synthetic dyes. William Perkin, a student of the organic chemistry August Hoffman at the Royal College of Chemistry at London University, discovered a purple dye during his experiments on coal-tar compounds. Perkin realized that this invention would have great commercial value, because purple was a very rare and expensive dye at this time. He opened his own laboratory and began commercial production of the dye (Ronan 1982). By the end of the century, many companies had their own laboratories and employed scientists, engineers, and technicians. The great master of invention, Thomas Edison, obtained thousands of patents from his private laboratory in Menlo Park, N.J., including the electric light bulb (1879), the phonograph (1877), the stock ticker, and the duplex repeating telegraph (Burke 1995).

In the twentieth century, many new science–industry and government–industry collaborations produced more inventions and discoveries, such as the automobile, the airplane, plastics, synthetic fabrics, and computers. In most of these cases, governments funded the basic research that laid the foundations for practical applications and commercial products (Dickson 1995). For example, computers were developed in government laboratories to solve difficult problems in rocket telemetry. Private companies, such as IBM, Apple, Dell, and Microsoft, have invested a great deal of money in computers and information technology, but the basic ideas were developed by academic scientists. The biotechnology industry follows a similar trend. Most of the important basic research, such as James Watson and Francis Cricke's discovery of the structure of DNA in 1953 and the development of recombinant DNA techniques, used government funds. For the most part, private biotechnology and pharmaceutical companies, such as Millennium Pharmaceuticals, Genentech, Amgen, and Monsanto, have capitalized on the basic research conducted by academic scientists. However, in recent years private companies are beginning to invest heavily in basic research. For example, Celera Genomics has sequenced the human and mouse genomes. (We consider genome sequence data to be basic rather than applied research.) We return to this issue further below.

To help ensure a smooth transfer of technology from the public to the private sector and to private university–industry collaborations, Congress passed an amendment to the patent laws known as the Bayh-Dole Act (1980), which was amended by the Technology Transfer Act (1986). These laws allow individuals and companies to commercialize research developed with the aid of government funds (Dreyfuss 2000). For example, if the National Institutes of Health (NIH) fund basic research in an academic setting relating to a new hypertension drug, a pharmaceutical company can use that data to develop a product and apply for a patent. To do this, the company and the university can sign a cooperative research and development agreement (CRADA), which would delineate the intellectual property rights of the company, the researchers, and the university.

Issues relating to intellectual property and university–industry collaboration were not clearly defined before these laws were passed. Prior to Bayh-Dole, over two dozen different policies pertained to intellectual property claims resulting from federal grants (LaFuze and Mims 1993, Lentz 1993). Many different institutions and individuals could make some claim to "own" the data generated, in part, by a government grant, including different researchers, technicians, different universities (if the research was conducted at different sites), private companies (if they funded any of the research), and private endowments (if they funded any research), as well as the government itself. The laws passed in the 1980s have helped those involved in research to define their roles in research and intellectual property rights. Although many university researchers believe that they "own" the data generated through their work, data ownership is determined by agreements faculty members have with institutions (Shamoo and Teaf 1990, Fields and Price 1993). Today, most universities have policies pertaining to intellectual property and require researchers to disclose potential inventions. In a typical arrangement, the university and the researcher may split the royalties from a patent on an invention developed at the university. For example, the University of Maryland, Baltimore, offers researchers a 50% share of royalties. Researchers who work for private industry usually must transfer part or all of their intellectual property rights to the company as a condition of employment.

One of the most significant effects of Bayh-Dole is that universities have become increasingly interested in patents and licenses (Bowie 1994). The rate of university patenting has increased dramatically, and universities have opened technology transfer offices designed to encourage patenting and to protect intellectual property rights (Dickson 1995). In the United States, research conducted in university laboratories constitutes the major output of basic research, with close to $20 billion annual investment mostly by the federal government (Shamoo 1989, Walsh et al. 1997). The Bayh-Dole Act was therefore a natural outgrowth of government policy to protect its investment and expedite its use for public good in promoting progress. To compensate for decreases in government or other sources of funding, many universities view intellectual property as a potential source of revenue. However, income generated from intellectual property has not yet become a significant component of the budget of most universities (Guston 2000). Income from royalties to universities is estimated at $350 million annually, representing about less than 2% of their total annual research budget (Waugaman and Porter 1992, Walsh et al. 1997). However, it is likely that universities will begin to realize increased revenues from intellectual property due to innovations in biotechnology, medicine, and information technology.

In recent years, universities have established technology transfer offices to boost their income from royalties related to patents and copyrights. Technology transfer offices usually consist of an officer familiar with intellectual property and technology transfer laws and guidelines who has access to an intellectual property attorney. Officers attempt to educate and train faculty members on measures designed to protect intellectual property, such as keeping dated and witnessed laboratory notebooks, rules on data sharing, and early filing of patents within the legal limit. Technology transfer officers also instruct researchers on the universities intellectual property policies and how to protect the university's interest in collaborative research with other investigators at other universities or in industry. Many of these financial interests of universities and the close ties between universities and industry raise ethical concerns about conflicts of interest (Rule and Shamoo 1997), which we discuss in chapter 7. Moreover, the interest of the university may collide with the interest of the faculty/inventor. The Bayh-Dole Act calls on the university to develop the invention and, if not, to turn the invention over to the inventor.

There are also some international treaties pertaining to intellectual property. The first international intellectual property treaty was the Paris Convention of 1883, which was adopted by 20 countries initially and has been adopted by many others since then. Other, recent important intellectual property treaties include the Agreement on Trade Related Aspects of Intellectual Property Rights (TRIPS), which was signed by 120 countries in 1994. Although a patent or a copyright grants legal protection only in the country in which it is issued, nations that abide by international intellectual property treaties honor each other's intellectual property laws. For example, a nation that abides by TRIPS does not allow the importation of pirated software or unauthorized generic drugs. However, TRIPS allows for some compulsory licensing addressing public safety or public health crises (Resnik 2001a). For example, a nation facing a devastating epidemic such as HIV/AIDS could use the compulsory licensing provisions of TRIPS to require a pharmaceutical company to license another company to manufacture HIV/AIDS medications.

As one can see from this brief history, the main rationale the people have offered for intellectual property protection is utilitarian: intellectual property laws promote social welfare by encouraging ingenuity and progress in science, technology, and the arts (Kuflik 1989). They encourage ingenuity and progress because they provide authors and inventors with economic incentives to produce original works and inventions and to share the products of their labor with the public. Without such protections, authors and inventors may decide to not pursue their original works or inventions or to keep them a secret (Foster and Shook 1993). When inventors are granted patents, the patent applications become public record, which enables other scientists and inventors to learn from their inventions. This allows researchers to share information while also granting them intellectual property rights. The intellectual property laws also protect the financial interests of businesses and therefore encourage business to invest in research and development (R&D). Businesses view R&D funding as risks that can be justified only if there is some expectation of a reasonable return on investment. Intellectual property laws enable businesses to take these risks by allowing them to control the products of their R&D investments (Resnik 2001a, Kuflik 1989).

Another type of justification for intellectual property comes directly from the work of John Locke (1764 [1980]), who was a strong defender of individual rights (i.e., a libertarian). According to Locke, all human beings have some inalienable rights relating to liberty of thought, action, and property. The main function of government is to protect these rights and prevent citizens from violating each other's rights. Thus, on the Lockean view, laws against theft can be justified on the grounds that they protect rights to personal property. We can acquire property, according to Locke, through original acquisition or transfer, such as through commercial transactions or gifts. Original acquisition of property occurs when one mixes or adds one's labor to a thing or common resource. For example, if we view the forest as a common resource, if I remove a piece of wood from the forest and carve it into a flute, then the flute becomes my property because I have added my labor to the wood. This libertarian approach implies that laws can be crafted to protect intellectual property rights and that people can acquire intellectual property through original acquisition or transfer. For example, one might acquire a new invention (e.g., a better mousetrap) by adding one's labor to previous ideas and inventions (e.g., the old mousetraps). One could acquire property rights to a song by using or putting together melodies, words, and harmonies from previous songs to make a new one (Resnik 2001a, Kuflik 1989).

Regardless of whether one adopts a utilitarian or a libertarian approach to intellectual property, the most basic theoretical issue with respect to intellectual property rights is finding the proper balance between public and private control of intellectual property. Most theorists agree that some form of private ownership is necessary in order to provide rewards and incentives to individuals and corporations, and most theorists agree that a public domain of information is needed to ensure that people have freely available resources to create new inventions and make new discoveries. But finding the proper balance between public and private control is not always easy, and that balance may change as new technologies, such as computers and recombinant DNA, emerge and social institutions, such corporations and universities, evolve. This is one reason why it is necessary to reevaluate and revise intellectual property laws as the situation warrants.

TYPES OF INTELLECTUAL PROPERTY

In this section we discuss four basic types of intellectual property recognized by U.S. law—patents, copyrights, trademarks, and trade secrets—and their relevance to sharing data in a research setting. We also discuss the status of data as a form of intellectual property.

Patents

Under U.S. law, a patent is a type of intellectual property granted by the Patent and Trademarks Office to an inventor. A patent gives inventors exclusive rights to prevent anyone else from using, making, or commercializing their inventions without their permission. Inventions may include machines, products of manufacture, methods or techniques, compositions of matter, or improvements on any of these. Individuals as well as corporations or the government can own patents. The length of a patent is 20 years from the filing date of the patent application (Kayton 1995). Patents are not renewable. Inventors can sell their patent rights, or they can grant others a license to use, make, or commercialize their inventions. In exchange for the licenses, the licensee may provide the licensor with royalties in the form of a one-time payment or a percentage of profits. An exclusive license is a license between the licensor and only one licensee. A nonexclusive license allows the licensor to license the invention to more than one licensee. Different companies often reach agreements allowing them to use, make, or commercialize each others' inventions, known as cross-licensing agreements (CLAs) and reach-through licensing agreements (RTLAs). These agreements enable companies to avoid costly and time-consuming patent infringement litigation.

Patent infringement occurs when someone makes, uses, or commercializes a patented invention without permission of the patent holder. If someone infringes a patent, the inventor can file an infringement claim with any U.S. federal court (U.S. Patent and Trade Office 2001, Foster and Shook 1993). The patent holder can sue the infringing party for damages and obtain an injunction requiring the infringing party to cease infringement. The party accused of infringement may challenge the patent, and the court will determine whether the patent is valid. Because all appeals in patent cases go to the same federal court, the Court of Appeals for the Federal Circuit in Washington, D.C., patent laws are uniform throughout the United States. Appeals of cases heard at this court, such as *Diamond v. Chakrabarty* (1980), can be heard by the Supreme Court. Research use is an important allowable use of an invention that is not patent infringement. An academic researcher can make or use an invention for research purposes only. However, the research use exemption does not apply to researchers who are attempting to develop commercial applications from patented items.

To obtain a U.S. patent, the inventor must file an application with the U.S. Patent and Trade Office. In deciding whether to award a patent, the office considers the following criteria (Foster and Shook 1993):

1. Product of human ingenuity: Is the invention a product of human ingenuity or a product of nature? Only products of human ingenuity can be patented. The courts have ruled that laws of nature, natural phenomena, mathematical formulas, and naturally occurring species are products of nature and cannot be patented. In a landmark case for the biotechnology industry, *Diamond v. Chakrabarty* (1980), the Supreme Court ruled that living things could be patented. The Court referred to an earlier patent case, *Funk Brothers Seed Co. v. Kalo Inculcant Co.* (1948) and stated that "anything under the sun made by man" is a human invention. Chakrabarty had filed a patent claim on a genetically modified bacterium useful in cleaning up oil spills. Prior to this case, the only living things that could be patented were hybrid species of plants protected by special plant patenting laws, such as the Plant Protection Act (1930). A lower court had rejected patent on the grounds that the genetically modified bacteria were not human inventions, but the Supreme Court negated this decision. This Court's decision paved the way for patenting many products of biotechnology and bioengineering, including genes, proteins, and transgenic animals (Resnik 2001a, Eisenberg 1995).
2. Novelty: The invention must be a new or innovative. It must not be previously patented or disclosed in a public document, such as a paper. If inventors publish their ideas (or someone else does) prior to filing a patent, this may prevent them from obtaining a patent on their inventions in most countries. However, the U.S. patent laws have a one-year grace period from publication to patent. Thus, in the United States, inventors can publish first and patent later. However, they may submit a provisional patent application with the U.S. Patent and Trade Office when they submit for publication, to protect their proprietary interest before filing a patent. Publication or any other means of conception such as an internal document can be used as evidence of the conception of an invention. An important characteristic for claiming priority of an invention is reduction to practice (see below). If two people both conceive of an invention at the same time, the person who is the first to reduce the invention to practice is awarded the patent on the invention. However, if two people both reduce their inventions to practice independently, regardless of the date of filing patent application, the person first to conceive the invention is awarded a patent. It is assumed that both have already filed the patent application.
3. Nonobviousness: The invention must not be obvious to a person trained in the relevant discipline or technical field. Whether an invention is or is not "obvious" is subject to a great deal of debate (Duft 1993).
4. Usefulness: The invention must serve some worthwhile practical use. "Trivial" uses, such as filling a landfill or as a subject of meditation, do not count as practical uses, nor do uses as research tools. For in-

stance, the U.S. Patent and Trade Office has recently ruled that basic genome sequence data is not in itself patentable; DNA patents must specify specific uses for DNA in drug development, diagnostics, or bioengineering (Resnik 2001a). If the invention has a military use or implications for national security, the U.S. government has the right to co-opt the invention and compensate the inventor, who may also sign a contract with the government.

5. Enabling description: Inventors must reduce their inventions to practice; that is, they must describe the invention in enough detail that someone trained in the relevant discipline or field could make and use the invention. This description of the patent becomes a public document and is part of the patenting "bargain."

Although the patent system encourages public disclosure in exchange for intellectual property rights, some corporations use the system not to develop new inventions but to prevent competing companies from developing new inventions (Resnik 2001a). For example, to secure the market for their trademarked drugs, large pharmaceutical companies have purchased patents on competing generic drugs owned by smaller companies. Other companies have developed "blocking" patents designed to prevent competitors from developing new products. For example, if a company is developing a new internal combustion engine, a competing company could block production of this engine by acquiring a patent on a part needed to make the engine.

Copyrights

Copyrights are exclusive rights granted by the U.S. government that allow the authors of original works to make copies of the work, make other works derived from the original work, perform or display the work, and distribute, sell, or rent copies of the work. People who perform any of these actions without the permission of copyright holders violate copyrights. Original works include written works, such as books, papers, software, databases, and poems; performances, such as plays or dances; audio-visual recordings, such as movies, music, photographs, and televisions shows; and artistic works, such as paintings and sculpture. A work can be original without being new or novel because the author is the first person to put the work into tangible form. A copyright extends for the lifetime of the author(s) plus 70 years, and may be renewed. To register copyright, one may file for a copyright with the U.S. Copyright Office at the Library of Congress. However, authors of original works have copyright protections even if they do not take this step. To ensure that others are aware of their claims to a copyright, many copyright holders write "copyright" on their original works, such as "Copyright © 2001 Shamoo and Resnik, all rights reserved." Copyrights protect original works but not the ideas expressed by those works (Office of Technology Assessment 1990, Chickering and Hartman 1980). Although it is illegal to sell copies of the book *Jurassic Park* without permission of the copyright holder, it is perfectly legal to discuss (or profit from) the ideas expressed in the book without the owner's permission.

Many copyright holders sell their rights to publishers or other distributors for a one-time fee or a percentage of profits. Work conducted for a business is generally considered "work for hire," and so copyrights belong to the business. The business may grant the employee some portion of copyrights as part of contract negotiations. Because academic research is not generally considered work for hire, academic researchers retain their copyrights unless they make specific deals with the university's technology transfer office.

One important exception to copyright law is the doctrine of fair use. According to this doctrine, it is permissible to copy portions of the author's work or even the whole work without his or her permission if the copying is for personal, educational, or research purposes and does not jeopardize the commercial value of the work (Foster and Shook 1993). For example, the doctrine of fair use allows a person to use a VCR to record a television show to watch later, but it does not allow a person to use a VCR to make or sell copies of the television show for a large audience. During the 1970s, the copying company Kinko's compiled, copied, and sold course packets—selections of readings from journals or books—for professors teaching university or college courses. Publishing companies sued Kinko's for copyright violations, and the courts ruled in their favor. Even though the use was for an educational purpose, it was not a fair use because it defrayed the commercial value of the published works. The recent dispute over the legality of the Napster web site illustrates the continuing evolution of the doctrine of fair use. Many companies from the recording industry sued Napster for copyright violation because the company was distributing copyrighted music over the Internet without permission. Also note that many types of knowledge, such as government documents, public records, weight conversion tables, temperature measures, calendars, known titles, phrases, and lists of ingredients, are considered to be in the public domain and are not copyrighted (Chickering and Hartman 1980).

Trademarks

A trademark is a distinctive symbol or mark, such as a name, phrase, device, stamp, logo, or figure, that businesses use to distinguish themselves. Some examples of trademarks include the name "Coca-Cola," the phrase "have it your way," the McDonald's arches, the Hot Wheels™ logo, and the Planter's peanut man. Trademarks are useful to businesses for marketing their goods and services, because they provide consumers with a way to easily recognize the business and its products. Trademarks are protected by state and federal laws and are important in commerce, but they play only a minimal role in research. To obtain federal trademark protection, a business may submit an application to the U.S. Patent and Trade Office. Trademarks are renewable indefinitely for 10-year periods (Office of Technology Assessment, 1990, Adler 1993, U.S. Patent and Trade Office 2001).

Trade Secrets

The forms of intellectual property discussed above—patents, copyrights, and trademarks—are rights granted by the government designed to promote the dissemination of information while protecting proprietary interests. The key policy issue in these forms of intellectual property is finding the proper balance of public and private control of information. Trade secrets, on the other hand, are designed to prevent information from becoming publicly available. The law recognizes trade secrets because they promote the interests of commerce and industry and can be more useful than other forms of intellectual property for some businesses (Foster and Shook 1993). For example, consider the formula for Coca-Cola, one of the best-guarded trade secrets. If the company had patented its formula when it invented Coca-Cola, then the patent would have expired decades ago and the company would have lost its share of the market for this product. As far as the company is concerned, it can make more money by keeping the formula a secret instead of patenting the formula. One reason why the company can do this is that the secret is well guarded and difficult to discover. Although many companies have manufactured products that taste similar to Coca-Cola, no company has manufactured a product that tastes just like "the real thing" because it is difficult to master all the subtle variations in ingredients and manufacturing processes the company employs. Other types of trade secrets may include other formulas, instruments, business plans, customer lists, and company policies. State laws protect trade secrets provided that the company makes an attempt to keep the secret and the secret has commercial value. Someone who discloses a trade secret to a competing business can be prosecuted under tort liability or for theft and can be fined up to and exceeding the monetary value of the secret.

The main problem with trade secrets is that they are difficult to protect. First, employees may disclose trade secrets either intentionally or inadvertently. Second, there are legal methods that competitors can use to discover trade secrets, such as reverse engineering. It is perfectly legal for another company to "reverse engineer" Coca-Cola by purchasing some of the product and analyzing it to determine how it is produced. Trade secrets are not protected if they are derived from independent research, open meetings, and a host of other methods. In the biotechnology industry, it is virtually impossible to keep trade secrets due to the open nature of biotechnology research and development. Most of the materials used in biotechnology are available to the public, such as organic compounds, organisms, common tools, and techniques. Thus, in biotechnology and pharmaceuticals, patents are generally a better form of intellectual property protection than are trade secrets (Resnik 2001a, Office of Technology Assessment 1990, Adler 1993).

The biotechnology and pharmaceutical industries have invested heavily in research and development (R&D) in the last two decades with the aim of developing patentable products, such as new drugs or biologics. Private investment in biomedical R&D in the United States rose from $2 billion per year in 1980 to $16 billion per year in 1990 and is probably now about $40 billion per year (data cited in Resnik 1999a). Most of the funding comes from pharmaceutical companies, which spent $26.4 billion on R&D in the United States in the year 2000 (Pharmaceuticals Manufacturers 2000). The number of biotechnology patents issued by the U.S. Patent and Trade Office rose from

3,378 in 1990 to 9,385 in 1997 (data cited in Glick 1997). The number of DNA patent applications received by the U.S. Patent and Trade Office rose from around 500 in 1994 to nearly 3,000 in 1999 (Enserink 2000). In deciding whether to develop a new product, a company must decide whether it will be able to obtain an adequate return on its investments. According to industry estimates, it takes $500 million of R&D and 10 years of testing to bring the average drug to the market (Pharmaceutical Manufacturers 2000). Many biotechnology products, such as proteins, genome sequence data, and transgenic organisms, also require investments on the scale of hundreds of millions of dollars (Glick 1997).

Data Sharing—Again

One final type of intellectual property to consider is research data. Although we discuss issues of data sharing in several places in this book, we revisit them here as well because the topic is so important. As we have already stressed, the sharing of data and other research resources is vital to the progress of science. But there are many reasons why researchers or research institutions might decide to not share data. One reason is that researchers or institutions may have a proprietary interest in research data. Suppose a researcher does animal toxicology studies on a drug that a pharmaceutical company is developing. She has a contract with the company and is employed by a university. Suppose a dispute arises over publishing the data: the researcher wants to publish but the company objects to publication. Who owns the data? The researcher? The company? Or the university? Or suppose a researcher obtains data at a university through a government grant and then leaves the university for a job at another institution. Can he take his data with him, or must it stay at the university? Clearly, many of the questions about sharing data can be framed in terms of ownership issues (Shamoo 1989, Shamoo and Teaf 1990).

There is certainly a sense in which one might view data as intellectual property, but there are no laws designed specifically to protect data. To treat data as intellectual property, one must therefore apply existing copyright, patent, trade secrecy, or tort laws to research data or enact specific institutional policies. For example, if one publishes research data in a journal or electronic database, one might use copyright protections to prevent other researchers from copying the data (Gardner and Rosenbaum 1998). In chapter 4 we mentioned that Celera Genomics is publishing its genome data but charges an access fee to commercial users, to the dismay of some (Marshal 2000b). This seems to be consistent with the doctrine of fair use, which would allow academic researchers to copy the published data for teaching or research purposes but would prevent unauthorized data copying for commercial purposes. If one publishes data as part of a patent application, on the other hand, the data become public record, and one would not be able to charge commercial users a fee for access to the data. Patent laws may allow inventors use of data, such as in developing a new drug, even if the laws do not give inventors ownership of the data themselves. For instance, many of human gene patent claims approved by the U.S. Patent and Trade Office pertain to use of genome sequence data in testing for genetic predispositions or in developing pharmaceuticals (Resnik 2001a).

Trade secrecy laws can provide companies with some ownership of data, provided that the data are properly protected trade secrets. For example, tobacco companies sought for many years to protect their research on nicotine's addictive properties under the cloak of trade secrecy (Resnik 1998b, Hurt and Robertson 1998). In the private sector, data are treated as "propriety information." The data submitted by private companies in support of a drug application to the Food and Drug Administration (FDA) are not made public, even after the drug has been approved. Although U.S. law protects this type of information, researchers may still face an ethical dilemma in situations where promoting the good of society requires them to break the law. For example, a scientist conducting secret research for a drug company who discovers a problem with the medication, which the company does not want to report to the FDA, must choose between abiding by the company's policies and serving the public good (Resnik 1998b).

Also note that specific contracts signed between researchers and universities or private companies may state or imply rules of data ownership and control. For example, CRADAs usually address issues of data control, and many private companies require researchers to sign contracts giving the company control over all data generated in its laboratories. On the other hand, there are some laws and regulations that require researchers receiving government funds to share data, such as the Freedom of Information Act and the NIH policy on data sharing (Fields and Price 1993, Cohen and Hahn 1999).

Although our opinions have no legal force, we offer the following principles as ethical guidance for data sharing (Shamoo and Teaf 1990), some of which have been mentioned in preceding chapters:

1. Researchers working on the same project *must* share data.
2. Researchers *must* share relevant data with committees and organizations in charge of overseeing research, such as institutional review boards, animal care and use committees, biological safety committees, radiation safety committees, data monitoring boards, the U.S. FDA, and conflict of interest committees.
3. Researchers should also share data and resources with colleagues in descending order of importance: (a) colleagues in the same laboratory, (b) colleagues in the same institution, (c) colleagues in the same discipline, (d) other colleagues conducting research or other scholarly activities, (e) the general public, including reporters, industry representatives, and citizen advocates.

To these we suggest adding the following principles:

4. No discriminatory restrictions should be placed on who can use and access the data based on expertise, nationality, race, sex, workplace, and so forth. Universities or their designees should have ownership of data for seven years subject to government access and audit when needed.

5. Raw data should be maintained in custody of the principal investigator or the university for seven years, subject to audit. The audit would reduce the need for returning to the original data.
6. There should be national and international databanks that are fully indexed for easy retrieval. Databanks should include published as well as unpublished data. Data published in the databanks that have been published elsewhere should be linked to the original publication.
7. Ethical rules for data sharing should not undermine legally valid rules that protect the confidentiality of medical records, criminal records, personnel files, and documents relating to national security.

ADDITIONAL ETHICAL CONCERNS

Before concluding this chapter, we return to some more fundamental issues in intellectual property. This first issue is the question of *who* has an ethically defensible claim to ownership of intellectual property; the second is the question of *what* ethically can be treated as intellectual property. Here we are not concerned with what the law does say about intellectual property but about what the law should say about intellectual property.

Who Has Intellectual Property Rights?

Consider an invention or an original work. Many different individuals and institutions may assert ownership claims over an invention, such as a transgenic mouse, or an original work, such as computer software. Who should be granted patent rights on the mouse or copyrights on the software? In many ways, this question parallels questions about authorship discussed in chapter 4, where we argued that authorship and accountability should go hand in hand: an author is someone who makes an important contribution and can be held publicly accountable for the research. If all authors have copyrights, then the question of who should have copyrights is the same as the question of who should be an author. One may argue that the same point applies to patent rights: an inventor, like an author, is someone who makes an important contribution to the invention and can be held accountable for the invention. That is, the inventor could describe the invention, explain how it works and what it does, and show how it is useful and original (Dreyfuss 2000). Interestingly, an invention often has more authors listed in the paper describing it than it has inventors listed on the patent application (Ducor 2000). One might speculate that these cases people are being listed as authors who do not deserve to be authors or people are not listed as inventors who deserve to be listed as inventors.

Although relying on some principle of accountability may settle many concerns about intellectual property rights, it does not address the role of "contributors" and any morally legitimate claims they may make to intellectual property. Because contributors do not, by definition, play a significant role in research, most of the intellectual property claims made by contributors relate to concerns about fairness, not to concerns about accountability. Consider the following examples:

- A lab technician carries out a great deal of the work in developing a patented mouse and is listed as an author on the paper but not as an inventor on the patent. Should the technician have any patent rights? If she has no patent rights, then should she not be listed as an author on the paper?
- A medicine man in the Amazon jungle teaches a team of botanists and pharmacologists about some of the healing powers of a native plant, and they develop a new drug by isolating and purifying a compound in the plant. Should the medicine man (or perhaps his community) be granted some share of royalties from the patent?
- An oncologist develops a valuable cancer cell line from cancerous tissue extracted from a patient's tumor. Should the cancer patient have intellectual property rights over commercial products from his tissue? (This example is based on the famous *Moore v. Regents of the University of California* [1990]. For further discussion, see Gold [1996]).
- A graphic artist develops images for a textbook and is listed a contributor but not as an author. Should she be granted a share of copyrights on the book?

Questions about "fairness" raise fundamental issues about how to allocate benefits and burdens. According to the libertarian approach exemplified by Locke, fairness is strictly a matter of contribution or merit: if you contribute something to project, than your fair share (i.e., your benefits) should be in proportion to your contribution. According to the utilitarian approach, on the other hand, what is fair is what best promotes society's good, and intellectual property principles and laws should promote the social good. Thus, it may follow, on this view, that it is fair not to allocate benefits, such as royalties, on the basis of contribution. The best way to maximize utility may be a system that rewards authors and inventors who are the first to create an original work or invention.

What Can Be Treated as Intellectual Property?

The final issue we consider in this chapter concerns the ethical or moral limitations on intellectual property. Are there some things that should not be treated as intellectual property? In recent years, many biological materials have been treated as intellectual property that were previously viewed as belonging to the public domain, such as organisms, cell lines, genes, and proteins, all of which biotechnology companies have now patented. Many people find the idea of "owning" products of nature to be morally or even religiously offensive or at least not in the best interests of science, medicine, and technology. In reflecting on these issues, we stress again the importance of the *Diamond v. Chakrabarty* (1980) decision and the Supreme Court's ruling that a human invention is "anything under the sun" made by man. The fundamental issue decided by the Court was drawing a line between a *product of nature*, which is not patentable, and a *product of human ingenuity*, which is patentable. One way of developing this distinction is to say that a product of human invention is something that does not exist in a natural state; it would not exist without human manipulation, control, refinement, analysis, and so on. For example, Benjamin Franklin discovered that lightning is static electricity, but he invented the lightning rod. Galileo discovered that Jupiter has moons, but he invented a type of telescope. This seems clear enough. However, consider some less clear-cut cases:

- Digitalis occurs naturally in the foxglove plant, but human beings can make an isolated and purified form of the compound, digoxin.
- Mice exist in nature, but human beings can create genetically altered mice with genes for specific human diseases, such as cancer or diabetes.
- Neural stems cells occur in the human body, but human beings can culture purified cell lines.
- The gene that codes for the protein erythropoietin occurs in the human body, but human beings can use recombinant DNA and molecular cloning techniques to produce mass quantities of an isolated and purified form of the protein.

While people may have a general sense of the difference between discovery and invention, the question we as a society face is how to draw the line between invention and discovery in difficult cases. In the examples above, the items in question are structurally and functionally similar, yet we may decide to call some discoveries and others inventions. To settle these issues, one might appeal to some metaphysical or scientific theory that uniquely divides the world into "products of nature" and "products of human invention." For instance, one could argue that inventions are produced by human beings and cannot exist without human intervention. The trouble with this suggestion is that if one takes a close look at the many different products of research and technology, one finds that all inventions and discoveries have human and natural causes. Moreover, these causes are interdependent and interacting. For example, many scientific laws and theories, such as the natural gas laws and general relativity, would not be known unless some human being had developed and confirmed them. These laws and theories may indeed reflect regularities in the world that are independent of human beings, but their discovery would not occur without human intervention. Furthermore, although artifacts and inventions result from human labor, they make use of natural resources and raw materials. For example, without steam there can be no steam engine, without electricity there can be no electric light bulb, and so forth. Our general point is simply this: questions about what can or cannot be treated as patentable often cannot be settled by the "facts" relating to humanity's interaction with the natural world. Therefore, we must appeal to ethical, political, or economic considerations to decide what is or is not patentable (Resnik 2001a).

In the debate about patenting biological materials, some of these concerns are as follows (Chapman 1999):

- Patenting treats living things or human beings as commercial products.

- Patenting violates the sanctity of nature or the human body.
- Patenting prevents people from gaining access to medications or diagnostic devices.
- Patenting co-opts our common genetic heritage; the gene pool belongs to everyone, not to individuals or corporations.

These concerns raise complex issues that we do not explore in depth here, but we encourage readers to consider arguments for and against various types of patenting as well as other forms of intellectual property in science and technology.

QUESTIONS FOR DISCUSSION

1. Do you think that people have a right to intellectual property?
2. Is it unethical to copy software without the copyright owner's permission?
3. If you are familiar with the Napster case, do you think the company acted unethically?
4. Should pharmaceutical companies be allowed to charge whatever price the market will bear for patented drugs? Should there be moral or political limits on drug prices?
5. Should developing nations violate international intellectual property agreements in order to make drugs available to patients with HIV/AIDS, dysentery, or malaria?
6. Do you have any objections to patenting DNA, cell lines, proteins, tissues, animals, or other human biological materials?
7. Would you have any objections to a patent on a genetically modified human?
8. Should scientists have free access to patented DNA for use in basic research?
9. Do you think that researchers, research institutions, and companies put too much emphasis on intellectual property?
10. Do you think that intellectual property undermines free inquiry, openness, and the academic ethos?

CASES FOR DISCUSSION

Case 1

A faculty member at a U.S. university met a very bright young postdoctoral fellow at a meeting in Germany. The postdoc was working for a company in Germany and had a new chemical entity that could be developed into a product to prevent one type of urinary tract infection. Animal testing had already been conducted, with very promising results. The postdoc then came to the United States to work for the university faculty member, with support from the German company. The German company, through its subsidiary in the United States, submitted an Investigational New Drug (IND) application to the FDA in order to start phase I clinical trials on humans. Later that year, a French company acquired the German company. In the meantime, the post-doc met a colleague at a meeting at a different U.S. university and collaborated to test the new chemical entity. They discovered a new modality to treat another disease with the same chemical entity.

At this time the faculty member's U.S. university was negotiating with the French/German company to have the research conducted at the university's facilities. From the start, the French/German company demanded sole proprietorship of the drug and wanted to control all of its aspects of research and development. The university then asked the postdoc to sign a visiting fellowship agreement assigning all intellectual property claims to the university. The postdoc refused, on the advice of the French/German company. Meanwhile, the German/French company filed for a patent alone without any mention of the part of the work conducted at the university.

- What should the university do? What should the university faculty member do?
- Who owns the patent? Is the patent application valid?
- What should each party have done in the first place?

Case 2

A university investigator is in hot pursuit of a project that received a medium-sized grant from the NIH. His grant depends on the use of reagents from an independent company. He has had a long and fruitful relationship with the company—he has given several seminars at the company, and his counterpart in the company has given several seminars at the university. Also, the investigator has earned a few thousand dollars annually from the company through consulting. He has signed a consultancy agreement with the company without clearance from the university. His agreement relinquishes all his intellectual property rights regarding the subject of the consultancy to the company.

The investigator asked the university to sign a material transfer agreement (MTA) so that he could start using the reagents. The university refused because the MTA gave too many rights to intellectual property to the company in exchange for the reagents. The university investigator was anxious to start his project and make progress so that he would be able to renew his grant. One day during his frequent seminars at the company, he was asked to sign the MTA agreement, and he did.

- What should the University do?
- What should the faculty member do?
- What should the company do?

Case 3

In early 1990s, a university faculty member was collaborating with a Danish company in a joint venture on a compound with a view toward clinical trials within a year. The company has already submitted a patent application on a portion of the project. In written correspondence between the university faculty member and her counterpart at the Danish company, both pledge full cooperation without mentioning anything about intellectual property.

A year later, the Danish company enlisted a U.S. company to conduct certain experiments. The university and the Danish and U.S. companies all entered into negotiation regarding intellectual property. The negotiations failed, and the university ordered the faculty member to stop any further collaboration.

- What should the faculty member do?
- What should the university do?
- What lessons are learned in this scenario?

Case 4

A faculty member at university A received an important material uniquely prepared by another faculty member at university B. The two have signed a Material Transfer Agreement (MTA) essentially sharing intellectual property. The faculty member at university A then modified the material and shipped it to a collaborator at university C. A few months later, the faculty member at university A prepared an abstract with the faculty member from university C. The faculty member at university B read the abstract and to his horror found that this is exactly the finding of his doctoral student.

- What should each one of them do?
- What should each university do?
- What should the graduate student do?

Case 5

A graduate student at a university was not able to obtain material as described in a paper published by a faculty member at another university. He wrote the faculty member for advice and received begrudging advice on how to do the procedure. After three more months of failure, he wrote to ask to see the lab notebook so that he could reproduce the data and stop wasting his time. His request was declined. What should the student do?

Case 6

A member of an NIH study section, while reviewing a grant proposal, realized she could do part of the proposed research faster and better with a method already available in her laboratory. Under normal conditions, she would not be conducting such research. After getting back to her laboratory, she gave the project to her most reliable postdoctoral fellow.

One year later, they submitted a paper to a prestigious journal. One of the reviewers was the investigator who wrote the original grant proposal. The original investigator has not yet published his paper on the subject because he has applied for a patent, which delayed writing of the paper. The original investigator complained to the U.S. Office of Research Integrity.

- What should Office of Research Integrity do?
- What should the reviewer do?
- Who should get the patent?

Case 7

An anthropologist and his team from a university have discovered a human skeleton in a national forest in Montana. Carbon dating shows that the skeleton is over 10,000 years old. Further study of the skeleton will prove to be extremely useful in determining human migration to the North American continent. However, a group representing Native Americans is taking legal action to have the skeleton returned to their custody. They say that the skeleton is one of their ancestors and should not be the object of scientific study.

- Who owns this skeleton?
- How should this dispute be settled?

Case 8

A biotech company is developing transgenic cows designed to produce milk nutritionally similar to the milk produced by human beings. They have applied for patents on the cows as well as other methods of producing human milk, including human lactation. Thus, they are seeking to patent women and their breasts.

- Should the company be allowed to patent any of these materials?
- What patent rights should the company have?

Case 9

A tissue collection and storage company has signed a contract with a medical school to collect human tissue for research purposes. The company plans to collect tissues from healthy and unhealthy human donors at the medical school. Tissue donors will sign an informed consent form giving the company their tissue. They will not receive any money for their tissue but will be informed that their tissue may benefit other people. Once the tissue is donated, it will be placed in a tissue bank. All personal identifiers linking the tissue to the donor will be removed. The company expects to profit by charging access to its tissue database. It also plans to patent valuable cell lines. The medical school will receive a portion of the profits. Do you see any ethical problems with this proposal?

7

Conflicts of Interest
and Scientific Objectivity

> Researchers and research institutions have a variety of financial, personal,
> and political interests that sometimes conflict with their professional, eth-
> ical, or legal obligations. These situations can create conflicts of interest
> or the appearance of conflicts of interest. This chapter discusses how con-
> flicts of interest affect research, how they are defined, and how they
> should be managed. It also describes how government agencies and re-
> search institutions have responded to conflicts of interest in research and
> describes some cases from science.

Individual scientists and research organizations daily encounter situations
where personal, financial, political, and other interests conflict with professional, ethical, or legal obligations or duties. Although conflicts of all types are
a normal part of human existence, some are called "conflicts of interest"
(COIs) because they involve conflicts between interests and duties. Most of
the concern with COIs arises because personal interests can undermine duties
relating to scientific objectivity (Shamoo 1992, 1993, Resnik 2001b). For example, a researcher with stock in a pharmaceutical company that sponsors his
research overestimates the clinical significance of his research on one of the
company's drugs, which drives up the price of his stock. An academic researcher in a National Institutes of Health (NIH) study section reviews a grant
from a competitor in the same field (Shamoo 1993). A scientist receives orders
not to publish results that are contrary to the interests of the company that
funds her research. A medical journal runs an advertisement for a new drug.
Other COIs may undermine other duties, such as the duty to protect human
subjects. For example, a physician-researcher receives $3,000 in patient care
costs per patient she recruits to be in a clinical trial. A university's institutional
review board (IRB) reviews a research proposal sponsored by a company that
has recently given $30 million to the university.

It is helpful to remember that a nation's ability to deal with problems, such
as COIs in research, are a sign of a stable democratic society with reasonable
public confidence in the system and the willingness of its population to abide
by its rules. From this perspective, the national will to deal with such issues is
an apparent luxury compared with the constraints presented by the poverty,
limited health care, genocide, war, and corruption that exist in many other
countries. Nonetheless, if a privileged society does not deal effectively with
COIs in research, the erosion of public confidence in science that may occur
can be extremely damaging and corrosive to democracy.

Defining Conflicts of Interest

The first step in understanding the issues in COIs is to define the phrase "conflict of interest." It will be useful to first examine a few paradigmatic cases of COI that arise for individuals:

- Legal: A lawyer has two clients with conflicting interests, such as a husband and wife who are getting a divorce (usually such representation is not allowed).
- Medical: A doctor goes on a Caribbean cruise sponsored by a pharmaceutical company.
- Research: A researcher conducts drug research funded by NIH while receiving $20,000 per year in consulting fees from the drug manufacturer.
- Political: A member of a zoning board owns 20 acres of land that may be rezoned for commercial use.
- Personal: A father is asked to referee his daughter's soccer game.

These cases contain important common elements: all of the individuals have interests that threaten their ability to carry out their primary duties or obligations. The lawyer has responsibilities to both of his clients and to the legal system to defend their legal rights, but his conflict may threaten his ability to do so. The doctor has an obligation to his patient to prescribe medications that will be in the patient's best interests, but he has a financial interest (relationship to the pharmaceutical company) that may threaten (or appear to threaten) his ability to do so. The researcher has an obligation to the NIH, the public, and colleagues in his field, but she has financial interest with the drug manufacturer that threatens her ability to perform her research objectively. The member of the zoning board has obligations to the voters and society to make decisions that promote the public good, but her financial interest (land) threatens or appears to threaten her ability to act in this fashion. The father has a duty to be a fair (or impartial) referee but he has a personal interest, his daughter. In situations like these, we begin to wonder whether the person with the conflict can or will fulfill his or her primary obligations. This brings us to the crux of the problem with COIs: they create ethical problems because they undermine trust (Resnik 1998b, Bradley 2000, DeAngelis 2000).

Throughout this book, we have shown that trust is very important in research: students must trust mentors or supervisors, principal investigators must trust subordinates, and colleagues must trust each other. Researchers must trust journals, granting agencies, and research institutions. Chapter 9 on human subjects discusses how research subjects must also trust researchers, and chapter 12 discusses how society must trust researchers. Because COIs can threaten or undermine trust, it is incumbent upon the research community to address these concerns.

A COI can undermine a person's ability to fulfill his or her duties in several different ways. First, a COI can affect a person's judgment or reasoning (Davis 1982, Shamoo 1993, Thompson 1993, Resnik 1998b, Bradley 2000). A person with a COI is like a thermometer that does not work properly. In some of these cases we might say that the person's judgments and decisions are biased; that is, they tend to be skewed in a particular pattern or direction that can be attributed to the particular interest. For example, the doctor may have a general tendency to overprescribe specific types of drugs manufactured by the pharmaceutical company. The father may fail to see fouls committed by his daughter's soccer team. Sometimes the problem is that the person is not only biased but also unreliable: a thermometer that registers a temperature that is higher and sometimes lower than the air temperature is unreliable. A lawyer with two clients with conflicting interests may sometimes make decisions that are unfair to one or the other client. The referee-father may favor his daughter's team or favor the other team in order to give the impression that he is impartial.

Second, a COI can affect motivation and behavior (Resnik 1998b, Porter 1993). A person with a COI may be perfectly capable of sound thinking but may fail to implement good judgment and reasoning due to temptations of that affect his or her motivation and behavior. For example, a zoning board member may know that it is not in the public's best interests to zone a piece of land for commercial use but may fail to act on this practical knowledge due to the temptation to cash in his 20 acres when it is rezoned. As a result, he may lobby for rezoning and vote for it. All people are tempted from time to time by a number of desires, but the problem with COIs, one might argue, is that they place people in situations where only people with extraordinary characters will not succumb to temptation.

Putting all of this together, we offer the following definition of a COI:

> Conflict of interest (for an individual): An individual has a conflict of interest when he or she has personal, financial, or political interests that undermine his or her ability to meet or fulfill his or her primary professional, ethical, or legal obligations.

In theory, it is fairly easy to define COIs, but in practice it is often difficult to determine (or know) whether a person has a COI, because we may not know how their personal, financial, or political interests are affecting (or will affect) their judgment, reasoning, motivation, or behavior. Many people with personal, financial, or political interests will acknowledge these interests but maintain that they have a great deal of integrity and will not allow their personal interests to undermine their ethical or legal responsibilities. How can we know which conflicts will affect the person and which will not? How much money does it take to affect reasoning or behavior? $10,000? $1,000? $100? We cannot address these difficult practical issues adequately here, but we will adopt a standard that we call the "reasonable person" standard: a person has a COI when a reasonable person with the relevant background, knowledge, or expertise would be affected in similar circumstances. Although some extraordinary people may be able to maintain their objectivity and integrity when faced with such conflicts, most people will succumb to biases or temptations. On the other hand, because the key issue in COI is trust, it is important to acknowledge that there are situations where we *do not know* that a COI exists but where we believe that trust is undermined because there is the perception or appearance of a COI. Thus, it is important to distinguish between apparent and actual or real COIs:

> Apparent conflict of interest (for an individual): An individual has an apparent conflict of interest when he or she has personal, financial, or political interests that do not undermine his or her ability to meet or fulfill his or her primary legal or ethical obligations, but that create the perception of a conflict.

These definitions also apply to scientific research. As discussed in chapter 2, scientists frequently have responsibilities to other members of the profession, clients, patients, students, society, adherence to professional standards, and ethical or legal standards of conduct. Scientists also have personal, financial, or political interests that could interfere with their ability to perform those duties. Many of these personal interests relate to career ambitions, such as the quest for reputation, fame, power, priority, funding, tenure, and promotion. These interests can affect scientific thinking, reasoning, motivation, and behavior. For example, a scientist who has stock options in a pharmaceutical company and is conducting research on that company's drugs has a responsibility to conduct objective (or unbiased) research. However, her financial interests may prevent her (or appear to prevent her) from fulfilling that responsibility; she may conduct research that is biased toward the company (or it may appear that her work is biased). Money or ambition can also interfere with a researcher's ability promote the rights and welfare of human subjects. A researcher with strong financial or personal interests in recruiting human subjects for a clinical trial may oversell the trial to his patients or take other steps to compromise the informed consent process. When students are supported by funds from industrial sponsors, conflicts may affect duties to the research profession, patients, and students (Blumenthal 1995). Virtually any area of research can be affected by COIs. Those that are most susceptible to the effects of COIs include objectives, design, methods, and analysis; publication; peer review; clinical trials; selection and recruitment of subjects; and funding (Spece et al. 1996, Bradley 2000, Resnik 2001b).

Because COIs can have such a great impact on scientific objectivity, they have been linked to scientific fraud and misconduct. For example, due to pressures to obtain funding, a scientist might fabricate or falsify data in a grant application or paper. Or perhaps a researcher working for a pharmaceutical company manipulates the data to make his results appear to be statistically or clinically significant. Indeed, money has played an important role in most of the cases of scientific misconduct (or alleged misconduct) discussed in chapter 5. On the other hand, because most scientists do not commit misconduct or fraud to promote their personal, financial, or political interests, we need to distinguish clearly between COIs and research misconduct: having a COI is not, in itself, research misconduct. However, a COI may be a risk factor for misconduct or fraud (U.S. Congress 1990).

The preceding discussion also allows us to understand why COIs are an important ethical concern in science and how the research community should address them. COIs are an important ethical problem because they may prevent scientists from fulfilling their professional obligations. Researchers with conflicts may fail to make objective judgments or decisions in research, publication, and peer review. Researchers may also fail to fulfill their duties to patients, clients, students, peers, or society. Thus, COIs can threaten the integrity of the entire research process. Just as important, COIs can undermine the trustworthiness of science by creating the perception (among peers or the public) that research is biased, unreliable, or morally tainted.

CONFLICTS OF COMMITMENT AND DUTY

It is important to distinguish between COIs and other types of conflicts that occur in research. Consider this example: a molecular biologist who is hired by a public university also consults with several private and public clients, including a biotechnology firm, a hospital, and the local health department. As a result, she often has a difficult time balancing her commitments to the university and to these other organizations. This is a type of situation known as a conflict of commitment (Resnik 1998b). A researcher who puzzles over whether to prepare his lecture or finish a paper would also have a conflict of commitment. Conflicts of commitment, unlike COIs, do not normally involve situations that compromise a person's thinking, reasoning, motivation, or behavior. They primarily have to do with the prudent and responsible management of time and effort. People with conflicts of commitment usually can manage their different commitments. However, if one cannot manage one's many different commitments, the responsible thing to do is to prioritize these commitments and eliminate some of them. Sometimes conflicts of commitments can lead to COIs. For example, a university scientist may become so involved with time-consuming consultations that she can no longer meet her professional, contractual, or other obligations (Davis 1995a).

There are also situations where duties conflict that are not COIs (Davis 1982). For example, a doctor may have to decide between respecting a patient's autonomy and promoting the patient's best interests when an otherwise healthy patient chooses to refuse life-saving medical care, such as refusal of dialysis. Or someone may have to choose between honoring a prior commitment to attend a meeting and taking care of some important business that just came up. A researcher may face a conflict between the duty to share data and the duty to respect intellectual property. Although conflicts of duties can lead to COIs when the person in question also has an interest in meeting a specific duty, COIs are not the same as conflicts of duty. COIs involve the collision between personal interests and duties, not conflicts among duties. For more on resolving conflicts of duty, see chapter 1.

MANAGING INDIVIDUAL CONFLICTS OF INTEREST

There are several ways to protect the integrity of the research process and promote trust in response to COIs. One strategy that has been adopted by many institutions is known as disclosure (McCary et al. 2000, Bradley 2000).

Researchers should disclose COIs and apparent COIs to the relevant parties. A relevant party would be someone in a supervisory role, who does not have a vested interest in the particular conflict situation, such as a department chair, section head, dean, or director. The person should have some degree of independence or objectivity. This is a useful strategy because it puts conflicts out in the open and allows people to assess them. For example, if a researcher discloses a COI in a paper, scientists may pay more careful attention to the paper's methods, results, and interpretations. The paper may demand some additional scrutiny, but it is not automatically invalidated (Resnik 1998b). Moreover, openness can promote trust because people are likely to be more suspicious and untrusting when they discover previously hidden conflicts than when the have access to them up front (Cho 1997). However, disclosure alone of COI may not be sufficient (Cech and Leonard 2001). A second strategy that has been adopted by many organizations is known as management of conflicts (McCary et al. 2000). According to this strategy, people with COIs disclose them to the relevant parties, who consult with other people to develop rules or policies for controlling the interests that are at stake. They may also decide to review these COIs on a regular basis and take additional steps to promote trust, if necessary.

Most research institutions have policies that require some form of disclosure of COIs, and many have methods for managing COIs (Cho et al. 2000). Fewer institutions make much use of a third strategy, known as avoidance. In this strategy, which is frequently used in government, law, and medicine, organizations make rules that prohibit specific situations that create COIs. For example, government ethics rules place limits on the amount of money a legislator may receive as a gift or honoraria. Medical ethics codes prohibit kickbacks and self-referrals. The NIH has COI rules for its study sections that prohibit scientists from reviewing grant proposals from colleagues at the same institution. COI avoidance may also occur when a person chooses to remove (or "recuse") himself or herself from the situation that creates the conflict, for example, when a reviewer for a journal declines to review a paper because of a personal bias against the authors. The attorney in the case mentioned above may decide not to represent one (or both) of his clients due to his COI.

Like disclosure and management of conflicts, conflict avoidance can promote integrity and trust. However, it sometimes can lead to outcomes that are worse (from a utilitarian point of view) than the outcomes that result from nonavoidance. For example, suppose that three fourths of the members of a zoning board own land that will be affected by their decision. If they all recuse themselves, the board either will lack a quorum and be unable to make a decision, or it will lack informed debate on the issue.

INSTITUTIONAL CONFLICTS OF INTEREST

It is important to realize that organizations or institutions can also have COIs. Consider the following situations:

- A television network decides to not broadcast a story that is unfavorable to a company because that company threatens to stop advertising on the network.
- A medical society endorses a medical product made by a company that donates a great deal of money to the society.
- A university's institutional review board approves a human research proposal over the objections of several members because a failure to approve the proposal could threaten a $5 million grant.
- A university disciplines a faculty member for speaking out on an environmental issue because several state legislators want him punished.
- A university is trying to silence a faculty member because he spoke against research conducted on his campus that in his opinion violates ethics.
- A university holds stock in a chemical plant but also hires employees who monitor its emissions.

These examples illustrate how institutions, including research institutions, government agencies, professional associations, and journals, can also have COIs and apparent COIs. These organizations, like individuals, often have collective duties to professionals, clients, students, patients, and the public. Their duties usually stem from their primary missions (or goals), such as research, education, and public service. Institutions, like individuals, may also have financial, political, or other interests that can adversely affect (or appear to affect) their ability to carry out these responsibilities. Although institutions do not "think," they do make collective decisions that result from the judgments, decisions, and actions of their members, and they do perform actions or behaviors. These decisions and actions occur through the various components of the organization's management structure, such as faculty members, committees, advisory boards, deans, vice presidents, and so on. Institutional COIs, like individual COIs, can also threaten the integrity or trustworthiness of research, except the damage may be more extensive because it may affect more researchers and members of the public (Association of Academic Health Centers 1994, Bradley 2000, Moses and Martin 2001). We define an institutional COI as follows:

> Conflict of interest (for an institution): An institution has a conflict of interest when its financial, political, or other interests threaten its ability to fulfill its professional, legal, ethical, or social responsibilities.

As with individual conflicts, the same three strategies to protect research integrity may apply: disclosure, conflict management, and avoidance. For some organizations, it may be enough to simply disclose the conflict; for others, avoidance may be the best option. We discuss institutional COIs at greater length in chapter 8.

To maintain some perspective on this topic, note that COIs are more or less unavoidable in society because all of us, including scientists, have interests that sometimes undermine (or are perceived to undermine) our responsibilities.

Unless one wants to become a hermit, the best option is to understand and respond to them in an honest, open, and ethical way. The next section helps to illustrate this point.

LIVING WITH CONFLICTS OF INTEREST

Although we believe that it is important to respond to individual and institutional COIs, it is not possible (or even desirable) to avoid all situations that can create COIs or apparent COIs. Individuals and institutions have many different duties and interests. Only a hermit could avoid all real and apparent COIs. Since most institutions need funding to continue to exist, it is doubtful that they can avoid real or apparent COIs as well. Given the ubiquity of real and apparent COIs, the best response is to take appropriate steps to disclose or manage these situations and to sometimes avoid these situations. Many situations in research that create COIs also have important benefits. For instance, intellectual property rights can create COIs but they can also encourage innovation and investment in research. From a utilitarian perspective, one might argue that society is best served by allowing researchers and research institutions to own intellectual property but to require individuals and institutions to make appropriate disclosures, and so on.

Lessons from Nonresearch Conflicts of Interest

Before presenting additional information on COIs in scientific research, it will be valuable to discuss how other sectors of society have responded to COIs. This discussion shows that science has much in common with other parts of our society. Moreover, the lessons from other disciplines will be informative for approaches to this difficult problem.

Concerns about COIs in scientific research are brand new compared with those in government. Aristotle, Democritus, and Confucius all conveyed the principle that government officials should be entrusted to serve the public faithfully. Adam Smith, the father of private enterprise, described his view of the priority of interests: "The wise and virtuous man is at all times willing that his own private interest should be sacrificed to the public interest of his own particular order or society [and] that the interest of his order or society should be sacrificed to the greater interest of the state or sovereignty" (quoted in Fleishman 1982, p. 34).

Concerns about COIs in government have existed for thousands of years, because government creates a conflict between civic duty and personal or financial interest. Trust is very important in government: the citizens must trust their elected and appointed officials. When citizens do not trust the government, they are more likely not to obey laws, not to pay their taxes, and not to vote in elections. Thomas Jefferson looked for "men who will not bend their politics to their purses, nor pursue measures by which they may profit, and then profit by their measures" (quoted in Fleishman 1982, p. 28).

Fleishman (1982) eloquently described the risk of self-interest to our democratic system of government: "Nothing—not errors of judgment, not waste, not inefficiency, not high taxes, not over-regulation, not even the loss of a war—so shakes representative government at its root as does a belief by the public that officials who govern act chiefly out of concern for private self-interest rather than for the public interest of those who elected them" (p. 27).

The potential for COI in the executive branch of government is especially clear, because of its responsibilities for the administration of billions of dollars in grants and contracts. Recognizing these risks, in 1962 the U.S. Congress passed the Bribery, Graft, and Conflict of Interest Act. Shortly thereafter, President Lyndon B. Johnson issued an executive order that prohibited the acceptance of gratuities and mandated the avoidance of actions that lead to the appearance of private gain, preferential treatment, impeding efficiency, or partiality or that in any other way adversely affected public confidence in the integrity of government (D'Agostino et al. 1988, National Contract Management Association 1989, Perkins 1961, Rauh 1961). In 1978, in the aftermath of the Watergate scandal, Congress enacted the Ethics in Government Act, which codified the need for financial disclosure and set penalties for violators (Williams 1985, p. 120).

Therefore, at least for executive branch employees of the U.S. government, there are clear COI prohibitions and criminal prosecution when employees of the federal government violate COI rules. However, what has not been dealt with effectively is what happens after a high-ranking official leaves government employment. At present, for example, a former Food and Drug Administration (FDA) official working for a pharmaceutical industry cannot deal with the FDA for a period of one year after leaving the position. However, he or she is permitted to give beneficial advice and contact information to the new employer.

Policies pertaining to the regulation of finance are generally designed to ensure the integrity of the system, prevent monopolistic practices, increase competition, improve efficiency, enhance quality of products, protect consumers, and improve overall economic well-being (McVea 1993). Two great financial institutions are directly involved in these issues: banking and the securities exchange. These institutions handle billions of dollars belonging to the public. The institutions and their stockbrokers and investment banker employees have tremendous fiduciary responsibilities that require the confidence and trust of the public. It is presumed that excessive regulations impede competition, efficiency, and consumer choice and result in higher costs for services and products. The challenge rises in finding a balance between the benefits of reasonable regulations and the harms of unnecessary controls. However, in any financial system, some regulation is essential, and in many instances the regulations pertain to COIs.

To what extent are the COI issues of finance and scientific research similar? To be sure, there is inequity in terms of the amount of money involved. Nevertheless, the worlds of wealth and investigation share some obvious common ground. Universities and industry routinely collaborate on projects and have mutual as well as different interests. Industrial progress increasingly depends upon basic research done at universities. And research institutions increasingly depend upon money from industry to support their research programs. The quest for support sometimes conflicts with such the goal of scientific independence and influences decision-making processes, both of individuals and of the institutions that employ them. These issues are covered more extensively in chapter 8.

Despite any such similarities in the institutions of finance and research, their obligations to the public are quite different. How important is confidentiality to the exercise of integrity in research? Examples of similarities of COIs in research to those in financial institutions include confidentiality of peer reviews of grants and manuscripts, promotion and tenure deliberations, and resisting temptations of "insider trading" on valuable information regarding relevant biotechnology companies. Violations of confidentiality in research have similar impact on public confidence and policies. Thus far, the management of COIs in university settings has been much less restrictive than that in the financial world (McCary et al. 2000, Cho et al. 2000).

Journalists find it as difficult to avoid COIs as any other group. Examples abound. *The Washington Post* wrote an editorial urging passage of the international General Agreement on Tariffs and Trade (GATT) without mentioning that the *Post* had sought and obtained special legislation attached to GATT designed to result in tens of million of dollars of direct benefit to the *Post* (Morton 1994, p. 52). The practice of paying large sums of money to well-known reporters is common knowledge. Cokie Roberts of *ABC News* was paid more than $12,000 to speak at a nonprofit event that was sponsored by a $4 billion company that distributes Toyotas (Kurtz 1996). George Will, a syndicated columnist, wrote a column against the newly proposed 100% tariffs on Japanese luxury cars but did not mention that his wife is a lobbyist for the Japan Automobile Manufacturers Association and was paid $198,721 in 1994 alone (Kurtz 1995).

Several newspapers, such as *The Wall Street Journal, The New York Times, The Washington Post,* and *The Chronicle for Higher Education,* have developed strict standards designed to minimize financial COIs. The Society of Professional Journalism (1991) has a code of ethics that states, "Journalists must be free of obligation to any interest other than the public's right to know the truth" (Sneed and Riffe 1991, p. 14). The code of ethics of the American Society of Newspaper Editors includes the statement that "[f]reedom from all obligations except that of fidelity to the public interest is vital" (Sneed and Riffe 1991, p. 14). These pronouncements make it clear that for journalists, the avoidance of COIs is crucial to meeting their obligations to the public.

What lessons can scientists learn from journalists? Would scientists make the same statement about the public's right to know the truth? That fidelity to the public interest is a primary central value? How high on scientists' priority list would these statements be? Do scientists' obligations to truth extend to the public or only to other scientists? To what extent are the public interest and the public's right to the truth compatible with the researcher's obligation for scientific integrity? Could the researcher's obligation to integrity conflict with acting in the public interest or providing truth to the public?

Lessons from Published Conflict of Interest Cases

Since World War II, the growth of science has been exponential. The United States alone spends over $200 billion annually on research and development, requiring a work force of more than half a million scientists and more than two million support personnel. With such large numbers, the culture of U.S. science reflects all of society's goods and ills. Scientists are human beings, no different than any other group. Furthermore, scientists often work in multiple functions. They may be involved in university teaching and research, private practice, private consulting, company ownership and equity, as well as simultaneous employment by a university and industry. As a result, scientists seem to be well placed for both conflicts of commitment and financial COIs (Korn 1993). Furthermore, as discussed above, universities themselves often have a financial stake in the outcome of research. This situation may place the interest of the inventor (i.e., researcher) in conflict with the university. Because of these factors, all of which involve and depend upon money, when problems of conflict occur today, they tend to be newsmakers. Public disclosures of problems, even though painful to some, provides public scrutiny.

The following five examples of COIs in research are presented primarily to illustrate the intertwining financial interests that either hinder scientific objectivity or are perceived as such by the citizens. Since these cases came to light, the NIH and National Science Foundation (NSF), along with universities, have promulgated better policies on COI disclosures. Additionally, the *Journal of the American Medical Association*, the *New England Journal of Medicine*, and the NIH now require their authors and researchers to disclose COIs. The last example is presented to show that COI is not always linked directly to financial interests.

Pharmatec and the University of Florida (U.S. Congress 1990)   In early 1980s, Dr. Boder, a professor at the University of Florida, invented a chemical delivery system (CDS) to carry drugs directly to the brain. Dr. Boder entered into an exclusive license agreement with a corporation to form a new start-up company, Pharmatec, with an initial investment of $6 million. Dr. Boder was to receive $1 million of the $6 million to develop and further test the CDS. Dr. Boder's time was then divided in a complicated fashion among the university and Pharmatec. Dr. Boder was also the Vice President and Director of Pharmatec, as well as the Chairman of the Department of Medicinal Chemistry at the Florida College of Pharmacy. The Dean of the College of Pharmacy was given 1,000 shares of stock. Dr. Boder hired three other College of Pharmacy faculty members to work for Pharmatec, who also received stocks from the company, as did some additional key administrators of the college. The dean, Dr. Boder, and other faculty members of the college became members of Pharmatec's Advisory Board.

One of the advisory board members, Dr. Sloan, an associate professor in the college, raised concerns regarding the safety of the CDS because of its structural similarity to a hemotoxin, MPTP. He suggested that, to ensure safety to students and faculty researchers at the college, the compound should be tested on primates. Dr. Sloan approached the dean and others and made presentations at conferences about the possibility of a toxicological effect. There was considerable delay before any toxicological tests were conducted, with the result that Dr. Sloan resigned from the advisory board. It is alleged that his career suffered from the incident.

The U.S. congressional report states: "The story of Pharmatec demonstrates how the financial interests of universities and their faculty can conflict with such important scientific questions as the safe conduct of research as well as the fair treatment of faculty" (p. 14).

t-PA: A Multicenter Trial (U.S. Congress 1990)   Each year 700,000 patients suffer from myocardial infarction. During the 1980s, the NIH funded research at medical centers across the country to evaluate thrombolytic agents such as t-PA that have the potential for dissolving blood clots. The clinical trials were to compare t-PA, which had not yet been approved by the FDA, with streptokinase (SK), which had been FDA approved for intracoronary administration. t-PA is a product of Genentech Corporation. In 1985, the *New England Journal of Medicine* published a paper showing that t-PA was twice as effective as SK in dissolving blood clots. No data were presented indicating the lack of difference between t-PA and SK in ventricular function, an important indicator with bearing on mortality. Also not reported was the fact that five of the coauthors owned stocks in Genentech. Two years later, the data on ventricular function was publicly revealed. Members of the NIH Safety and Data Monitoring Committee expressed concerns about the t-PA results. NIH dissolved the committee and formed a new one that included only one member from the former committee. Genentech stocks rose and fell precipitously, depending on the latest news about t-PA. Later, it became known that 13 of the researchers involved in the nationwide t-PA studies owned stocks in Genentech.

At roughly the same time as the U.S. studies, two European groups had been conducting clinical trials comparing SK and t-PA. Based upon large populations of 12,000 and 20,000 patients, they published their findings. One report published in the journal *Lancet* showed that SK alone reduced mortality by 12% and that SK plus aspirin reduced mortality by 42%. In 1987 an FDA advisory committee decided to recommend approval of SK for use in dissolving blood clots, but not t-PA. This action resulted in an uproar from the business community. Subsequently, the FDA reversed its decision on t-PA and approved it.

This case illustrates the impact that COIs can have on the general public and on public institutions when university scientists enter the private arena, becoming stockholders in companies whose product they are evaluating.

The Retin A Acne Case (U.S. Congress 1990)   Retin A is a cream product of Johnson and Johnson Corporation. In 1988, the *Journal of the American Medical Association (JAMA)* published an article and an editorial claiming that Retin A "could reverse wrinkles and other damage caused by photo-aging." After the article, about 1.2 million tubes of Retin A were sold in one month, compared with less than 0.25 million for the same month a year earlier. Later a reporter disclosed that the author of the *JAMA* editorial and one of the authors of the research article received financial compensations from Johnson and Johnson. Furthermore, it was subsequently determined that the safety of Retin A had been exaggerated and that the study had not been well controlled for bias because of the absence of a double-blind design. Also, an NIH consensus conference has concluded that the safety and effectiveness of Retin A have not yet been established.

This case illustrates the impact COIs can have on the objectivity of scientists. Moreover, it illustrates that public confidence in our scientists and scientific institutions such as scientific journals can be undermined by COI or the appearance of a COI.

Clinical Trials of Therapeutic Drugs for Myocardial Infarction (Porter 1992)   In 1983 Thomas Chalmers evaluated 145 clinical trials of the therapeutic drugs of myocardial infarction. He placed each study in one of three levels of bias control. Highly controlled studies included those that were randomized and blinded. Partly controlled studies included those that were randomized but not blinded. The category of no controls included those that were neither randomized nor blinded. He found that the effectiveness of the new drugs was inversely related to the degree of bias control. When the bias control was categorized as highly, partly, or not controlled, the drugs were effective only 9%, 24%, and 58% of the time, respectively. This example illustrates that even though there was no direct financial interest for the investigator, investigators' bias for their sponsor or their own success as a researcher can seriously corrupt the results.

Concerns about such practices prompted the American Medical Association's Council on Scientific Affairs and Council on Ethical and Judicial Affairs to make the following statement: "For the clinical investigator who has an economic interest in the outcome of his or her research, objectivity is especially difficult. Economic incentives may introduce subtle biases into the way research is conducted, analyzed, or reported, and these biases can escape detection by even careful peer review" (quoted in Porter 1992, p. 159).

Familial Hypercholesteremia and the Nobel Prize (Shamoo 1992)   Michael Brown and Joseph Goldstein were awarded the Nobel Prize in Physiology and Medicine in 1985 for discoveries related to the elucidation of the mechanism of familial hypercholesteremia (FH), which in part enhanced the understanding of the larger problem of atherosclerosis. The mechanism could not have been determined without three crucial and separate discoveries related to issues of genetics, receptor dysfunction, and blood-cell relationships. Brown and Goldstein made the discovery that the disorder is caused by the receptor on the cell membrane, but Avedis Khachadurian made the other two discoveries, made before that of Brown and Goldstein. As early as 1964, Khachadurian showed that FH was due to a single Mendelian gene disorder. Additionally, at least four years before the Brown and Goldstein publications, Khachadurian discovered that the disorder was not located within the cell and would therefore be revealed in some interaction between the blood and the cell. Thus, although Khachadurian made two of the three key discoveries, the Nobel Prize was awarded to Brown and Goldstein.

An investigation of the literature showed that there was a consistent pattern by Brown and Goldstein in not quoting Khachadurian's work in the 1970s and early 1980s (Shamoo 1992). However, after receiving the Nobel Prize, Brown and Goldstein as well as others gave clear recognition to the importance of Khachadurian's discoveries. For example, Myant's 1990 book referred to Khachadurian's 1964 key findings as follows: "This work, a landmark in the development of our understanding of FH, is worth placing on record" (p. 403). Brown and Goldstein wrote the foreword for Myant's book.

The importance of this case can be seen in the remarks of Philip Siekevitz, a leading U.S. scientist at Rockefeller University: "The intense competition for recognition by peers and by the general public, for prizes, for commercial gain, is slowly eroding the scientific ethic. . . . And if this ethos is disappearing, then the citation indices no longer reflect worth but a lack of the scientific communitas. The future of the scientific endeavor depends on regaining the scientific soul" (quoted in Shamoo 1992, p. 72).

Advisory Groups and Conflict of Interest

It is taken as an article of faith that "advisory groups" render objective opinions regarding important public policy issues and the relative worth of projects for funding, in the form of advisory councils, advisory boards, study sections, and review panels. The U.S. government widely uses advisory groups for policy and funding decisions. The reliance on such groups is primarily based on two premises: expertise in the subject area and objectivity. Shamoo (1993) conducted an analysis of 10 years (1979–1989) of funding decisions of grant applications of members of the advisory councils of the NIH, and found that members of the advisory groups received nearly twice the percentage of grants funded despite the fact that their merit ratings by the study sections were the same as those for the rest of the grant applicants.

THE MANAGEMENT OF SCIENTIFIC CONFLICT OF INTEREST

Association for Academic Health Centers

Despite increasing concerns about scientific COIs in the 1980s from both the congress and the general public, due in part to cases such as those described above, universities were generally reluctant to take a leadership role in tackling the issue and being accountable for the actions of their employees (Bradley 1995). In 1994, following a series of congressional hearings and media revelations related to the erosion of scientific objectivity and the potential loss of public confidence in the scientific process, the Association for Academic Health Centers (AAHC) issued a document entitled *Conflict of Interest in Institutional Decision-Making*.

The AAHC document called for the preservation of the traditional missions of teaching, research, and service during this period of increasing funding from industry. Oversight procedures would play a key role in this effort. It further called for full and accurate disclosure of potential COIs, on the part of both university employees and the institutions themselves. Although it suggested no criteria for minimum disclosure, the AAHC pointed out that some states and universities required disclosure of leadership positions in a company, investments of more than $25,000 in any work-related company, corporate ownership of at least 10%, annual consultation agreements paying more than $5,000, and any research involvement with industry at all. Additionally, the disclosure should hold not only for the university personnel themselves, but also for those related by blood and for close relationships outside the family. At the institutional level, disclosure should pertain to those who have decision-making authority and extend to the making of investment decisions involving companies with faculty interests. The AAHC guidelines also called for the prompt publication of the results of research, fairness in the allocation of the financial benefits of intellectual property, and the administration of patent issues in the public interest. They also deal with the free utilization of knowledge by students and the conduct of sponsored research under the terms of university policies and in the same context as federal funds. Finally, COI should be avoided in the pursuit of the financial benefits of technology transfer.

The effect of these guidelines is uncertain. The AAHC has no authority to control the behavior of its membership. There is little evidence of voluntary compliance by the members of the AAHC. On the contrary, one's impression is that because these principles were published, academic health centers have been competing with a vengeance for industrial funding. Nevertheless, these guidelines have helped stimulate the discussion of approaches to COIs. Their breadth of coverage can serve as a framework by which to compare the management of COIs by organizations that do have the ability to control the behavior of their membership.

Federal Conflict of Interest Policies

In July 1995, after a prolonged period of revisions and redrafting (Warsh 1989, Pramik 1990, Zurer 1990), the NIH and NSF both issued final rulings under the heading "Objectivity in Research; Investigatory Financial Disclosure Policy; Final Rule and Notice" (42 CFR Part 50; 45 CFR Part 64). The essence of the NIH ruling is the minimal requirement for the disclosure of any financial COI in the form of a $10,000 equity interest by investigators or their immediate family members in any organization whose products are related to the research of the investigators. The scope and wording of the disclosure statement and the monitoring of financial COI are left to the individual research institutions that receive federal funding. All universities and other research institutions have subsequently issued their own guidelines fulfilling these requirements.

The FDA has also issued its own requirements for COI policies. Its policy covers the same issues as the NIH and the NSF, but its requirements are directed toward participating institutions rather than their individual employees.

Recently, the U.S. Public Health Service (PHS) issued some draft interim guidelines on COIs (PHS 2000a). These guidelines were crafted after a conference on COIs in clinical research sponsored by the PHS, NIH, and FDA in the fall of 2000. This conference was initiated in response to growing concerns about COIs in clinical trials and relationships between clinical investigators and the pharmaceutical industry (Shamoo 1999, Angell 2000, 2001, Bodenheimer 2000, Hilts 2000, Agnew 2000). The guidelines outline responsibilities for research institutions, investigators, and IRBs. Institutions should

- collect information on COIs and to relay that information to concerned parties, such as IRBs
- develop COI policies and form committees to review COIs
- develop educational programs on COIs
- become aware of their own COIs and take steps to manage them
- establish independent oversight committees to manage institutional COIs

The guidelines also recommend that investigators consider carefully the impact of COIs and make relevant disclosures, and take part in educational programs on COIs. IRB members are encouraged to disclose COIs, to have policies and procedures for managing its own COIs, to pay greater attention to COIs in clinical trials, to develop policies or mechanisms for minimizing the impact of COIs in clinical trials (PHS 2000a). These policies are very recent, and we do not yet know their effect on research. So far, the reaction among research institutions has been less than favorable (Marshall 2001).

The Conflict of Interest Policy at the University of Maryland, Baltimore

The policies of the University of Maryland, Baltimore (UMB), are an example of how institutions have met these responsibilities. The policies, available at the web site for this book, were in response to a 1996 legislative act that encourages institutions of higher education to increase their financial resources through various arrangements with industry, including collaborative research and development. Such relationships must avoid violations of the law, as determined by the Maryland State Ethics Commission. Like the NIH policy, UMB's guiding principles revolve around the fundamental principle of disclosure. However, the scope of UMB's frame of reference, like that of many other institutions, is broader than that of the NIH. Its principles include an open academic environment, research that is appropriate for an academic environment, the freedom to publish, the avoidance of misuse of students and employees, the routine use of university resources for purposes of teaching and research (not commercial purposes), and the monitoring and management of the outside interests of employees in ways that are consistent with their primary commitment to the mission of UMB.

UMB has chosen to monitor these relationships through an appointed

Conflict of Interest Officer. Each faculty member is required to complete a form that identifies any relationships with "an entity engaged in research or development, or an entity having a direct interest in the outcome of research or development. . . ." The forms are reviewed by the appropriate chair or division head and by the dean for their approval. The Conflict of Interest Officer reviews those relationships that are identified as potential COIs. The Vice President for Academic Affairs makes the decision about whether a given relationship represents a "harmful interest." When a relationship is confirmed as a harmful interest, under two defined circumstances the Board of Regents allows the relationship to continue. One circumstance is that the success of the research or development activity depends not only upon the employee's participation, but also upon the financial interest or employment of the employee. For example, a waiver could be granted for a project that would fail without a particular university scientist's investment in, or simultaneous employment by, a biotech company. The other circumstance is when a given COI can be managed in ways that are consistent with the purposes of the relevant provisions of the law. These legal provisions deal with constraints related to the acceptance of gifts and honoraria, advocacy representation by an employee to the Board of Regents on behalf of a corporation, and the misuse of one's position for personal gain. University employees who seek waivers must make a formal request that is acted upon by the Vice President for Academic Affairs. Individuals whose requests are disapproved must discontinue their relationships within a reasonable time or risk losing employment by the university.

CONCLUDING REMARKS

Recall our earlier remarks about living with COIs. All of the policies and rules discussed above recognize that COIs will occur in research and that many of them cannot be avoided. The policies attempt to strike some balance between accountability and freedom in the conduct of research. On the one hand, it is important to have rules that promote accountability, because these rules help ensure the objectivity, integrity, and trustworthiness of research. On the other hand, excessive and highly strict rules can impede research by interfering with scientific creativity and innovation, by undercutting financial rewards, or by impeding the funding of research. Clearly, we need rules and policies that address COIs in research. But how should we craft them and implement them? These are not easy questions to answer. Deciding how to respond to COIs raises ethical dilemmas for researchers, research institutions, government agencies, and businesses. Almost all parties agree that any policy must involve an education component. Researchers should help students and colleagues understand what COIs are, how they can occur, why they create serious problems relating to objectivity and integrity in research, and how best to respond to them.

COIs vary a great deal in their degree of seriousness. The spectrum of COIs ranges from the benign and trivial to unethical and criminal misconduct. Policies such as those discussed above attempt to provide a balance between regulatory accountability and the freedom necessary to conduct research. Considering the complexity of our society, the increased financial underpinning of COIs, and the heightened demands of the public for greater public accountability, how good are these policies? How close do the guidelines of the Association for Academic Health Centers come to ideal guidelines? Should accountability be enforced?

In today's society, it is difficult to imagine the scientific process without some sort of mechanisms that deal with the issues of misconduct and COIs. One view of how to proceed is to cultivate an improved moral culture that attracts idealistic individuals with high ethical standards to the scientific enterprise. Another view is that scientists, like everyone else, are subject to frustrated dreams, resentments, and hopes for fulfillment, and that the best we can do in these circumstances is to work hard to foster, especially for scientists in training, an understanding of the crucial importance of scientific integrity and its relationship to the day-to-day processes of science. And we also need a reasonable system of accountability. Fortunately, no system is perfect, and we can therefore avoid the concern expressed by T.S. Elliott: "Perfect System, No need for good people."

QUESTIONS FOR DISCUSSION

1. The approaches to the management of COIs in science appear to rely primarily on disclosure, without the severe penalties that can be levied for violations of COI policies in finance or government. Considering the goals of science and other dissimilarities between science and the other disciplines, do you believe the differences in management are warranted?
2. Can you think of situations where scientists should remove themselves from a COI situation?
3. Should some COIs be prohibited? Which ones?
4. What is the difference between an actual and an apparent COI? Does it matter?
5. How much money (or stock, etc.) has to be at stake before a person has a COI?
6. How are COIs are risk factor for misconduct?
7. How important is COI to science? Should it be viewed as just another issue of life, no more or less important than others? Or, given the importance of integrity in science, should it be viewed as a crucial issue for scientists?
8. What is the best approach to sensitize young scientists to the predicament of COI? To approach established scientists?
9. Can you give an example of scientific COIs from your own experience or that you have heard about? How was it dealt with it? How should it have been dealt with?
10. How do you evaluate the process for managing COIs? Do you view it as primarily preventive or primarily remedial? Is it fair to the in-

dividual scientists? To the research institutions? To the public? Do you think that existing policies favor one group over others? Can you think of any changes that would improve the procedures?

11. In the world of finance, confidentiality is a key aspect in managing COIs. How important is confidentiality to integrity in research?

12. Journalists believe that the public's right to know the truth is all-encompassing. Should the same be true for scientists? Journalistic codes of ethics state that fidelity to the public interest is a primary value. Should the same be true for scientists? What bearing do these questions have on COIs in science?

13. Analyze the case "Pharmatec and the University of Florida," discussed in this chapter. Consider the primary and secondary interests, the type of COI that occurred, and how it would have been managed under the several COI policies presented above.

14. Consider the case "tPA: A Multicenter Trial," described in this chapter, and how it would have been managed under the several COI policies presented above. What are the most important differences between this case and the case in question 13?

15. In the cases "Clinical Trials of Therapeutic Drugs for Myocardial Infarction" and "Familial Hypercholesteremia and the Nobel Prize," what do you think are the likely primary and secondary interests?

CASES FOR DISCUSSION

Case 1

A faculty member of a midwestern university has a postdoctoral fellow who had been working for three years on one aspect of a new drug that has just been approved by the FDA. The drug company pays the mentor $5,000 per year consulting fees. This year, the company is sponsoring a three-day conference in San Francisco, all expenses paid. The conference brings together approximately 15 scientists from around the country who are leaders in research on this drug. Their job is to speak to 300 invited guests, physicians who are potential prescribers of the drug. All the physicians' expenses are paid. The speakers will each receive a $3,000 honorarium. The faculty member accepts the invitation, and the postdoctoral fellow hears about it by accident. He informs his mentor that he has new data indicating that the drug may have serious side effects. The mentor points out that the work is not yet published and that she will deal only with the published data for now.

- Under the terms of the COI policies described above, is this a COI?
- If the answer is yes, what is the COI, what type is it, and who has it?
- Are there COIs in this case that are not covered by the policies?
- Thinking back to chapter 3, is this a case of misconduct?
- Should the mentor have done anything differently up to the point that the postdoctoral fellow told her about the new data? What should the mentor and postdoctoral fellow do now?

Case 2

A senior researcher in a major research university has two grants from NIH and research contracts from two different large pharmaceutical companies. She also serves on the National Institute of Heart and Lung Advisory Board and one of the FDA's advisory panels. Her work pertains to drugs that lower cholesterol. The FDA panel that she is on was convened to decide whether to recommend the final approval of a drug for consumer use. The drug is manufactured by one of the two companies with which she has a contract. However, the contract has nothing to do with this particular drug. Prior to the deliberations, she disclosed her research contract as a COI and proceeded to participate in the panel. She was one of those who voted to recommend approval of the drug, but the recommendation would have passed anyway, without her vote.

- Is this really a COI case? Was it necessary for the senior researcher to have disclosed her contract with the company as a COI?
- Should the FDA have allowed her to deliberate on this panel?
- Despite the fact that she was allowed to participate on the panel, do you think she can deliberate without being unduly influenced by the contract she holds?
- Should universities encourage or discourage their researchers from placing themselves in such positions?

Case 3

A well-known researcher with 30 years of service at NIH had been a leading proponent of a drug to be used for insulin-resistant diabetes. During those years, he had amassed a great deal of data on the drug that supported his position. However, the scientific literature contains a number of other reports that warn of the drug's serious side effects. The researcher also serves on the FDA advisory panel that decided the fate of the drug. His only connection to the drug manufacturer was that he received $4,000 annually in consultant fees and presented a few seminars. The FDA panel unanimously voted to recommend the drug to the market. Three months later the NIH researcher took a position with the company as director of their diabetes studies. He received a large increase in salary, which nicely complemented his retirement salary from NIH.

- Is there a problem here, or does this case merely represent a trouble-free example of how the scientific marketplace works?
- Should the researcher have done anything differently?
- What are your comments about the interests and positions of NIH and FDA, and what, if any, actions they should take?

Case 4

A junior scientist at a university made a major discovery for a new anti–breast cancer drug. With the help of the university's Office of Research Development, she applied for a patent and established an agreement that splits the profits between her and the university. The new drug had the potential for bringing in millions of dollars for both parties. Using venture capital, the university formed a start-up company. The junior scientist and her department chair were on the board of directors. Other board members included several university administrators and a few employees of the venture capital company. The patent was awarded few years later. The start-up company still has not made any profits, but it is very close to marketing the drug.

The junior scientist, while at a conference, heard that a researcher at another university has come up with a drug very close in structure to hers, but one that is much more effective and has fewer side effects. The inventor of the new drug plans not to patent his drug but instead to place the information in the public domain. A different group of venture capitalists formed a new company to manufacture the drug as quickly as possible. The junior scientist, with prodding from her venture capitalists, is now thinking about challenging the new company with a lawsuit on the basis of patent infringement. The patent battle could delay and may eventually prevent the new company from ever producing the new drug.

- What are the COIs in this case, and who is experiencing them?
- Because NIH funds have not been used for this research, should the NIH and university COI policies be applied to this case? If so, what impact would these policies have?
- At this point in the case, what should the interested parties do?

Case 5

A member of an NIH study section was the primary reviewer of a grant proposal submitted by a very close personal friend and colleague. The extent of their relationship was well known among the close-knit research community, and the primary reviewer chose not to recuse himself. He proceeded to review the proposal and gave it his highest ranking. During the deliberation, another member of the study section raised the issue of the perception of COI. The chair of the study section and the reviewer in question rejected the implications of the comments, pointing out that the member's signature on the COI declaration was sufficient indication of his ability to make an objective judgment. Additionally, the NIH scientific review administrator said that study section members were obligated and expected to put personal relationships aside as part of their commitment to an objective evaluation. The study section proceeded with the overall approval of the grant proposal. However, the administrator informed the chairman of the department in question that she has the right to go through the formal appeal process.

- Was the scientific review administrator justified in making the statement about expected objectivity? What should the policy be in such circumstances? Should personal friendships ever be considered as a disqualifier for an objective review?
- Should the member of the study section in question have done anything differently?

- Was the other member of the study section justified in bringing the subject of COI?

Case 6

A member of an NIH study section has been asked to review a grant proposal submitted by a direct competitor to her own research. They are both working on practically the same project and are very familiar with each other's strengths and weaknesses. Their mutual animosity is common knowledge; during scientific conferences, their exchanges almost amount to shouting matches. The reviewer prepared a very thoughtful and lengthy evaluation. She highly criticized the proposal and gave it a poor rating. The proposal received an overall average rating, which removed it from consideration for funding.

- Under the terms of existing federal or university COI policies, does this represent a COI?
- Given the general awareness of their competitive positions and their mutual animosity, was the scientific review administrator justified in not intervening? In selecting the reviewer in the first place?
- Should the member of the study section have done anything differently?

Case 7

A newly appointed bright and industrious assistant professor became a member of an NIH study section. Her research was in a new area of x-ray diffraction of membrane proteins. She was the primary reviewer of a grant proposal from a senior department chair at a different university. She recommended the rejection of the proposal, and the committee concurred. A few months later, the chair whose grant was turned down got the bad news. The chair reviewed the membership of the study section and noticed that one member—the reviewer in question—was someone he had rejected for a job in his department. The chair wrote to the scientific review administrator and expressed his concern, particularly if the assistant professor was one of the two primary reviewers. The administrator confirmed with the reviewer the truth of the chair's statement about the job application. After assessing the notes of the deliberations, the administrator dismissed the complaint.

- Is there a COI in this case? If so, is it within the scope of any of the COI policies discussed in this chapter?
- Was the chair's concern reasonable? Is there any reason why the assistant professor should have acted differently?
- Was the administrator justified in his actions? Were there other options that the administrator might have taken?

Case 8

A well-known researcher was ready to publish some important findings made after three years of work with his two postdoctoral fellows. The findings clearly add a new and crucial dimension to the activity of a receptor discovered six years ago by someone in India. However, the original discovery is not well known in the United States. The two postdoctoral fellows wrote the paper with a clear citation to the earlier, foundational discovery made by the Indian scientist. The senior researcher admonished the two postdocs for not recognizing the originality and importance of their discovery. His viewpoint was, "Why dilute the impact of your paper? Why publicize someone else's work unnecessarily?"

- What are the COIs in this case? Do they fall within the scope of COI policies?
- Is this a case of COI, scientific misconduct, or both?
- At this point in the development of the case, what options should the two postdoctoral fellows consider? What should be their guidelines for decision making?

Case 9

A senior staff scientist and section chief at NIH outsourced a portion of her research with a subcontract to a junior researcher at a nearby university. The subcontract was $150,000 per year for five years. Although the research was a component of the NIH researcher's work, it was to be carried out independently. After two years, the university researcher wrote a paper without using the name of the NIH scientist as a coauthor. The NIH scientist received a draft of the paper and asked for her name to be added, because the research had been her conception, even though she had not contributed to the work.

- Does this case represent a COI, or is it merely a dispute about authorship?
- If you think it involves a COI, what type of COI is it? Does it fall under the category of any of the conflict of interest policies mentioned in this chapter?

Case 10

A university scientist/ethicist who is often cited by the national media on issues related to research on human subjects is called by a journalist from a major newspaper in a distant city. The journalist wants to know what he thought of the letters just received from the FDA and OPRR warning his university about their continued and frequent failure to comply with federal regulations. The letters in question had been addressed to a university vice president, who happens to chair a search committee formed three months ago to find a top-level assistant on research affairs. Two weeks ago the scientist/ethicist had applied, with many others, for the job.

- Is the COI fairly obvious here? Does it fall under the umbrella of any COI policies?
- What should the scientist/ethicist do? Should he tell the journalist about his application? Should he inform the vice president of the journalist's request for his opinion? Should he give the interview off the record or find a reason not to give the interview at all?

- Is there any reason for the scientist/ethicist to consider the university's interests as more important than his own? The public's right to be informed as more important than his own interests?

Case 11

A clinical researcher receives $3,200 per patient from a drug company to enroll patients in a clinical trial of a new hypertension medication. The money covers patient care costs and administrative costs for the duration of the study and includes a $200 finder's fee. After the initial screening and enrollment, patients will make a total of eleven 15-minute office visits during the study. At each visit, nurses will take blood, record vital signs, and ask them questions about their hypertension. The clinician will do a physical exam.

- Is this financial arrangement a COI or apparent COI?
- Should it be prohibited?
- During the informed consent process, should patients be told about the clinician's financial interests?

Case 12

A clinical researcher has partial ownership of a patent on a new gene therapy technique. Her work is being funded by a biotech company, which owns the other part of the patent. She also has stock in the company. She plans to use her patented technique in clinical trials for gene therapy to treat breast cancer. If her cure works, she will make millions of dollars, and so will the company. Even if the cure doesn't work, she still may make a great deal of money if the value of her stock rises.

- Does the researcher have any COIs or apparent COIs?
- Should any of these financial relationships be prohibited or avoided?

8

Collaboration between Academia and Private Industry

The petroleum industry was hatched in a very modern symbiosis of business acumen and scientific ingenuity. In the 1850s, George Bissell, a Dartmouth College graduate in his early thirties who had enjoyed a checkered career as a reporter, Greek professor, school principal, and lawyer, had the inspired intuition that the rock oil plentiful in western Pennsylvania was more likely than coal oil to yield a first-rate illuminant. To test this novel proposition, he organized the Pennsylvania Rock-Oil Company, leasing land along Oil Creek, a tributary of the Allegheny River, and sending a specimen of local oil to be analyzed by one of the most renowned chemists of the day, Professor Benjamin Silliman, Jr. of Yale. In his landmark 1855 report, Silliman vindicated Bissel's hunch that this oil could be distilled to produce a fine illuminant, plus a host of other useful products. Now the Pennsylvania Rock-Oil Company faced a single, seemingly insurmountable obstacle: how to find sizable quantities of petroleum to turn Professor Silliman's findings into spendable cash. (Chernow 1998, p. 74)

This chapter examines some of the ethical dilemmas and issues arising from relationships between higher learning institutions and private industry, including conflicts of interest, research bias, suppression of research, secrecy, and the threat to academic values, such as openness, objectivity, freedom of inquiry, and the pursuit of knowledge for its own sake. The chapter also provides an overview of the historical, social, and economic aspects of the academic–industry interface and addresses some policies for ensuring that this relationship benefits researchers, universities, industry, and society.

THE DEVELOPING RELATIONSHIP BETWEEN SCIENCE AND INDUSTRY

Although the times have changed and much more money is at stake, nineteenth-century scientist-entrepreneurs such as Bissell and Silliman have much in common with their contemporary counterparts, such as Craig Venter, the head of Celera Genomics Corporation. The ingredients are the same: a well-known scientist from a well-known institution invents a product or develops a process that can be used by large number of people and hopes to make a lot of money from it. In Venter's case, he became frustrated with academic science and launched his own company and research program. Venter's key innovation was the "shotgun" approach to genome sequencing, which stands in sharp contrast to the traditional, and slower, "clone by clone" method. Venter has

raised several hundred million dollars in venture capital to use this approach
to sequence mouse, fruit fly, and human genomes. The company sequenced
the human genome for about $300 million. The shotgun approach breaks apart
an entire genome, uses automated sequencing machines to sequence different
fragments, and then uses supercomputers to put all the parts back together
again (Marshall 1999d). Although Venter and academic researchers have
clashed over issues related to data access, release, and control, Celera Genomics
and the publicly funded Human Genome Project (HGP) collaborated to produce a complete sequence of the human genome, which was published in *Science* and *Nature* on February 16, 2001 (Venter et al. 2001, Robert 2001). However, clashes between the two groups remain, with some HGP researchers
accusing Celera of relying on the HGP's data and methods (Wade 2001). Although the company has yet to turn a profit, its earnings have increased
steadily and it has sold over $1 billion in stock. Because most of the human
genome is now available on the Internet, Celera, located in Rockville, MD,
plans to make most of its money from selling genomics information services
(Celera Genomics 2001).

As noted in chapter 6 on intellectual property, the collaboration between
Watt and Bolton on the development of the steam engine in the late 1700s set
the example for future science–industry ventures. The modern industrial laboratory was developed in mid-nineteenth-century Germany, when the dye industry hired chemists to invent and produce synthetic dyes. The development
of the petroleum industry, as exemplified by the contributions of Bissell and
Silliman, followed a similar pattern. Business leaders began to realize the economic value of applying scientific methods and concepts to solving technical
and practical problems. Science became a commodity (Dickson 1988). Thus,
the first marriages between science and industry took place outside of the university setting, in private laboratories, businesses, or research centers.

This is still a very important aspect of the science–industry relationship.
Pharmaceutical companies, biotechnology companies, food companies, seed
companies, software companies, chemical companies, automotive companies,
and electronics companies all conduct a great deal of research outside of the
university setting. In 1995, the United States spent $170 billion on research
and development (R&D). Private industry funded 59.4% of that total, followed by the federal government at 35.5% and other organizations, such as
private foundations or universities, at 5.1%. If one looks at who actually performs research, in 1995, private industry performed 70% of all R&D, followed by federal laboratories and universities, each at about 13% (Jaffe 1996).
It is likely that these percentages have changed somewhat since 1995, given
the trend toward privatization that started in the 1980s. Although the federal
government funded $90 billion worth of R&D in the United States in the year
2000 (Malakoff 2001), it is likely that private industry funded more than 60%
of R&D, or roughly $125 billion. Because we have seen a tremendous increase
in private biotechnology laboratories in the 1990s, it is also likely that private
industry performed more than 70% of R&D in the year 2000.

An important and at that time unusual marriage between science and private industry began in 1920s at the University of Wisconsin, when Professor Henry Steenbock discovered that he could activate vitamin D by irradiating food. He patented his discovery, hoping to benefit his own university and ensure quality of the manufacturing process (Bowie 1994). The Board of Regents of the University of Wisconsin rejected Dr. Steenbock's offer to accept any funds from the invention or from any private philanthropic organization. A group headed by some of the school's alumni started a nonprofit foundation, the Wisconsin Alumni Research Foundation (WARF), to fund further R&D. WARF was responsible for thousands of patent disclosures, hundreds of license agreements, and incomes of millions of dollars to the foundation (Bowie 1994). The foundation gave 15% of invention royalties to the inventor and 85% to the foundation in order to disburse research grants to university faculties. Although WARF was formally not part of the University of Wisconsin, it was for all practical purposes a part of the university, because university officials controlled the foundation, and its functions were comingled with university functions. To make money, WARF attempted to obtain monopolistic control over vitamin D synthesis and negotiated and enforced narrow license agreements that prevented poor people from having access to vitamin D. For example, WARF claimed that its patent applied to vitamin D produced by sunlight, and WARF refused to license other companies to use their vitamin D irradiation process to develop other food products, such as oleomargarine (Bowie 1994).

To understand the significance of the change in universities represented by the patenting of research conducted at universities, one must place universities in their social and historical context. Since ancient times, there were schools of higher learning, such as Plato's Academy or Aristotle's Lyceum. There were also schools that provided students with training for priesthood. But these schools were highly exclusive and did not affect many students. The birth of universities took place during the thirteenth and fourteenth centuries in Europe. During the Crusades of the early 1100s, Europeans reclaimed territory that had been occupied by the Islamic Empire during the middle ages. They discovered hundreds of ancient Greek, Roman, and Islamic texts on a variety of subjects, including law, medicine, biology, physics, mathematics, philosophy, logic, optics, history, and alchemy. Much of this knowledge consisted of ancient texts, such as Ptolemy's *Almagest* and most of Aristotle's scientific works, which Europeans had "lost" during the Dark Ages but which had been preserved for posterity by Islamic scholars. The "new" knowledge also included original works by Islamic scientists, such as Avicenna, Alhazen, and Averroes.

Because these texts were written in Arabic, Europeans had to translate them into Latin or the vernacular. Once these new works became available, European students were eager to learn them. Because these students were not familiar with these texts, they hired scholars to help them read and interpret them. The first university was a law school established in Bologna, Italy, in 1158. The students hired the teachers, set the rules, established residencies, and procured books (Burke 1995). A school of theology was established in

Paris in 1200. During the next century, universities were established in Germany, England, Spain, and the Netherlands. The first subjects taught in universities included civil law, cannon law, theology, medicine, and "the arts" (i.e., geometry, music, astronomy, and mathematics). Other scientific subjects, such as biology, chemistry, and physics, were not taught in universities until much later (Goldstein 1980).

An important point of the development of universities is that education was the main reason why universities were established. Universities did not even begin to emphasize research until the 1500s, when the University of Padua in Italy became known as a haven for scholarly exchange, free thought, and intellectual development. The "modern" university system, consisting of professors, instructors, doctoral students, masters-level students, and undergraduate students, did not emerge until the nineteenth century in Germany. The "commercialized" university, that is, a university with strong intellectual property interests and ties to private industry, is a relatively recent development. For hundreds of years, universities emphasized academic norms such as openness, free inquiry, and the pursuit of knowledge for its own sake. Business norms, such as secrecy, directed inquiry, and the pursuit of knowledge for the sake of profit, simply were not part of the university culture until the twentieth century.

Before World War II, the U.S. government did not invest heavily in research. Indeed, in the 1930s Bell Laboratories conducted more basic research than any university (Dickson 1988). During the war, the government began funding large-scale research programs, such as the Manhattan Project and the development of radar, jet airplanes, and computers. After World War II, it became clear to many people involved in government and in science policy that science and technology helped the Allies win the war and that continued investment in R&D would be a key pillar in national security and defense (Dickson 1988, Guston 2000). Federal investments in R&D grew from less than $1 billion in 1947 (or less than 0.3% of the gross national product) to $3.45 billion in 1957 (or 0.8% of the gross national product). A crucial turning point occurred in 1957, when the Soviet Union launched Sputnik, convincing many politicians that America was in grave danger of losing its scientific and technological edge over the Russians. From that period, federal funding of R&D grew steadily at 5–10% a year, and the government made more extensive use of scientific advisors. Federal support of R&D climbed to $26 billion in 1965 and then leveled off from 1966–1976, but then climbed again to $40 billion in 1985 (Dickson 1988). During this period, the federal government became the leading sponsor of R&D in the United States, but this pattern changed in the 1980s, as private industry increased its investments in R&D. In 1980, private industry and the federal government each sponsored about 48% of research, but the percentage has shifted, and private industry is now once again the leading sponsor of R&D (Jaffe 1996).

After World War II, universities and colleges began to proliferate and expand around the United States, fueled by an increasing number of students seeking higher education. The G.I. bill allowed soldiers returning from the war to obtain an education during the 1940s and 1950s, and the baby boom generation increased enrollments during the 1960s and 1970s. Throughout the United States, state governments helped fund expansion of the higher education system, and the federal government contributed by funding R&D. However, many state colleges and universities began facing financial difficulties in the 1970s due to increasing enrollments but insufficient or shrinking state funds (Bowie 1994). In response, these institutions sought to increase revenues from traditional sources, such as tuition, fees, and donations from alumni. Universities (and to a lesser extent colleges) also began to try to obtain additional revenues from sources related to R&D, such as grants, contracts, entrepreneurial activities, and intellectual property rights. These very same economic pressures exist today and help explain why universities have become increasingly involved in commercial activities (Bok 1994). At the same time, many academic leaders have sought to expand their institutions and enhance their economic strength and overall status by building ties to the private sector. Public and private institutions have both taken a strong interest since the 1970s in increasing revenues related to research activities.

Important initiatives were implemented in the 1970s, included the University Cooperative Research Projects Program and the Industry-University Cooperative Research Centers Programs, administered by the National Science Foundation (NSF). These efforts created dozens of centers to enhance multidisciplinary areas of research in all of the sciences. During the 1970s and 1980s, universities began more actively pursing patents and developed technology transfer offices (Dickson 1988).

The twentieth century has also seen several different eras in private R&D investments. For example, during the 1940s, companies invested heavily in the development of vacuum tubes and television. During the 1950s and 1960s, companies sponsored a great deal of R&D on transistors, semiconductors, and pharmaceuticals. The 1970s and 1980s saw massive R&D investments in integrated circuits and computer hardware and software. By the 1980s, biotechnology became the rage (Teitelman 1994). The molecular biology revolution that began in the 1970s was the catalyst for the private industry investment in biotechnology. For industry to tap the scientific basis of and develop this new field, it realized it needed collaboration with university-based researchers. It began when the West German chemical company Hoechst G.A. invested $70 million in a joint venture with Massachusetts General Hospital (MGH) affiliated with Harvard Medical School (Bowie 1994). MGH was to hold all patent rights of any discovery, but Hoechst would have first rights to any commercial products.

The true first major corporate investment in a university came in 1974, when Monsanto Company and Harvard Medical School entered into a 12-year joint venture whereby Harvard received $23 million for research and Monsanto received all of the patent rights from the venture. Also, Monsanto received first look at the results prior to publication. The university formed a committee to "protect academic freedom" and the "public good" (Culliton 1977) to review publication delays. The Harvard/Monsanto agreement was kept confidential until 1985, reflecting the university's discomfort at that time with collaboration with industry.

In 1981, Edwin Whitehead, president of Technicon, a medical diagnostics company, made a $120 million contribution to establish The Whitehead Institute at the Massachusetts Institute of Technology (MIT). The mission of the institute was to conduct biomedical research with potential applications in medicine and biotechnology. Whitehead himself retained control of faculty appointments at the institute. Faculty also held appointments at MIT. When the institute was formed, faculty at MIT objected to the commercial ties between the university and private corporations and the potential conflicts of interest. Despite these concerns, researchers at the institute have made important contributions to basic and applied biomedical science (Teitelman 1994).

In 1982, Monsanto negotiated an agreement with Washington University in St. Louis, Missouri. Monsanto gave $23.5 million to Washington University Medical School for research in the area of biotechnology. The agreement stipulated that royalties from patents and licenses would be split three ways among the university, the medical school, and the principal investigator's laboratory, but none would be paid directly to the investigator (Bowie 1994). It was claimed that excluding investigators from receiving royalties would avoid conflicts of interest among the faculty members. Monsanto received first rights of refusal to patents and the right to review publications. In 1994, Scripps University entered a $20 million per year agreement with the Swiss pharmaceutical company Sandoz. Under this arrangement, Sandoz funded research conducted at Scripps in exchange for first-refusal rights to almost half of Scripp's research results (Beardsley 1994).

The next example of corporate investment into a university illustrates how the instability of the corporate model can affect academic life. The Italian drug company FIDIA planned to give Georgetown University $3 million a year for 20 years (a total of $60 million) for research on neuroscience, to be housed in an institute within the university (Bowie 1994). The institute would primarily be devoted to basic research. FIDIA presumably would have received in return a strong connection to the best and brightest in this field, credibility, and the first rights of refusal on patents. Unfortunately, FIDIA filed for bankruptcy in Italy, and its contributions to Georgetown were reduced to a few million dollars. The university had to downscale its efforts to build its program and hire investigators.

In response to the rapid growth of the biotechnology and university–industry partnerships in the field, *Scientific American*, not known as a radical journal, published an article titled "Big-Time Biology" (Beardsley 1994). The article raised serious concerns regarding the rapid growth of biological sciences into an industry and how it is affecting university culture. An example to illustrate the modern complex relationship between private gains, universities, and researchers (Ready 1999) involves Dennis Selkoe, a researcher at Harvard Medical School who founded California-based Athena Neurosciences. The company is based on Selkoe's own research and has already earned him millions of dollars. Athena Neurosciences manufactures a controversial blood test for Alzheimer's disease. Without disclosing his relationship to the company, he was one of the endorsers of a National Institutes of Health (NIH) report for the new Alzheimer test. A Harvard panel concluded that he did not violate the university's conflict of interest policy, but he did agree to publish a disclosure statement in the same journal that published his original work. Apparently, Selkoe routinely wrote about Alzheimer's disease without reporting his affiliation with Athena. He also had a $50,000 per year consulting contract and served on the board of directors. As another example, in 1997 the University of California at Irvine found out that their cancer researchers had failed to inform the FDA of a side effect of a drug they had developed. These researchers had investments in the company that hoped to sell the drug (Ready 1999). The university shut down the laboratory.

These examples illustrate the benefits and risks associated with blurring the lines between industry and academia. The amount of funding from industry to university research is on the rise, and universities themselves are engaged in building their own corporations by joint ventures and equity arrangements. In 1997, U.S. corporations spent $1.7 billion on university research (Shenk 1999). The survey data available from 1994 indicate that 90% of companies involved in life sciences had relationships with university research; 59% of those corporations supported university research directly, at about $1.5 billion, accounting for 11.7% of all R&D funding at universities (Blumenthal et al. 1996a). The survey further indicates that over 60% of companies involved in university research received patents and products from the data generated. According to Dustira (1992), industry support to R&D in the biomedical field rose from 31% in 1980 to 46% in 1990, while at the same time the contributions of the NIH dropped from 40% to 32%.

The Association of University Technology Managers (AUTM), representing over 300 university and research institutions, claimed that in 1998 alone, 364 start-up companies resulted from technology transfer activities within these institutions. The total number of start-up companies since 1980 now exceeds 2,500 (Press and Washburn 2000). AUTM also claims that these technology transfer activities generated $34 billion in 1998, supporting 280,000 American jobs. If one looks only at the global impact of the biotechnology industry, it is clear that this industry is becoming a new force in the world's economy, supporting millions of high-paying jobs and promoting economic activity, investment, and development (Enriquez 1998). The political economy of the twenty-first century will undoubtedly be shaped by biotechnology (Carey et al. 1997).

This brief review illustrates the many ways that university–industry relationships can affect research and educational activities. Individual researchers may use contracts or grants from private companies to conduct research, hold conferences or workshops, or develop educational materials. They may also hold stock or equity in companies, share patents with companies, or receive honoraria, salary, or fees from companies. Institutions engage in similar activities: they receive grants and contracts, hold stock and equity, hold patents, and receive fees. In addition, institutions also receive contributions to their endowments and from companies and form joint ventures.

ACADEMIC VALUES VERSUS BUSINESS VALUES

Numerous tensions have arisen in the marriage between business and academia. Universities and businesses traditionally have emphasized different values or norms (Bowie 1994, Davis 1995b, Resnik 1999a,b, Dickson 1988). Below are some examples:

- The main goals of institutions of higher learning are to educate students; to advance human knowledge through research, scholarship, and creative activities; and to conduct public service. Private, for-profit corporations, on the other hand, aim to maximize profits and to produce goods and services. Nonprofit corporations also seek to produce goods and services, and they seek financial growth and stability.
- Higher learning institutions emphasize openness and the free exchange of data and ideas. Private corporations, on the other hand, often use secrecy to protect confidential business information and proprietary interests.
- Higher learning institutions emphasize academic freedom, free speech, and free thought. Private corporations, on the other hand, conduct research for specific purposes and may impose restrictions on public communications to protect the interests of the corporation.
- Higher learning institutions emphasize honesty and objectivity in research. Private corporations may endorse and promote these values in principle, but also as a means of complying with the law, for enhancing market share, or for ensuring the quality of goods and services.
- Higher learning institutions emphasize knowledge for its own sake; corporations emphasize the utilization of knowledge for the sake of profit or other practical goals.
- In capitalistic countries, private corporations compete with different companies on the free market. To compete on the market, corporations must produce high-quality goods and services; invest wisely in technology, equity, infrastructure, and R&D; and make effective use of human, financial, and technical resources. Higher learning institutions, on the other hand, have not traditionally competed with each other in the free market. Many of these institutions are subsidized by government funds and have monopolistic control over local markets.
- Private corporations have obligations to stockholders, customers, employees, the government, and the community. Higher learning institutions have obligations to students, faculty, staff, alumni, the government, and the community.

Can this marriage work or is it doomed to failure? Will private interests corrupt universities? To answer these questions, it will be useful to review some of the benefits and harms of collaborations between academic institutions and private corporations.

POSSIBLE BENEFITS OF COLLABORATION BETWEEN ACADEMIA AND PRIVATE INDUSTRY

Benefits to Academic Institutions

It should be apparent to the reader that universities and colleges benefit financially from relationships with industry. Private corporations and private interests provide billions of dollars for universities to conduct research; develop courses, educational materials, and curricula; hire faculty and staff; build laboratories and facilities; acquire tools and instruments; hold workshops and conferences; and even enroll students. Academic institutions also benefit from the knowledge and expertise obtained from the private sector, which can be useful in generating ideas for research or education. For example, a professor teaching a course in bioengineering may consult with leaders in the private sector to help prepare his students for real-world problems. Many institutions also appoint people from the private sector to boards and committees in order to obtain advice in preparing students for careers in business, industry, or the various professions. Industry leaders often provide key advice on research and education as consultants to colleges and universities.

Benefits to Industry

Industry benefits from having access to university facilities, equipment, and researchers. Although many companies already hire their own excellent researchers and have state-of-the-art facilities and equipment, universities also still have economically valuable resources. Although research has become increasingly privatized in the last two decades, many of the world's top researchers are still employed by universities, not by private companies. Corporations may also benefit from good publicity and visibility in their association with universities or colleges.

Benefits to Society

Society benefits from this private investment in academic institutions, which have helped to expand and support universities, have created higher paying jobs, and have contributed to economic development. Society also benefits from the goods and services produced by academic–industry collaborations, such as new drugs, medical devices, information technologies, and so forth. And society benefits from the increases in productivity that result from academic–business collaborations. The increased productivity is evident from a survey indicating that industry-supported university research produced four times more patents per dollar than did industry research and increased the rate of the technology transfer from laboratory to useful products (Blumenthal et al. 1986, 1996a,b). Francisco J. Ayala, a prominent biologist and once a member of a presidential committee on science and technology, stated that biotechnology is "contributing to the economic welfare of the nation, and it has by and large benefited academic progress. The benefits have far outstripped harms that may have occurred" (quoted in Beardsley 1994, p. 93).

POSSIBLE HARMS OF COLLABORATION BETWEEN ACADEMIA AND PRIVATE INDUSTRY

Individual Conflicts of Interest

Chapter 7 discussed conflicts of interest (COIs) in detail, which we briefly revisit here. Chapter 7 focused mostly on the COIs for individual researchers arising from their relationships to industry. Some of these include funding or research through contracts or grants, ownership of stock or equity, intellectual property rights, honoraria, consulting agreements, fees for enrolling patients in clinical trials, and gifts from industry. All of these COIs can undermine the researcher's primary obligations to the university, to his or her profession, and to society by compromising the objectivity of research. Even if COIs do not actually create biases in research, they can still undermine trust by creating the appearance of bias. Thus, it is important to address apparent COIs as well. Chapter 7 also discussed strategies for managing individual COIs, such as disclosure, monitoring, and prohibition or avoidance.

Institutional COIs

As also discussed in chapter 7, it is now widely recognized that research institutions can also have COIs that undermine objectivity and trust. An institution of higher education may have COIs in its obligations students, faculty, alumni, and the community that are affected by its relationships with industry. These COIs can affect the institution's decisions, policies, and actions and can undermine trust in the institution (Resnik and Shamoo 2001). The following situations can create COIs or apparent COIs for universities:

- University investments in corporations that sponsor research at the university: For example, if a university or university foundation owns a significant percentage of equity or stock in a drug company, this financial interest may affect its ability to conduct objective reviews of research proposals submitted by the company. It could also lead the university to agree to suppress research results that are unfavorable to the company, in order to protect its investment in the company. In the tragic death of human gene therapy patient Jessie Gelsinger, many commentators argued that the University of Pennsylvania and James Wilson both had COIs in this case. Wilson and the university both owned stock in a company that had founded Genovo. The company contributed $4 million per year to help form the Human Gene Therapy Institute, which sponsored the clinical trial in which Gelsinger died (Marshall 2000d). One way of dealing with this type of COI is to prohibit a university (or college) from having significant shares of stock or equity in companies that sponsor research at the university. Others have suggested that universities can place these investments in a blind trust to minimize the COI (Moses and Martin 2001).

- University intellectual property interests: As mentioned above, many universities now own patents and copyrights. This type of financial interest could affect the university's decision making if the university can take steps to increase the value of its intellectual property. For example, if the university and a professor both own a patent on a new medical device, the university may not provide an objective review of the professor's research if this adversely affects the value of the patent. In the Gelsinger case, Wilson and the University of Pennsylvania had patents on gene therapy techniques used the study.
- University–industry joint ventures: Research institutes, such as the Human Gene Therapy Institute and the Whitehead Institute, described above, are becoming increasingly common. Although some commentators have argued that these institutions can help minimize university COIs by serving as intermediaries between universities and corporations, these institutes can have their own COIs because they have their own financial interests (Moses and Martin 2001).

University Institutional Review Boards

Most universities (and some colleges) that conduct research on human subjects sponsor institutional review boards (IRBs), which are charged with task of approving, reviewing, and monitoring research to protect patients from harm and promote the rights and dignity of patients. The vast majority of people who are appointed to IRBs are employees of the institution. Although IRBs are required to have noninstitutional members, most IRBs are composed of 20% or less of these noninstitutional members. Having a high percentage of people on the IRB who are also employees of the institution creates a potential COI for the IRB and the institution, especially when a great deal of money is a stake (Francis 1996, Shamoo 1999, Agnew 2000). IRB members may feel pressure to approve proposals that are already been funded by a government agency or private corporation. One way to minimize this COI is for the IRB to review proposals before they get funded, but the drawback of this suggestion is that it could triple the work of a committee that is already overburdened.

Increased Secrecy in Academia

Problems with data sharing and suppression of research related to relationships with industry have been discussed above. Private corporations view research as proprietary information, and they often prohibit researchers from discussing data, ideas, or results prior to publication (Rosenberg 1996). The work by Blumenthal et al. (1996a,b, 1997) shows that researchers are under some pressure to not share data and to delay or stop publication in order to protect intellectual property or honor obligations to private companies. Betty Dong's case, discussed below, illustrates how companies may attempt to suppress unfavorable results. This climate of secrecy can have a detrimental impact on students as well, who may become involved in secret research that they cannot discuss with other students or professors. As mentioned several times above, openness is vital to scientific progress and is one of the most important academic norms. Some fear secrecy will have broad effects on research and academic life. On the other hand, some argue that academic researchers may influence industry to promote greater openness in industry-sponsored research (Davis 1991). So far, it does not appear the academic researchers are winning the battle for openness. Moreover, many researchers may not feel that they can criticize the industry's secrecy policies because they do not want to jeopardize their own funding or risk the wrath of university administrators. Some commentators have also pointed out that researchers have reasons to keep data and results confidential even if they are not receiving funds from industry. In any case, the conflict between secrecy and openness in research bears watching. We need to find ways to promote openness while protecting private interests. In discussing cases of how secrecy has prevailed to the determent of research progress, Steven Rosenberg remarked, "This is the real dark side of science" (quoted in Press and Wasburn 2000, p. 42).

Diversion of University Resources from Basic to Applied R&D

Although many universities emphasize applied research as a part of their mission, basic research should not be neglected in order to achieve short-term economic or practical goals (Brown 2000, Zolla-Parker 1994, Bowie 1994). If corporations can influence academic appointments, they can increase the percentage of faculty who conduct applied research at a university, and faculty interests can have a trickle-down effect on graduate and postdoctoral students. As corporate funds continue to flow into a university, it may lose its commitment to basic research and knowledge for its own sake and may become more interested in applications and profits. The curriculum can also become transformed from one that emphasizes education in critical thinking and the liberal arts to one that emphasizes the training of students for careers in business, industry, or the professions. Talented faculty who might normally be involved in teaching may be encouraged to conduct research so the university can increase its revenues from contracts and grants (Brown 2000). Corporate dollars can transform an academic institution into a private laboratory and technical training school.

Research Bias

Because private corporations are interested in producing and marketing specific products to enhance the profit, market share, and stock value of the corporations, they may influence the process of research to ensure "favorable" outcomes (Crossen 1994, Resnik, 1999b, 2001b). For example, if a study is not supporting a conclusion that is favorable to the company, the company can withdraw funding. Once a study is completed, a company may try to prevent unfavorable results from being published. A company may also attempt to manipulate or misrepresent data to produce a favorable result, or discredit research that is "unfavorable" to its products. Although research bias can occur in the public or private sector, the economic incentives to conduct biased research are stronger in the private sector and therefore pose a hazard for university–industry relationships. Moreover, the penalties for bias, such as loss of funding or tenure or a damaged reputation, are potentially more damaging to academic researchers than to private researchers or corporations.

For an example of research bias related to industry, consider the controversy over calcium-channel blockers. In 1995, Psaty et al. published results of a population-based case–control study of hypertensive patients and the risk of myocardial infarction associated with calcium-channel blockers versus beta-blockers versus diuretics. With 335 cases and 1,395 controls, they found that the risk of myocardial infarction was increased by 60% among users of calcium-channel blockers with or without diuretics. With 384 cases and 1,108 controls, they found that the use of calcium-channel blockers was associated with about a 60% increase in the risk for myocardial infarction compared with beta-blockers. Because the study was supported by federal funds, several pharmaceutical companies who manufacture beta-blockers requested all of the documents, including original data, under the Freedom of Information Act (Deyo et al. 1997). The companies hired several academic consultants to analyze the research, and the consultants wrote scathing critiques of the study. The companies even attempted to interfere with the publication of the article (Deyo et al. 1997).

Following the controversy of calcium-channel blockers, Stelfox et al. (1998), conducted a survey of literature published from March 1995 through September 1996 on the subject. They demonstrated a strong association between authors supporting the safety of calcium-channel blockers and their financial ties with pharmaceutical companies. Stelfox et al. classified the authors into three categories: critical, neutral, and supportive of the safety of calcium-channel blockers. They found that 96% of supportive authors had ties with the manufacturer, compared with 60% and 37% of neutral and critical authors, respectively. Earlier, Davidson (1986) obtained similar results that demonstrated a link between industry funding sources and favorable outcomes for new therapies.

Subsequent research has demonstrated a strong connection between sources of funding and research results. Cho and Bero (1996) and Cho (1998) found that the overwhelming percentage of articles with drug-company support (9%) favor the company's drug, compared with those without drug-company support (79%). Friedberg (1999) reported that only 5% of new cancer drug studies sponsored by the company developing the new drug reached unfavorable conclusions, compared with 38% of studies on the same drugs sponsored by other organizations. In the dispute over second-hand smoke, articles sponsored by the tobacco industry indicated that second-hand smoke has no ill health effects, whereas studies sponsored by other organizations supported the opposite conclusion (Bero et al. 1994). The tobacco industry also blocked research (Hilts 1994) and the publication of unfavorable results (Wadman 1996). Rochon et al. (1994) found that the industry-sponsored research on nonsteroidal anti-inflammatory drugs (NSAIDS) favored these medications as opposed to control drugs.

In 1995, the Boots Company made Dr. Betty Dong, clinical pharmacologist at the University of California, San Francisco, withdraw a paper on drugs used to treat hypothyroidism that had been accepted for publication in the *Journal of the American Medical Association* (*JAMA*). Boots had funded her research in the hopes that she could show that its product, Synthroid, was superior to three generic alternatives. Synthroid is a brand name for levothyroxine, which was manufactured in 1987 by Flint Laboratories and later bought by the Boots pharmaceutical company and then by the Knoll pharmaceutical company. The sale of Synthroid generated nearly $500 million dollars annually (Weiss 1997). To Boots's surprise, Dong showed that several generic drugs were just as safe and effective as Synthroid and also less expensive. Boots responded by trying to change her report, and the company spent several years trying to discredit her research. Because Dong had signed an agreement with Boots not to publish the results without written consent from the company, Boots invoked this clause in the contract to prevent Dong from publishing the paper in *JAMA* (Wadman 1996). In the meantime, the company published a more favorable article in another journal (Weiss 1997, Altman 1997, Shenk 1999). To avoid a lawsuit, Dong withdrew her submission from *JAMA*. Two years later, the *New England Journal of Medicine* published her findings.

Shenk (1999) recites several cases where corporate sponsors of research derailed the publication of adverse findings: Nancy Olivieri, a University of Toronto researcher, who was threatened by the Canadian drug manufacturer Apotex if she published her results on drug L1; David Kern, a Brown University researcher, who was pressured by a local company and his own university to not publish his data on lung disease related to the company's plant; Curt Furberg, a hypertension researcher, resigned from a research program on calcium-channel blockers funded by Sandoz in order to avoid tempering his data. Bodenheimer (2000) discusses concerns about the relationship between academia and the pharmaceutical industry and addresses problems with the use of ghostwriters by industry. As mentioned in chapter 4, some companies hire professional writers to write research manuscripts but list physicians or scientists as authors.

CONCLUSION: MANAGING THE UNIVERSITY–INDUSTRY RELATIONSHIP

To summarize the preceding section, there are benefits as well as risks in university–industry relationships. While we may appear to have stressed the negative aspects of this relationship, we would like to temper this impression. As noted above, there are many benefits of the university–industry interface. Moreover, it is hard to imagine how the modern research enterprise could proceed without some type of collaboration between academia and industry. For the last few hundreds years, ties between universities and private corporations have been growing stronger as research has increased in its practical relevance, economic and commercial value, complexity, and cost. Changes in the financial and economic aspects of research have transformed universities from institutions of that focus on education and "pure" research to institutions that also have commercial ties and interests and conduct "applied" research. Although it is important to preserve and promote values traditionally associated with academic institutions, such as openness, objectivity, freedom of inquiry, and the pursuit of knowledge for its own sake, it is not realistic to expect that we can return to an earlier era. Instead of romanticizing about the "good old days" or bemoaning the "corrupt" nature of the current system, we should develop practical policies for ensuring that university–industry relationships benefit both parties as well as society.

Based on the discussion in this chapter as well as preceding ones, we recommend the following guidelines for university–industry relationships (for further discussion, see Rule and Shamoo 1997, Resnik and Shamoo 2001):

1. Develop and implement strategies for managing individual and institutional COIs: Disclosure is the first step in dealing with COIs, but as Krimsky et al. (1996a,b) found, many researchers do not disclose COIs. Some authors, such as Cho (1998), believe that disclosure is not sufficient. Individuals can take steps to avoid COIs by obtaining multiple sources of funding for research, refusing to hold stock or equity in companies that sponsor research, not taking honoraria or consulting fees, not accepting patient recruitment fees over and above administrative costs, refusing certain types of gifts, and so on. We also believe that disclosure may sometimes be insufficient. However, because it not realistic to expect that universities or individuals can avoid all COIs in research, decisions to prohibit or avoid a COI must be made on a case-by-case basis by considering the strength of the COI as well as the benefits and harms created by the situation. Despite this, the research community should consider prohibiting certain financial relationships such as owning equity in small corporations while conducting its clinical trials. Because the federal government does not set very restrictive COI rules for obtaining grants, universities have a variety of COI policies (McCary et al. 2000). Harvard Medical School has some of the strictest guidelines. Harvard allows researchers to have no more than $20,000 in stocks in corporation where they are involved in studying their products. Also, they cannot receive more than $10,000 in royalties or consulting fees from companies that sponsor their research. Harvard recently contemplated drastically relaxing its COI rules at a time of great concern about COIs (Mangan, 2000). The reports indicated that Harvard was contemplating increasing equity to $100,000 or 0.5% of corporation's value. The move by Harvard brought a raft of criticism (Mangan, 2000, O'Harrow Jr., 2000; Angell, 2000). Later, Harvard backed down and announced that it will not change its COI (O'Harrow Jr, 2000). The Harvard example, illustrates the powerful lure of industry money even for a highly endowed and reputable institution. Cho (1997) argues that the first moral obligation of a researcher is to the

integrity of research, and the obligation to financial interest should be secondary.

2. Develop COI committees to manage COIs: Most research institutions use existing administrative hierarchies (e.g. department chair, section head, director, dean, etc.) for managing COIs of its employees. The U.S. Public Health Service (PHS) (2000) has recommended that universities also appointment committees to manage COIs, especially those that require more than mere disclosure. Both the PHS and Moses and Martin (2001) also suggest that each university develop a committee to manage its own COIs as an institution.

3. Where possible, take steps to dilute COIs, such as placing investments in blind trusts, pursuing multiple sources of funding, developing separate research institutes, and so on: Although these steps will not eliminate COIs, they may help minimize their impact.

4. Ensure that research conducted at universities is not suppressed: Time and again, problems have arisen when private corporations have suppressed research. Although companies should be able to control research conducted in private laboratories, and they should have some input into the publication of any research they sponsor, research conducted at universities should not be barred from the public domain. One way that universities can take an active approach to this problem is require that researchers who conduct their work in university facilities do not sign contracts granting companies the right to stop publication of the results.

5. Be especially wary of involving students in secret research conducted for industry: Students enroll in universities for education and career advancement and should not be exploited as a cheap source of labor for commercial research. Because students should be allowed to discuss their work with their colleagues and teachers, no student master's or doctoral thesis should involve secret research.

6. Develop intellectual property policies that protect the rights of researchers as well as the interests of the university, industry, and the public, and provide researchers with proper legal counsel so they will be more willing to share data while they are filing for a patent: Agreements between universities and industry, such as Cooperative Research and Development Agreements, should address concerns about date sharing and management related to intellectual property.

QUESTIONS FOR DISCUSSION

1. What do you think of the development of university–industry relationships in the twentieth century?

2. What kind of university–industry relationship would you like to see in the twenty-first century?

3. Give some examples from your own experience of university–industry relationships that were acceptable and not acceptable to you.

4. Are there or should there be different moral limits in industry, academia, or society?
5. Can you give some examples of benefits to academia from industry, and vice versa, that are not listed in this chapter?
6. What proposals do you have for managing university–industry relationships?

CASE STUDIES

Case 1

A biotechnology company is giving $2 million for three years to a researcher at a university to test his new diagnostic device on patients for an FDA-approved protocol. The researcher is one of the few experts in the field. The researcher and his department chair are both on the company's scientific advisory board. They both receive payments of $5,000/year for this service.

- What are your concerns about this arrangement?
- Should the COI committee be involved?
- How would you manage the issue, if any management is needed?

Case 2

A large pharmaceutical company awards a $6 million contract for three years to a researcher at a university to conduct trials on patients. The company's proposed conditions are as follows:

a. Six months' delay in publication of research outcomes
b. First rights of patenting of the discoveries
c. The researcher serves on their scientific advisory board
d. The researcher will conduct the research

- What is the role of the university in this arrangement?
- Should the university accept the terms as they are offered or make a counteroffer? What should the counteroffer be?
- How would you manage the conflict, if one exists?

Case 3

A large pharmaceutical company pays a researcher at a university consulting fees of $10,000 per year, and once or twice a year an honoraria of about $3,000 to give a talk. The same researcher also serves on one of the FDA advisory councils.

- Do you have any concerns? What are they?
- How should these concerns, if any, be managed?

Case 4

A fifth year graduate student about to receive her doctoral degree discovers through gossip at a national meeting that her research has been tapped by a company. After talking to her mentor, she learns he has been discussing patents and obtaining a contract to develop the discovery into a patent. The student was told that all this would occur in the future and that she has nothing to do with it. She was also told that her data will earn her the Ph.D. she sought and that is what the work was for.

- Do you see any problem?
- Does the student have any grievance toward his mentor?
- What should the student do, if anything?
- How you would have dealt with this situation if you were the mentor?

Case 5

Five large industrial plants near a university are planning to give $12 million each to endow a Center for Environmental Science (CES). The total gift to the university will be $60 million. As a condition of the gift, the companies require the following:

a. The CES will have a governing board consisting of 10 members of academia and industry; five members of the board will represent the companies giving the gift.
b. The governing board will have the power to appoint a director of the CES and will also approve all faculty appointments to the CES.
c. The governing board will also have the power to approve course development activities, conferences, guest lectureships, as well as research projects sponsored by the CES.

- Do you see any problems with this arrangement?
- Should the university accept this gift?

9

The Use of Human Subjects in Research

This chapter discusses the history of human experimentation, with special attention to cases that have helped to shape ethical codes and policies. It discusses important codes, such as the Nuremberg Code and the Declaration of Helsinki, and it provides an overview of U.S. federal regulations. The chapter also addresses some key concepts and principles in human research, such as informed consent, risk/benefit ratios, minimal risk, research versus therapy, and vulnerable populations.

The use of human subjects in research came into sharp focus during the Nuremberg war crimes trials, when the world discovered the atrocities committed by Nazi doctors and scientists on tens of thousands of prisoners held in concentration camps. While these tribunals were unfolding, the American Medical Association (AMA) was developing a set of principles to be followed in experiments using human subjects (Advisory Committee 1995). After the tribunals concluded, in 1947 the research community adopted the world's first international code for research on human subjects, the Nuremberg Code (quoted in Advisory Committee 1995, p. 103). The code emphasizes the importance of fully informed and voluntary consent of research subjects, minimization of harms and risks to subjects, scientific validity of research design, and the social value of the research. Since Nuremberg, there have also been many documented cases of unethical or questionable research conducted in the United States and other countries (Capron 1989; Beauchamp and Childress 1994; Advisory Council 1995). There have also been many ethical controversies in human subjects research, such as the use of placebos in research, the nature and practice of informed consent, and research on vulnerable populations, such as children, prisoners, and the mentally ill (Shamoo and Irving 1993, Egilman et al. 1998 a,b). As a result, various federal agencies and scientific and professional associations have developed regulations and codes governing human subjects research, and there has been a great deal of discussion and debate about ethical standards that should govern the use of humans in research (Levine 1988, Pence 1996). This chapter reviews these regulations after providing a historical and philosophical perspective on these issues.

HISTORICAL BACKGROUND: HUMAN EXPERIMENTATION BEFORE WORLD WAR II

Alexander Morgan Capron (1989) has observed that "the darkest moments in medical annals have involved abuses of human research subjects" (p. 127). A brief survey of the history of human subjects research supports this view. Before the Scientific Revolution (circa 1500–1700 AD), medicine was an observational rather than an experimental science. Medical research was based on the teaching of Hippocrates (460–377 BC), the father of scientific medicine. Hippocrates developed theories and principles that explained diseases in terms of natural rather than supernatural causes. According to his teachings, health was a state of balance among the four humors of the body, blood, phlegm, yellow bile, and black bile. Disease occurs when the body becomes out of balance as the result of too much or too little of one or more humors. The goal of medicine is to use various treatments and therapies to restore the body's proper balance. For example, Hippocratic physicians believed that bloodletting could restore health by eliminating excess blood.

Hippocrates' method was observational rather experimental because he did not use controlled interventions (or experiments) to obtain medical knowledge. Instead, Hippocrates gathered knowledge through careful observation of disease conditions, signs, symptoms, and cures. He also developed detailed case histories. The Hippocatic physicians believed in the body's ability to heal itself, and they tended to prescribe nonaggressive and noninterventional therapies, such as special diets, herbal medications, exercise, massage, baths, and prayer. The Hippocratic School developed a code of medical ethics that emphasized the importance of promoting the welfare of the individual patient. Two of the Hippocratic Oath's key tenets, which evolved hundreds of years after his death, are to keep patients from harm and injustice ("do no harm") and to benefit the sick. Although Hippocratic physicians sought to improve medical knowledge, their code of ethics and their philosophy of medicine implied that medical advances would occur slowly and would not sacrifice the welfare of the individual patient for scientific progress (Porter 1997).

This conservative approach to medical research began to change during the Scientific Revolution, as physicians such as Paracelsus (1493–1542), Andreas Vesalius (1514–1614), and William Harvey (1578–1657) (Harvey 1628 [1993]) challenged medical dogmas and sought to apply the new experimental method to medicine. However, these physicians still did not conduct many controlled experiments on human beings. Although Paracelsus, Vesalius, and Harvey dissected human bodies, they did not gain their knowledge of anatomy from experiments on living human beings. While Harvey conducted some experiments on human beings, his experiments were relatively benign and noninvasive. For example, he used a tourniquet to demonstrate the direction of the flow of blood in human veins, and he measured pulse and blood pressure. He conducted his more invasive procedures, such as vivisections, on animals. As physicians began to apply the experimental method to medicine, experiments on human beings became more common and more risky. One famous eighteenth-century experiment conducted by the English physician Edward Jenner (1749–1823) illustrates some recurring ethical concerns. Jenner observed that dairymaids who developed cowpox did not develop smallpox. He hypothesized that cowpox provided an inoculation against smallpox. To test his hypothesis, he inoculated James Phipps, an eight-year-old boy, with some material from a cowpox pustule. The boy developed a slight fever but suffered no other ill effects. Six weeks after this inoculation, Jenner exposed Phipps to the smallpox virus and he did not develop the disease (Porter 1997).

During the nineteenth century, experiments on human beings became even more common. For example, William Beaumont (1785–1853) treated Alexis St. Martin for a bullet wound in the stomach. The wound healed but left a hole in the stomach. Beaumont hired Martin as a servant and used him as an experimental subject, because he could observe the process of digestion through the hole in Martin's stomach (Pence 1995). During the twentieth century, physicians began to accept the germ theory of disease developed by Louis Pasteur (1822–1896) and Robert Koch (1843–1910). Despite Pasteur's unquestioned place in science, there are now historical studies indicating that his behavior was not above ethical reproach. For example, Pasteur treated a patient for rabies without first ensuring the safety of the treatment in animal experiments (Geison 1978). The surgeon Joseph Lister (1827–1912) performed a variety of experiments to develop and test antiseptic methods in medicine. For instance, Lister observed that carbolic acid was effective at reducing infections among cattle, and he hypothesized that this compound has antiseptic properties. To test his idea, he applied lint soaked in carbolic acid and linseed oil to a boy's wound. He also took measures to prevent germs from entering the wound. The boy, James Greenlees, did not develop an infection. Lister applied his method to dozens of other cases of compound fractures and amputations and published his results in *Lancet* in 1867 (Porter 1997).

One of the most disturbing experiments in the United States before World War II took place in 1874 in Cincinnati, when Robert Bartholomew inserted electrodes into the brain of Mary Rafferty, a 30-year-old "feeble-minded" patient who was dying of terminal cancer, which had spread to her scalp. Bartholomew saw a research opportunity and for several hours electrically stimulated Rafferty's brain and recorded her responses, which were often cries of pain (Lederer 1995).

Many of the human experiments were inspired by the work of Pasteur and Koch, who developed vaccines for bacterial infections. To implement this methodology, researchers needed to establish a link between a pathogen and a disease, isolate a disease pathogen, develop a vaccine, and then test the vaccine. In 1895, Henry Heiman, a New York pediatrician, infected two mentally retarded boys, 4 and 16 years old, with gonorrhea. In 1897, the Italian researcher Giuseppe Sanerilli injected yellow fever bacteria into five subjects without their consent in order to test its virulence. All five subjects became severely ill, although none died (Lederer 1995). Many physicians, including William Osler, condemned this experiment. In his textbook *The Principles and Practice of Medicine* (1898), Osler discussed Sanerilli's experiments as well as some other studies of yellow fever.

U.S. Army physician Walter Reed and his colleagues in Cuba conducted the most famous yellow fever experiments around 1900. Yellow fever had become a major health problem for military operations in Cuba, the Caribbean, and Central America. At the time, researchers hypothesized that yellow fever was transmitted to humans by the *Aedes aegypti* mosquito. Because there were no animal models for the disease, human subjects were required to study its transmission. The risks of being a human subject were great, because medicine had no cure for the disease, which often resulted in death. Two investigators working with Walter Reed, James Carroll and Jesse Lazear, allowed themselves to be bitten by mosquitoes in order to test the hypothesis. Reed had also agreed to participate in these experiments, but he was in Washington when his colleagues exposed themselves to the disease. Both colleagues contracted yellow fever, and Lazear died from the disease. After Lazear died, Reed decided not to use himself as an experimental subject, but he continued experimenting on human beings to develop a vaccine. Because the risks of being an experimental subject were so great, Reed and his colleagues had volunteers sign written contracts stating that they understand the risks of the experiment and that they agree to participate. Volunteers were also given $100 in gold and free medical care for their participation. Although other researchers obtained undocumented informed consent from subjects, this is believed to be the first case of the documentation of informed consent in research. Research subjects who participated in subsequent yellow fever experiments came to be regarded as heroes and martyrs. Surviving volunteers (all soldiers) received gold medals and government pensions (Lederer 1995).

One important theme of human experimentation before World War II is that many of the subjects were from vulnerable populations: children, mentally ill people, poor people, prisoners, minorities, and hopelessly ill people. As noted above, Bartholomew's subject was "feeble-minded." In 1911, Hideyo Noguchi of the Rockefeller Institute used orphans and hospital patients as experimental subjects for developing a diagnostic test for syphilis. Noguchi injected his subjects with an inactive solution of the causative agent of syphilis, which produced a skin reaction in subjects with syphilis but no reaction in neutral controls. Many leaders of medical research were outraged by Noguchi's use of healthy subjects in his experiment. In 1915, Joseph Goldberger, an investigator for the U.S. Public Health Service, attempted to induce the disease pellagra in male prisoners in Mississippi by placing them on a diet of meat, cornmeal, and molasses. He was able to prove pellagra is a nutritional deficiency resulting from this diet. The governor of Mississippi granted the prisoners pardons for their participation (Lederer 1995).

Before World War II, physicians and surgeons had ambivalent attitudes toward human experimentation. On the one hand, most physicians accepted the Hippocratic idea that they should not harm their patients. Claude Bernard restated the principle in his *Introduction to the Study of Experimental Medicine* (1865 [1957]). According to Bernard, physicians should never perform on man an "experiment, which might be harmful to him to any extent, even though the result might be wholly advantageous to science (p. 101)." On the other hand, physicians regarded many risky and untested interventions as therapeutic and believed that it was sometimes necessary to try these treatments in order to benefit the patient. While physicians condemned many of the unethical experiments that were brought to their attention, they also had a strong commitment to medical research and experimentation and did not want to place any burdensome restrictions on research. While most physicians thought that self-experimentation was noble and virtuous, they did not think that informed consent was always necessary. Indeed, most physicians at the time thought that it was more important to avoid harming the research subject than to obtain the subject's consent. For many years the AMA considered adopting a code of ethics for research on human subjects, but it did not adopt one until 1946 (Lederer 1995).

In 1900 Prussia was the first nation in the world to formalize the prohibition of medical interventions other than for therapeutic purposes (Capron 1989). The Prussian directive required that consent be given and that prospective subjects be informed of adverse consequences. It also excluded minors from research. These directives were not given in a vacuum or without a cause: they came as a reaction to numerous and repeated abuses of patients in medical research. For example, the discoverer of the bacillus strain that causes leprosy, Amauer Hansen (1841–1912), carried out an appalling experiment on an unwitting 33-year-old woman when he twice pricked her eye with a needle contaminated by nodules of a leprous patient (Bean 1977). Hansen was later merely reprimanded.

The conduct of Walter Reed and his colleagues stands in sharp contrast to some egregious examples discussed above. Reed was one of the medical officers during the construction of the Panama Canal. The project required a great deal of manpower, but numerous workers were dying from yellow fever. Reed developed a vaccine for yellow fever and tested it on the canal workers. None of Dr. Reed's 22 subjects who contracted yellow fever died from it, and thousands of workers were able to avoid the infection. Reed demonstrated a genuine concern for the welfare of his fellow human beings and for informed consent (Bean 1977). Reed himself prepared English and Spanish versions of a contract signed by each individual volunteer. Dr. Reed's informed consent document and the process he followed were exemplary and are considered by some to be as good as today's methods and documents. Although some scholars claimed that the ethical/legal doctrine of informed consent evolved in the 1950s and 1960s (Advisory Committee 1995), Reed's work shows that he followed this paradigm before it became more broadly accepted.

In the early 1900s, the eugenics movement flourished in Europe and in the United States (for further discussion, see chapter 11). In the 1930s, one Canadian province and 28 states in the United States passed laws requiring the sterilization of the criminally insane, presumed "feeble-minded," psychopathic personalities, and the mentally ill (Proctor 1988, Ollove 2001). By late 1930s, California alone had sterilized 13,000 persons, and the U.S. total is estimated to be between 30,000 and 100,000 persons (Proctor 1988, Ollove 2001). The state of Virginia in the early twentieth century was a leader in sterilization efforts. The *Baltimore Sun* reporter Michael Ollove chronicled the ordeal of a Virginian who was sterilized for being "feeble-minded." Later, this Virginian became a soldier, winning the Purple Heart, the Bronze Star, and Prisoner of War honors during World War II (Ollove 2001). The eugenics movement helped provide impetus for the Nazi atrocities committed in World War II. Hitler was a strong advocate of eugenics, and he believed it was necessary to control human breeding in order to prevent the Aryan race from being corrupted by inferior races, such as the Jews and Gypsies.

HISTORICAL BACKGROUND: HUMAN EXPERIMENTATION AFTER WORLD WAR II

The Nazi experiments conducted on human beings stand out as clearly the worst experiments ever performed on human subjects. None of the subjects gave informed consent, and thousands of subjects were maimed or killed. Many of the experiments were not scientifically well designed or conducted by personnel with appropriate scientific or medical qualifications. Moreover, these experiments were planned, organized, and conducted by government officials. Subjects included Jews, homosexuals, convicted criminals, Russian officers, and Polish dissidents. Some of the experiments included the following (Pence 1995, Caplan 1988, 1992, Proctor 1988, Müller-Hill 1992):

- Hypothermia studies where naked subjects were placed in freezing cold water
- Decompression studies where subjects were exposed to air pressures equivalent to the pressures found at an altitude of 70,000 feet
- Wound healing studies, where subjects were shot, stabbed, injected with glass or shrapnel, or otherwise harmed to study how their wounds healed
- Vaccination and infection studies, where subjects were intentionally infected with diseases, such as typhus, staphylococcus, malaria, and tetanus, in order to test the effectiveness of vaccines and treatments
- Josef Mengel's (1911–1979) experiments designed to change eye color, which resulted in blindness
- Mengel's human endurance experiments, where subjects were exposed to high levels of electricity and radiation
- Mengel's twin studies: exchanging blood between identical twins, forcing fraternal twins to have sex to produce children, creating conjoined twins by sewing twins together at the back, placing children in virtual isolation from birth to test the role of nature and nurture in human development

By mid-twentieth century, human experiments, ethical and otherwise, were becoming more common, but the research community had not put a great deal of thought into the ethics of human subjects research. Although some physicians, most notably Claude Bernard (1813–1878) and William Osler (1849–1919), had written about the ethics of human experimentation, and the AMA had drafted some documents on human experimentation, there were no well-established ethical codes for experimentation on human subjects before 1947. This is one reason why the Nuremberg Code has an important place in history: it was the first internationally recognized code of ethics for human research.

Although the Nuremberg Code did help to define and clarify some standards for the ethical conduct of human experiments, many abuses took place after the code was adopted. Some of these ethical problems in research were discussed by Henry Beecher (1904–1976) in an exposé he published in the *New England Journal of Medicine* in 1966. Beecher described 22 studies with ethical violations, including the now well-known Tuskegee syphilis study, the Willowbrook hepatitis experiments, and the Jewish chronic disease case study. The Tuskegee study took place from 1932 to 1972 in a public health clinic in Tuskegee, Alabama. The purpose of the study was to follow the natural etiology of later-stage syphilis in African-American men. Six hundred subjects were enrolled in the study, which was funded by the U.S. Department of Health. The subjects were divided between an "experimental" group of 399 subjects with untreated syphilis and a "control" group of subjects without syphilis. The initial plan was to conduct the study for one year, but it lasted nearly 40 years. The subjects who participated in the study were not told that they had syphilis, that they were not receiving a medically proven treatment for syphilis, or that they were participating in an experiment. Subjects with syphilis only knew that they had "bad blood" and could receive medical treatment for their condition, which consisted of nothing more than medical examinations. Subjects also received free hot lunches and free burials. An effective treatment for syphilis, penicillin, became available in the 1940s, but the subjects were not given this medication. The study not only had ethical problems, but also had scientific flaws: key personnel changed from year to year, there were no written protocols, and records were poorly kept. Even though Beecher brought the study to the attention of the public, it was not stopped until Peter Buxton, who worked for the U.S. Public Health Service, reported the story to the Associated Press. The story soon became front-page news, and a congressional investigation followed. In 1973, the U.S. government agreed to an out-of-court settlement with families of the research subjects, who had filed a class-action lawsuit (Jones 1981, Pence 1995). In 1997, the Clinton administration issued an official apology on behalf of the U.S. government.

The Willowbrook hepatitis experiments were conducted at Willowbrook State School in Willowbrook, New York, from 1956 to 1980. A team of researchers, led by Saul Krugman and Joan Giles, began a long-range study of viral hepatitis in this institution for mentally retarded children. Viral hepatitis was endemic at Willowbrook: most children who entered Willowbrook became infected within 6–12 months of admission. Although the disease is usually not life threatening, it can cause permanent liver damage. Victims of the disease usually have flulike symptoms, such as fever, fatigue, and nausea. The disease is transmitted orally through contact with feces or body secretions. In their research, Krugman and Giles infected healthy subjects with viral hepatitis. This allowed them to study the natural progression of the disease, including its incubation period, and to test the effectiveness of gamma globulin in preventing or treating the disease. They collected over 25,000 serum samples from more than 700 subjects. The two researchers justified their study on the grounds that it offered therapeutic benefits to the subjects: the children in the study would receive excellent medical care, they would avoid exposure to other diseases, and they would acquire immunity against more potent forms of hepatitis. Krugman and Giles obtained written informed consent from parents, although some critics have charged that the parents did not understand the nature of the study. Krugman and Giles also obtained appropriate approvals for their study: the study was approved by the New York State Department of Mental Hygiene, the New York State Department of Mental Health, and the human experimentation committees at the New York University School of Medicine and the Willowbrook School (Munson 1992).

The Jewish chronic disease case study took place in Brooklyn, New York, in 1964. In this case, researchers introduced live cancer cells into 22 unsuspecting patients (Faden and Beauchamp 1986). The purpose of the study was to learn more about the transplant rejection process. Previous studies had indicated that healthy subjects and subjects with cancer have different immune responses to cancer cells: healthy subjects reject those cells immediately, whereas cancer patients have a delayed rejection response. Researchers claimed that they obtained informed consent, but they did not document the consent. They claimed that there was no need for documentation because the procedures they were performing were no more dangerous than other procedures performed in treating cancer patients. Investigators also did not tell the subjects that they would receive cancer cells, in order to avoid frightening them unnecessarily (Levine 1988).

Besides these historically significant cases from the history of biomedical research, there have also been some noteworthy cases in social science research. One of the methodological problems with social science experiments is that researchers can influence the very phenomena that they are attempting to study. If human subjects know that they are participating in behavioral experiments, they may change their behavior from what it would have been otherwise. To get around this bias, many social science researchers believe that it is sometimes necessary to deceive human subjects about the experiments in which they are participating. This is precisely what Stanley Milgram did in his 1960s experiments relating to obedience to authority. In one of these experiments, Milgram used two subjects, a "teacher" and a "learner." The teacher was led to believe that the purpose of the experiment was to test the effects of punishment on learning. The teacher provided the learner with information that the learner was supposed to recall. If the learner failed to learn the information, the teacher was instructed to give the learner an electric shock. The severity of the shock could be increased to "dangerous" levels. In some designs, teachers and learners were in different rooms; in other designs, teachers and learners could see each other. In reality, the learners never received an electric shock, and they faked agony and discomfort. Milgram was attempting to learn more about whether the teachers would obey the authorities—the researchers who were telling them to shock the learners (Milgram 1974). At the end of each session, Milgram debriefed his subjects and told them the real purpose of the experiment. Many of the teachers said that they suffered psychological harm as a result of these experiments because they realized that they were willing to do something that they considered immoral (Soble 1978).

Another noteworthy case of deception in social science research took place in Wichita, Kansas in the 1954. During these experiments, investigators secretly recorded the deliberations of six different juries in order to gain a better understanding of how juries make their decisions. The judges of the Tenth Judicial Circuit and the attorneys in the cases approved of the study, although the litigants were not told about the study. When this study came to light, the integrity of the jury system was cast in doubt. In 1955, a subcommittee of the Senate Judiciary Committee held hearings to assess the impact of this research on the jury system. As a result of these hearings, Congress adopted a law forbidding the recording of jury deliberations (Katz 1972).

Three more recent cases have contributed to the history of human experimentation. The Human Radiation Experiments took place in the United States from 1944 to 1974, during the cold war era (Advisory Committee 1995). These experiments were funded and conducted by U.S. government officials or people associated with government institutions on over 4,000 unsuspecting citizens and military personnel. Many of these experiments violated standards of informed consent and presented serious harms or risks to the subjects. Most of these experiments were conducted in order to aid U.S. cold war efforts by providing information about how radiation affects human health. Most of these studies used radioactive tracers and did not result in significant harm to the subjects. However, several of the studies that involved children exposed them to an increased lifetime cancer risk, and several studies caused death shortly after the administration of radiation. Moreover, they found that the exposure to radon from the dust of underground uranium mines caused at least several hundred miners' deaths from lung cancer, and other miners had an elevated risk of cancer. Furthermore, inhabitants of Marshal Islands developed thyroid cancer from U.S. hydrogen bomb tests. The military rationale for these experiments is that they might help the United States "win" a nuclear war or at least become better prepared to survive a war.

In 1994, the Clinton administration began declassifying documents related to these experiments and appointed a commission to develop a report on this research. The commission issued its report in 1995. Although the commission openly discussed some ethical problems with the research, it also found that most studies contributed to advances in medicine and public health (Advisory Committee 1995, Moreno 1999, Beauchamp 1996, Guttman 1998). It also judged the experiments according to the standards that existed at the time that they were conducted: according to the commission, most of these experiments did not violate existing ethical or scientific standards. Nevertheless, as Welsome (1999) observed: "Almost without exception, the subjects were the poor, the powerless, and the sick—the very people who count most on the government to protect them" (p. 7). Some of the more noteworthy studies that came to light that may have violated the existing ethical standards included the following:

- Researchers at Vanderbilt University in the late 1940s gave pregnant women radioactive iron to study the effects of radiation on fetal development; a follow-up study found that children from these women had a higher than normal cancer rate.

- In Oregon State Prison from 1963 to 1971, researchers x-rayed the testicles of 67 male prisoners, who were mostly African Americans, to study the effects of radiation on sperm function.
- During the late 1950s, researchers at Columbia University gave 12 terminally ill cancer patients radioactive calcium and strontium to study how human tissues absorb radioactive material.
- Researchers released a cloud of radioactive iodine over eastern Washington State to observe the effects of radioactive fallout.
- From the 1940s to the 1960s, researchers injected encapsulated radium into the nostrils of over 1,500 military personnel; many developed nosebleeds and severe headaches after exposure.

Perhaps the most troubling aspect of these studies is that most of them took place after the international community had approved the Nuremberg Code, and many of them took place after the Declaration of Helsinki (1964). It is ironic that the U.S. government, which had been so outspoken in its criticism of Nazi research, would also sponsor human experiments that many would consider unethical (Egilman et al. 1998a,b).

During the 1990s, the research community learned about a variety of ethically questionable studies on mentally ill patients. The national media also covered many of these stories. As a result, the National Bioethics Advisory Commission (NBAC) issued a report recommending changes in federal regulations on research on people with mental disorders (NBAC 1998). Many of these problems originally came to light through a series of articles at a conference held in 1995 (Shamoo 1997c) and a series of articles in journals (Shamoo and Irving 1993, Shamoo and Keay 1996, Shamoo et al. 1997). This was followed by a major series of articles in the *Boston Globe* (Kong and Whitaker 1998). Many of these research projects were "washout" studies. A washout study is a protocol for testing a new drug that requires a subject to stop taking a medication for a period of time so that it no longer has any significant pharmacological effects. The purpose of the washout period is to conduct a controlled clinical trial and reduce biases due to drug interactions. After the washout period, the protocol randomly assigns patients to groups that are administered an existing treatment or a new drug. The protocols may also include a placebo control group. In some washout studies, the harms to subjects are fairly minimal, especially if the washout period is short and subjects are carefully monitored under inpatient settings.

However, in the studies that many people regarded as unethical, the subjects were taking medications for depression, schizophrenia, and other serious mental disorders. One study of washout research with schizophrenia patients found that many subjects suffered the effects of withdrawal from medications and experienced relapses, which could include increased psychosis or rehospitalization (Wyatt 1986, Baldessarini and Viguera 1995, Gilbert et al. 1995, Wyatt et al. 1999). As a result, more than 10% of subjects dropped out of these studies (Shamoo and Keay 1996, Shamoo et al. 1997) for variety of reasons. Because 10% of schizophrenics commit suicide, a relapse of this disease can be very dangerous. In 1991, Craig Aller, a patient with schizophrenia at the University of California at Los Angeles, and his family argued that he suffered permanent brain damage due to a relapse caused by a medication washout as part of his participation in the research protocol conducted for that purpose (Aller and Aller 1997). Another patient in this study allegedly committed suicide (Aller and Aller 1997). In some of these studies, researchers asked the subjects to consent, but critics questioned whether the patients were capable of giving informed consent (Shamoo and Keay 1996). Many of these experiments did not mention informed consent. Other experiments that were criticized include studies whereby mentally ill subjects were given ketamine to induce psychosis and delusions, to study the mechanism of the disease, and healthy children 6-12 years old were given fenfluramine (an obesity drug) to test whether they were prone to violence (Sharav and Shamoo 2000)—children were selected for these studies because their siblings were incarcerated.

Our last example concerns the HIV/AIDS research in developing nations. A controversy over this research erupted when Peter Lurie and Sidney Wolfe (1997) published an article in the *New England Journal of Medicine* attacking the use of placebo controls in studies on the perinatal transmission of HIV in developing nations. Lurie and Wolfe said that these studies violated the international codes of research ethics because they did not provide subjects with an effective therapy. Subjects in the placebo groups received no medication for preventing the perinatal transmission of HIV, even though a treatment regimen, the AIDS Clinical Trials Group (ACTG) 076 protocol, was proven effective in reducing the transmission of HIV from a mother to her newborn child during pregnancy and lactation during clinical trials in Western nations. In the United States, it would be regarded as unethical to give HIV-infected pregnant women a placebo, because they could instead be placed on the ACTG 076 protocol. Critics said that these trials constituted a double standard: how could a study that would be considered unethical in the developed world be considered ethical in the developing world? Opponents of the studies also argued that the methods of informed consent used in these studies were not very effective and that most subjects probably did not understand that they might receive a placebo; proponents, on the other hand, defended the studies on the grounds that their design was required in order to produce useful results (Varmus and Satcher 1997).

Although the ACTG 076 protocol is effective, it uses $800 of zidovudine (AZT), which is 10 times more money than most people in developing nations can afford to spend on health care. To help combat the HIV/AIDS pandemic, it is important to develop medications and treatments that are effective and inexpensive. To achieve this goal, researchers gave subjects 10% of the AZT used in the ACTG 076 protocol. A placebo control group was required, according to the researchers, in order to prove whether such a small dose of AZT is more effective than a placebo. Other study designs that do not use a placebo could be implemented, but it would take more time and effort to determine whether such low doses of AZT are effective if one does not include a placebo control group, because these studies would require more subjects in order to achieve the desired level of statistical significance. Proponents also pointed out that different concepts of informed consent may apply in different countries (Resnik 1998c). One important outcome of this dispute is that the World Medical Association decided to revise its Declaration of Helsinki (2000) in order to address issues relating to research in developing nations.

ETHICAL DILEMMAS AND PRINCIPLES

The discussison below outlines some of the key ethical dilemmas and principles relating to all human subjects research.

The Good of the Individual versus the Good of Society

In many ways, human experimentation raises a classic ethical dilemma addressed by moral philosophers since antiquity—the good of the individual versus the good of society. According to all of the moral theories discussed in chapter 1, human beings have moral worth and we should respect and promote the rights and welfare of individual human beings. On the other hand, most theories also stress the importance of promoting social welfare. Scientific and medical research can promote many important goals that enhance social welfare, such as human health, education, control of the environment, agriculture, and so on. It is important to use human subjects in research in order to gain scientific and medical knowledge, but this also places people at risk and may violate their dignity or rights. Thus, a central ethical question in all human subjects research is how to protect the rights and welfare of human subjects without compromising the scientific validity or social value of the research. Different authors have responded to this dilemma in different ways. Those who take a very conservative approach argue that we should never compromise human dignity, rights, or welfare for the sake of research (Jonas 1992). Others take a more progressive approach and argue that although it is important to protect human subjects, to advance research we must sometimes give the interests of society precedence over the interests of individuals (Lasagna 1992).

This tension between the individual and society occurs in many different aspects of research ethics. For instance, most people would hold that it is acceptable to use a human being in research if he or she gives informed consent. Informed consent respects the rights and welfare of the individual. But it is often difficult for patients to understand the benefits and risks of participating in a study, or the nature of the study and its scientific importance. A variety of influences may also affect the subject's ability to make a perfectly free choice, such as the hope of a cure, money, and family expectations. Those who place a high priority on protecting individuals will insist on the high standard of informed consent in research, while those who do not want to undermine research may be willing to accept standards of informed consent that are less demanding, claiming that they are more realistic. We may have no research subjects at all if we insist that subjects be *completely* informed and uninfluenced by any coercive factors (Inglefinger 1972).

In some types of research, such as social science experiments, it may not be possible to achieve unbiased results if subjects are informed of the nature of the research, because the subjects may change their behavior if they know what hypothesis the experiment is trying to test. In his study on obedience to authority, Milgram maintained that he needed to deceive his subjects in order to obtain unbiased results. Although his experiments may have obtained socially important results, they caused some psychological harm to the individual subjects. One might also argue that these experiments violated the dignity of the subjects because subjects were manipulated and deceived (Sobel 1978).

Similar dilemmas arise in the use of experimental and control groups in research. Suppose a clinical trial is testing a new type of HIV treatment regimen. Subjects are randomized into two groups: one group receives the standard HIV regimen, which includes a combination of several antiretroviral drugs; another group receives a different combination of drugs, which includes a new drug. If the study starts to yield positive results, at what point should researchers stop the study and make the new treatment regimen available to all patients? If the trial is stopped too soon, then it may not generate statistically significant and useful data; if the trial is stopped too late, then many patients may fail to benefit from a new and effective therapy. Similar issues arise when the clinical trial uses a placebo group as the control group: the use of a placebo control group may enhance the scientific validity of a study at the expense of the welfare of those individuals who receive placebos, such as the subjects in the Tuskegee study. Many ethical dilemmas related to the methodology of clinical trials involve conflicts between the good of the individual and the good of society (Freedman 1987, Schaffner 1986, Kopelman 1986).

Weighing Risks versus Benefits

Human experimentation also raises ethical issues relating to the risks and benefits to individuals and society. In any research protocol, one must ask whether the benefits of the research outweigh the risks to the individual (Levine 1988). Risk is a function of both the *probability* and the *magnitude* of the harm: a study that has only 2% probability of causing death may be deemed very risky due to the severity of this harm, whereas a study that has a 60% probability of causing a side effect such as dizziness or headache may be deemed not very risky due to the relatively benign nature of the harms. In contrast, most benefits are not usually analyzed in probabilistic terms. We believe the concept of "opportunity" could fill this conceptual role: an opportunity is a function of the probability and magnitude of a benefit. A study that has only a small probability of a great benefit, such as a cure from a fatal illness, may be judged as presenting a great opportunity, whereas a study that has a high probability of a minimal benefit may be judged as presenting only a moderate opportunity.

Although assessments of statistical probabilities are empirical or scientific judgments, evaluations of harms or benefits are ethical or value judgments (Kopelman 2000). Therefore, ethical decision making is essential to all risk/benefit calculations. For example, phase I clinical trials often raise important risk/benefit questions. In many of these studies, researchers test drugs on healthy or diseased subjects in order to estimate their toxic effects. Diseased subjects have a small possibility of obtaining a medical benefit (Miller 2000). Usually, healthy research subjects are paid for their participation, so they derive some benefit from participation. Subjects also provide their informed consent, so this is not usually the main issue. The issue often boils down to this: what level of harm should a subject be allowed to withstand in the name of research? Most would agree that phase I studies on healthy subjects should not be conducted if there is even a small probability of death, but what about other harmful effects, such as cancer, kidney failure, or allergic shock? A similar problem arose recently when the U.S. Environmental Protection Agency (EPA) had to decide whether they should approve studies testing the effects of pesticides on healthy subjects (Robertson and Gorovitz 2000).

In medicine, there is also a long and honorable history of self-experimentation. One could view self-experimentation as a highly altruistic act and morally praiseworthy. However, are there limits on the risks that a researcher may take in the name of science? A few years ago a group of researchers said they would test an HIV/AIDS vaccine on themselves (Associated Press 1997). Although this is certainly a worthy cause, one might argue that these researchers should not be allowed to take the risk of contracting HIV/AIDS. Even when risks are not likely to be great, controversies can still arise if the subjects are not likely to derive any benefits from research participation and they cannot provide adequate informed consent. For example, one might argue that Phase I clinical trials on children are morally problematic because children cannot provide informed consent, they are not likely to benefit from participation, and they may be harmed.

To focus questions about risks and benefits, U.S. federal regulations use the concept of "minimal risk." The Common Rule, which applies to research funded by the NIH or other federal agencies, defines minimal risk as follows: "[T]he probability and magnitude of harm or discomfort anticipated in the research are not greater in and of themselves than those ordinarily encountered in daily life or during the performance of routine physical or psychological examinations or tests" (*Federal Register* 1991, 56.102.i). Although this idea may seem to be clear, it glosses over the obvious observation that risks ordinarily encountered in daily life may vary a great deal between and among populations: a child born in Sudan faces in his ordinary life the risk of malaria, yellow fever, hepatitis, dysentery, and civil war, whereas a child born in the United States does not ordinarily encounter these risks (Kopelman 2000).

Just Distribution of Benefits and Harms

Human experimentation also raises important dilemmas in the distribution of benefits and harms. Although these issues have existed since human experiments first began, they have not received a great deal of attention in the literature so far (Kahn et al. 1998). The benefits of research participation may include access to new medications or treatments, knowledge about one's physical or mental condition, money, and even self-esteem. The harms include many different physical effects, ranging from relatively benign symptoms, such as dizziness or headache, to more serious effects, such as renal failure or even death. Research also may involve legal, financial, or psychosocial risks. For many years, researchers and policy makers have focused on the need to *protect* human subjects from harm. This attitude was an appropriate response to the harmful research studies discussed above, such as Tuskegee and Willowbrook, and many research policies and practices that did not protect some vulnerable subjects from harm.

A vulnerable subject can be defined as a research subject who cannot give adequate informed consent or cannot adequately promote his or her own interests. Vulnerable subjects include children, prisoners, desperately or terminally ill people, mentally ill people, and poor or illiterate people. In a sense, all sick patients are potentially vulnerable because they may be susceptible to the therapeutic misconception—the belief that the intervention can provide a medical benefit or cure even if it there is very little chance of obtaining either (Applebaum et al. 1987). Children have been and still are regarded as vulnerable subjects: researchers have taken a very protective attitude toward children, and there are many strict rules and guidelines for research on children. Issues regarding distributive justice have arisen in several areas of research, such as access to HIV/AIDS clinical trials, research on children, and inclusion of women in clinical research (Schuklenk 1998, Dresser 1992). These as well as many other cases involve questions about how we should distribute benefits and burdens in research.

Research versus Practice

An important conceptual issue that has a direct bearing on many of the difficult dilemmas in human experimentation is the distinction between *research* and *practice*. Health care professionals often perform interventions on patients that are innovative or unproven. For example, a surgeon may try a new surgical technique in performing an emergency trachiostomy, or a general internist may tailor her medication orders to meet the needs of her particular HIV patients and may use nonstandard doses or combinations of drugs. If these interventions were conducted in order to benefit the patient, they have a reasonable chance of benefiting the patient, and they are not part of a research study, then many would hold that these interventions are not research—they are simply innovative practices. As such, they do not need to conform to standards of research ethics, but they should be based on standards of acceptable practice. If, on the other hand, interventions are conducted to develop generalizable knowledge, then they may be regarded as research (National Commission 1979).

Although distinctions between research and practice make sense in the abstract, they become blurry in concrete cases. For example, consider the case of Baby Fae, an infant born with a defective heart who received a baboon heart when no human hearts were available (Pence 1995). The cross-species transplant (or xenograft) was conducted despite very low odds of success. She lived with a baboon heart from October 26 to November 15, 1984. Clearly, this was a highly innovative procedure that probably benefited transplant science much more than it benefited the patient. Or consider the birth of Louise Brown, the world's first test tube baby, in 1978. No one had performed in vitro fertilization in human beings before she was conceived. An obstetrician, Patrick Steptoe, performed this procedure in order to benefit his patient, Lesley Brown, who was suffering from fertility problems (Pence 1995).

One might argue that innovations in practice, such as the cases of Baby Fae and Louise Brown, should be viewed as research and should be regulated as such. To protect patients/subjects and as well as biomedical science, these innovations in practice should be developed into formal research protocols. Indeed, some research ethics codes, such as the Helsinki Declaration (2000), encourage clinicians to conduct their innovations as research protocols. However, because innovations in medical practice are fairly commonplace and often benefit patients, and clinicians often would rather avoid the administrative burden of developing a protocol and submitting it to an IRB for review, it will continue to be difficult to compel clinicians to meet this ethical standard (King 1995).

The influential Belmont Report (National Commission 1979) and other codes of human research ethics, such as that of the Council for the International Organization of Medical Sciences (CIOMS 1993), have adopted a balanced approach. According to this balancing view, some fundamental principles of research ethics, often in harmony, may conflict in various cases. To settle these conflicts, one must weigh and consider these different ethical principles in light of the facts, and there is no set formula for ranking these principles or settling these conflicts. Below is a list of the principles governing the ethics of human experimentation, derived from several sources (National Commission 1979, Levine 1988, Beauchamp and Childress 1994, Emanuel et al. 2000):

1. Informed Consent: When subjects are capable of making decisions that involve a degree of complexity or risk, researchers should obtain informed consent. When subjects lack the capacity to make such decisions, researchers should obtain informed consent from a legally authorized representative. Subjects should be able to withdraw from a study at any time for any reason.

2. Respect for Persons: Researchers should respect the privacy, dignity, and rights of research subjects, and they should take steps to protect confidentiality.

3. Beneficence: Researchers should attempt to minimize the harms and risks of research participation, maximize benefits to subjects, and strive for a justifiable risk/benefit ratio. Researchers should not conduct experiments that have a high probability of causing death, nor should they not harm subjects in order to benefit society. Researchers should be prepared to end experiments in order to protect subjects from harm.

4. Social Value: Researchers should conduct experiments that have scientific, medical, or social worth; they should not use human beings in frivolous research.

5. Justice: Researchers should promote a fair and equitable distribution of benefits and harms in research. Subjects should not be excluded from participation in research without a sound moral, legal, or scientific justification.

6. Protection for Vulnerable Subjects: Researchers should take extra precautions when dealing with vulnerable subjects to avoid harm or exploitation.

7. Scientific Validity: Research protocols should be scientifically well designed; experiments should yield results that are replicable and statistically significant. Researchers should strive to eliminate biases and should disclose and/or avoid conflicts of interest. Research personnel should have the appropriate scientific or medical qualifications. Research institutions should have the appropriate resources, procedures, and safeguards.

8. Data Monitoring: Researchers should monitor data to promote the welfare of subjects and ensure scientific validity, and should continually report harms, benefits, and unanticipated problems in implementing the protocol.

Many of these principles are implied or expressed in well-known research ethics codes. We believe that these principles (or some very similar set of principles) should play a key role the ethical evaluation of research.

HUMAN RESEARCH ETHICS CODES

As discussed above, the Nuremberg Code (1949) was the first internationally recognized code of human research ethics. The code emphasizes the importance of informed consent and includes provisions for minimizing risk to subjects, justifying risks in terms of benefits, and meeting standards of scientific validity and social worth. But there are many issues that the Nuremberg Code did not address. For instance, it contains no discussion of confidentiality, justice, or research on subjects who cannot provide informed consent. Although the Nuremberg Code has great historical significance, other codes also play an important role in guiding contemporary international research.

During its 1964 meeting in Helsinki, the World Medical Association issued a set of important guidelines to further define and augment the protection of human subjects used in research. The document came to be known as the Helsinki Declaration, and has since been revised, mostly recently in 2000. The declaration reaffirms many of the ideas set forth in the Nuremberg Code and also discusses subjects who cannot give informed consent, confidentiality, justice, and exploitation. The declaration holds that subjects who cannot provide informed consent can still participate in research if consent is obtained through a legally authorized representative.

One of the most controversial parts of the declaration has been its discussion of the distinction between *research* and *therapy*. The declaration acknowledges that physicians often conduct research while providing therapy, but it also holds that the physician's obligations to patients are paramount. The most recent version of the declaration includes a provision about providing subjects with the best current prophylactic, diagnostic, and therapeutic methods. According to this latest version of the declaration, the controversial HIV trials mentioned above would been regarded as unethical because they used placebo control groups even though a proven prophylactic method existed.

In the last decades of the twentieth century, many national and international professional associations, such as the American Medical Association, the British Medical Association, the American Psychological Association, the American Anthropological Association, the American Sociological Association, the World Health Organization, and CIOMS, have adopted position statements on research ethics as well as research ethics codes.

HUMAN RESEARCH ETHICS REGULATIONS

Although codes of research ethics are important in their own right and have a great deal of moral authority, they do not have the persuasive force of the regulations that have been adopted by various countries. The first steps toward developing human research regulations in the United States took place in 1953, when the National Institutes of Health (NIH) opened an intramural research operation called Clinical Center. The Clinical Center was in charge of overseeing human experiments conducted at the NIH's intramural campus in Bethesda, Maryland, and reviewed protocols in order to avoid "unusual hazards" to subjects before proceeding with experiments (Capron 1989, Hoppe 1996, Advisory Committee 1995). Late in 1965, the National Advisory Health Council, at the prodding of then NIH Director James Shannon, issued the first prior review requirement for the use of human subjects in proposed research (Capron 1989). In 1966, this action prompted the Surgeon General of the U.S. Public Health Service to generalize prior peer review requirement to all NIH-funded research on human subjects. The Food and Drug Administration (FDA) in 1971 issued its own similar regulations for testing new drugs and medical devices.

In 1974, the United States enacted the National Research Act, which required that the Department of Health, Education, and Welfare (DHEW), a precursor to the current Department of Health and Human Services (DHHS), codify all of its policies into a single regulation (45 Code of Federal Regulations 64 or 45 CFR 46). These regulations required each research institution that conducts intramural or extramural research funded by the DHEW to establish or use an Institutional Review Board (IRB) to review and pass judgment on the acceptability of the proposed research according to the detailed requirements listed in the regulations. The regulations set forth rules for IRB composition, decision making, oversight, and documentation. IRBs should comprise people from different backgrounds, including scientific and nonscientific members, male and females members, as well as members from within the institution and members from the local community. In 1976, the NIH also developed the Office for Protection from Research Risks to provide oversight for human subjects research. This office was recently renamed the Office for Human Research Protection (OHRP) and relocated to report directly to the DHHS, in order to provide it with stronger, more independent, and broader governing authority.

In 1979, the first presidentially appointed commission on human experimentation, the National Commission for the Protection of Human Subjects of Biomedical and Behavioral Research, known simply as the National Commission, issued its report, known as the Belmont Report. The 1974 National Research Act mandated the formation of the National Commission in response to the public outcry over revelations of abuse of human subjects in research, such as the Tuskegee study. One of the important effects of this report was major revisions in federal human research regulations. In 1978, the DHEW revised its regulations to add additional protection for pregnant women, fetuses, in vitro fertilization, and prisoners. From 1981 to 1986, changes in U.S. regulations included revisions to DHEW's regulations for IRB responsibilities and procedures, changes in the FDA regulations to bring them in line with DHEW regulations, further protections for children, and a proposed federal common policy for the protection of human research subjects (Advisory Committee 1995, p. 676).

In 1991, the U.S. government issued a final federal policy known as the Common Rule, which was adopted by 16 agencies and departments (Common Rule 1991). However, three federal departments, including the EPA, never adopted the Common Rule. The FDA adopted rules similar to the Common Rule that apply to privately funded research conducted to support applications for new drugs or medical devices submitted to FDA. However, these rules have some potential regulatory loopholes or gaps pertaining to human subjects research, because privately funded research that is not conducted in support of an application for a new drug or medical device is not covered by any existing federal regulations. This is in contrast to the National Animal Welfare Act, which covers use of all animals in research. In order to close this regulatory gap and provide uniform protection for human subjects, Jay Katz was the first to suggest in 1973 that the United States govern the use of *all* human subjects in research (Final Report 1973, Katz 1993, 1996, Shamoo and O'Sullivan 1998, Shamoo 2000).

In the fall of 1995, President Clinton appointed the National Bioethics Advisory Commission (NBAC) to examine bioethical issues in human research and medical practice. Several federal agencies, members of Congress, and various patient and consumer advocacy groups had called for the formation of such a commission to address ongoing issues and concerns. Since its formation, the NBAC has issued reports on human cloning, embryonic stem cell research, gene therapy research, and research on people with mental disorders.

INSTITUTIONAL REVIEW BOARDS

Although the federal human research regulations have been revised many times since 1978, their basic tenor has not changed. These regulations all require IRB oversight and review of research protocols. Although research institutions are charged with assuring to the federal government that human research meets specific requirements, IRBs are charged with fulfilling these institutional responsibilities. IRBs have the full authority to review and approve or disapprove research protocols, to require modifications of protocols, to monitor informed consent, to gather information on adverse events, to stop experiments, to examine conflicts of interest, and to require adherence to federal and local, institutional requirements.

Most IRBs consist of 15–25 members who are employees of the research institution and one nonscientist member from the community. Critics have claimed that these situations can raise conflict of interest issues for IRB members (Cho and Billings 1997, Shamoo 1999) as discussed above and in chapter 7. An IRB or its members may face some pressure to accept a proposal so that the institution can obtain a grant or other source of funding. IRBs often face enormous workloads and unrealistic deadlines. Demands to accelerate or streamline the review process can affect the quality of IRB review. To do its job well, an IRB must often take some time to carefully review protocols and discuss key issues, but this can slow down a process that researchers and institutions would like to accelerate. IRBs also often have trouble recruiting qualified and committed members, because membership on an IRB can place heavy demands on a person's time. In response to these and other problems, many commentators, as well as the NBAC, have recommended some structural changes in IRBs, but no significant changes have occurred to date (Moreno et al. 1998, Inspector General 1998).

To ensure that institutions comply with federal regulations, IRBs usually consider the following questions and issues when reviewing research proposals:

(1) Is it research? Research is defined by federal regulations as a systematic investigation that contributes to generalizable knowledge (Common Rule 1991 §102d, or 45 CFR 46 §102d). When the regulations were republished in the *Federal Register* as the Common Rule, they were given the new number 28012 with the same subsections (e.g., §102d) as the 45 CFR 46, however. If the goal of the intervention is entirely therapeutic, then it may not be research. Medicine includes many "experimental therapies" that are not treated as research. Students often conduct educational projects designed to teach research methods and techniques that may not be considered to be research.

(2) Is it human subjects research? Research may involve human tissues but not human subjects. A human subject is a "living individual about whom an investigator . . . obtains data through interaction or intervention with the individual or identifiable private information" (Common Rule 1991 §102f). Research on stored human tissue is not covered by current federal regulations and presents IRBs with some important ethical and policy dilemmas. Several organizations, including the NBAC, have made some recommendations concerning research on stored human tissue (Clayton et al. 1995). We would recommend that IRBs evaluate protocols for human tissue research according to the same standards used to evaluate human subjects research.

(3) Does the research require IRB approval? Federal regulations do not require that all research conducted using federal funds be reviewed by an IRB. For example, educational research, research relating to existing, publicly available data if subjects cannot be identified directly or through links, research that evaluates public benefit programs, and food quality research do not require IRB review.

(4) Does the research require full IRB review? Some types of research qualify for expedited review, such as research that has only minimal risk or involves only minor changes to an existing protocol. "Minimal risk" is defined as follows: "[T]he probability and magnitude of the harm or discomfort anticipated in the research are no greater in and of themselves than those ordinarily encountered in daily life or in routine physical or psychological examinations or tests" (Common Rule 1991 §102i).

(5) Are risks minimized? There are many different risks in research, including physiological, psychosocial, financial, and legal risks. If a proposal is judged as "more than minimal risk," then an IRB needs to ask whether the research proposals take appropriate steps to minimize these risks.

(6) Are the risks justified in relation to the benefits? Even proposals that involve a great deal of risk may be judged ethical if the IRB decides that the risks are justified in relation to the benefits to the subject and to society. Benefits to subjects include medical as well as psychosocial benefits (participation itself may be a benefit). Benefits to society may include advancement of knowledge.

(7) Is selection of subjects equitable? To satisfy the demands of justice and equitability, the IRB needs to ask whether the proposal will exclude certain types of subjects and why. Federal regulations require that research proposals provide a sound scientific, moral, or legal reason for excluding specific populations from a study (59 *Federal Register* 14508). Very often researchers can provide a sound scientific rationale; for example, there is no good reason for including men in a study of ovarian cancer or minors in a study of osteoporosis. A valid moral rationale for excluding subjects would be to protect those subjects or a third party, such as a fetus. Federal regulations pertaining to protection of fetuses require researchers to exclude pregnant women from studies that involve significant risks to the fetus (45 CFR 46, subpart B).

(8) How will subjects be recruited? IRBs address this question to promote equitable subject selection and to avoid potential coercion, deception, or exploitation. IRBs usually review advertisements to ensure that are not deceptive or coercive.

(9) Is confidentiality protected? All federal regulations require researchers to take adequate steps to protect patient confidentiality (Common Rule 1991 §111a7). Most investigators protect confidentiality by removing personal identifiers from published data and keeping the original data under lock and key for several years before destroying it. Some kinds of research may pose special problems for confidentiality. Researchers may also have legal or ethical obligations to break confidentiality in some circumstances, such as when dealing with information relating to child abuse or domestic violence.

(10) Is informed consent required? In most protocols, researchers should

obtain informed consent from subjects or their legally appointed representatives. In cases where consent is given by a representative, the IRB may also require that the subject assent to the research, if it is in the subject's interests to provide assent. However, there are some notable exceptions to this policy. For example, investigators do not have to obtain informed consent for research on public benefit programs. IRBs may also approve exceptions to standard informed consent requirements if obtaining informed consent would invalidate or bias their research, for example, in social science experiments (§116c). IRBs must then provide full justification for their exception.

(11) Does informed consent need to be documented? Federal regulations require that informed consent be documented except in cases when the research is judged to be minimal risk, the principal harm arising from the research would be potential breach of confidentiality, and the only record linking the subject to the research would be the informed consent document itself (§117c). In cases where the research subject is not able to sign an informed consent form, the legally appointed representative must sign the form.

(12) Is informed consent adequate? IRBs take a careful look at the *process* of obtaining informed consent. IRBs are concerned about the quality and integrity of the process as well as fairness and potential exploitation or coercion. Although IRBs often spend a great deal of time examining the informed consent form to make sure that it covers everything that needs to be discussed, and that it is understandable and well written, informed consent should be much more than just signing a form. It should be an ongoing conversation between researchers and subjects about the benefits and risks of research participation (Veatch 1987). Federal regulations provide details about information that must be included in informed consent (Common Rule 1991, §116), including information about the purpose of the research, its duration, and relevant procedures; the number of subjects enrolled; foreseeable risks, costs, or discomforts; possible benefits; alternative treatments; confidentiality protections; any compensation for injuries; payment for participation (if any); ability of the subjects to refuse or withdraw at any time without any penalty; ability of the researchers to withdraw subjects to protect them from harm; potential disclosure of significant findings to subjects or their representatives during the study; and whom to contact. Also, IRBs must be satisfied that enrolled subjects can comprehend the information given to them. If the subjects are decisionally impaired, then arrangements should be made for determining their legally appointed representatives.

(13) Are any safeguards required to protect vulnerable subjects? Safeguards that may help protect vulnerable subjects could include provisions to promote adequate informed consent, such as using legally appointed representatives if the subjects cannot give consent. IRBs may also need to include members with some knowledge of the needs and interests of these vulnerable populations. For example, to review research on prisoners, an IRB must have a member who is qualified to represent the interests of prisoners. The federal government has other protections for vulnerable subjects, which are discussed below.

(14) Is the protocol scientifically valid? The IRB should also ensure that research proposals meet appropriate standards of scientific validity, because poorly designed studies expose subjects to research risks without the promise of obtaining useful results (Levine 1988). An IRB may consider statistical issues, such as sample size, sampling biases, and surrogate end points. The IRB may consider conceptual issues related to research design, such as the merits of quantitative versus qualitative research and using the "intent to treat" model in clinical research. Although it is very important for research protocols to meet the highest standards of scientific rigor, this requirement may sometimes conflict with other ethical principles, as discussed above. Randomized, controlled clinical trials have become the "gold standard" for clinical research, but they have generated a great deal of controversy relating to the use of placebo controls as well as rules for starting or stopping clinical trials. The IRB may also need to consider whether there is adequate empirical data for proceeding with a study, such as data from previous animal or human studies. If the research is part of a clinical trial to generate data to support an application to the FDA, then the IRB will want to know whether the study is a phase I, phase II, or phase III study, whether it is an expanded access or human use trial, and so on.

(15) How will the data be monitored to protect subjects from risks and ensure the validity of the results? It is very important for IRBs to continually monitor clinical trials to learn about potential benefits, problems with the protocol, and adverse events, such as unanticipated harms, including death. Adverse events need to be reported to the IRB, which will report them to the appropriate agency. IRBs may establish boards to monitor results and determine whether trials should be discontinued.

(16) Are there any conflicts of interest? Chapter 7 discusses conflicts of interests in detail, and these conflicts can occur in human experimentation research as well. Federal regulations require researchers to disclose conflicts of interest to the government (see 21 CFR 54, 60 *Federal Register* 35810). Clinical researchers may have a variety of financial interests in research, including private funding, stock, salary, and economic incentives to recruit subjects into clinical trials: to encourage investigators to recruit research subjects, companies may pay them a fee for each subject recruited or patient care costs over and above what it costs to provide care for the patient (Spece et al. 1996).

(17) Are there any collaborating institutions? A great deal of research today involves collaboration among many different researchers at different institutions. The IRB needs to ensure that this collaboration does not harm subjects and that other institutions abide by the relevant regulations and guidelines. International research collaboration has become especially controversial, because researchers in different countries may abide by different ethical standards (Macklin 1999).

PROTECTING VULNERABLE SUBJECTS

Mentally Disabled Research Subjects

Mentally ill or mentally disabled subjects may have impaired decision-making abilities and may be unable to promote their own interests. Throughout history, mentally ill or mentally disabled people have received unfair and even inhumane treatment, including being subjected to forced hospitalization and sterilization. Nazi eugenics and racial purification policies began with programs to prevent mentally ill or disabled people from reproducing. In the past, mentally ill research subjects have not been accorded the same protection as other research subjects (Shamoo and O'Sullivan 1998, Shamoo 2000). Both the Belmont Report (National Commission 1979) and the President's Commission for the Study of Ethical Problems in Medicine and Biomedical and Behavioral Research (1983) recognized that mentally disabled people should be treated as vulnerable or potentially vulnerable research subjects. (We distinguish here between mental illness and mental disability to emphasize that mental illnesses, such as depression, are different from mental disabilities, such as dyslexia or mental retardation. A mental illness may or may not cause a patient to be mentally disabled.)

Decision-making ability depends on at least four conditions: (1) overall mental status (consciousness, memory, orientation, reasoning ability, judgment), (2) the ability to communicate a choice, (3) a stable set of values or preferences, and (4) the ability to comprehend or understand the consequences of a decision. Mentally disabled patients may lack the ability to meet any or all of these conditions. The more severe and chronic the mental disorder, the more likely the impairment of decisional capability. Patients with schizophrenia, manic depression, major depression, and anxiety disorders may represent the most likely group with problems related to decisional capacity. Decision-making ability can be compromised even further when decisionally impaired subjects are confined in an institution, due to potential coercive factors in that environment.

Although both the National Commission and the President's Commissions recommended extra protections for the mentally disabled, the federal government did not issue special regulations on the mentally disabled as a separate subpart of 45 CFR 46 when it revised this document, due to insufficient advocacy for the mentally ill at that time (Shamoo and Irving 1993). The Common Rule (1991) discusses added protections for the mentally disabled as part of the IRB composition: "If an IRB regularly reviews research that involves a vulnerable category of subjects, such as children, prisoners, pregnant women, or handicapped or mentally disabled persons, consideration shall be given to the inclusion of one or more individuals who are knowledgeable about and experienced in working with these subjects" (§107a).

At present, what constitutes an acceptable degree of risk when mentally disabled individual is enrolled in research as a subject can be interpreted differently by various IRBs. The continuing controversies regarding this vulnerable group are due in part to this lack of clarity of the guidelines. For example, some researchers argue that the washout studies discussed in this chapter pose an acceptable degree of risk, while others argue that these studies expose subjects to unacceptable research risks.

The NBAC spent two years studying ethical issues in research on the mentally ill or disabled and filed a report in 1998. In its executive summary, the report recommends the following:

1. IRBs that review protocols for research on mentally ill or disabled subjects should include at least two members familiar with these disorders and with the needs and concerns of the population being studied.
2. For research protocols with greater than minimal risk, IRBs should require independent, qualified professionals to assess the potential subject's decision-making ability.
3. For research that involves greater than minimal risk and offers no prospect of direct medical benefits to subjects, the protocol should be referred to a national Special Standing Panel for a decision, unless the subject has a valid legally appointed representative to act on his/her behalf.

Children

Federal regulations 45 CFR part 46 subpart D, "Additional Protections for Children" recognize the limited ability of children to comprehend the nature of their participation and they require a parent, guardian, or legally authorized representative to provide informed consent for research participation. An affirmative sign of approval (or assent) from the child may also be required for a child to participate in research, provided that the child can provide assent and assent is in the child's best interests. The federal regulations require IRBs to classify a research proposal on children into one of four categories:

1. Minimal risk research: This category, discussed above, is the same for all human subjects, whether children or adults.
2. Greater than minimal risk research with the prospect of direct medical benefit to the child: For research in this category, IRBs must consider whether the research risk can be justified in light of anticipated benefits to the subject, the risks/benefit relationship to the subject as compared to alternative treatments, and assent of the subject is secured.
3. Greater than minimal risk with no prospect of direct medical benefits to the child: For research in this category, IRBs must consider whether the risk is a minor increase over minimal risk, the protocol is within the scope of medical and other procedures the subject may experience, the procedure produces generalizable knowledge, and assent of the child is secured. The term "minor increase over minimal risk" is vague and not defined by the federal regulations.
4. Greater than minor increase over minimal risk with no prospect of direct medical benefits to the child: Research with children under this

category can be considered under certain circumstances and after referral to the Secretary, DHHS. The secretary can approve the research protocol if the research outcome can be shown to contribute to our understanding of pediatric conditions and improve the general welfare of children.

Before 1998, all drugs were tested on children on a voluntary basis, and very little research on children was done. The pharmaceutical industry avoided extensive research with children for fear of liability. The ethical issues in the use of children in research became more critical because of two actions taken in 1997 and 1998 by the federal government. In 1997, President Clinton ordered changes in testing drugs and biological products that are usually used for children. Drugs and biological products are normally tested on adults despite the fact that some are used widely in children without any tests conducted on children. The scientific literature clearly indicates that drugs affect children differently than adults and not necessarily only in a dose-related way. By the end of 1998, the FDA mandated that the pharmaceutical industry test drugs and biological products on children if they are to be used in children. The logic behind this regulation is the same as that requiring the inclusion of women and minorities in research trials (Tauer 1999). This new ruling gave rise to an ethical dilemma between the norms of promoting justice and protecting vulnerable populations: how can one help ensure that pediatric treatments are safe and effective without threatening the well-being of children? Many medications have been tested only on adults, not on children. When pediatricians prescribe these medications for children, they must do so on an "off-label" basis (i.e., the drug as labeled is not officially appproved for children), and they often have to make guesses about appropriate doses and schedules. One might argue that we have been overly protective when it comes to enrolling children in research and that we need to take steps to reverse this trend (Tauer 1999).

Prisoners

Prior to the National Commission's report in 1979, the use of prisoners in research was common. Although prisoners can make free choices, most people would agree that the highly coercive prison environment undermines their ability to do so. Current federal regulations reflect the National Commission's recommendation for special restrictions on the recruitment and use of this population as human subjects in research. Prisoners are compensated for discomfort and time spent in research. The normal compensation package for adults outside the prison could be regarded as coercive and exploitative in the prison environment because most prisoners would prefer research participation to the daily boredom of prison life. One might argue that most prisoners would not participate in research if they were not in prison. There are also problems with maintaining confidentiality in the prison environment. In his book *Acres of Skin*, Hornblum (1998) chronicles how in the 1960s and 1970s researchers used the skin on the backs of prisoners to test numerous drugs and perfumes for toxicity and cancer causation. The experiments were conducted at Holmesburg Prison in Philadelphia, by University of Pennsylvania researchers. The records of these experiments are "lost." Several ethical issues came to light: subjects received payment and coercion, housing for the experiment was better than that provided for other prisoners, the human contacts during the experiments may have been unduly coercive, and informed consent was barely informative.

The federal regulations provide for *additional* safeguards for prisoners when they are enrolled as research subjects. Research protocols may involve prisoners only if (1) the research is of minimal risk related to the causes, effects, and process of incarceration; or if (2) the study is of the prison and inmates as an institution; or if (3) the research is on conditions of prisoners as a class; or if (4) the research is therapeutic with potential benefits to the prisoner subject (45 CFR 46, subpart C). If the research is nontherapeutic, the Secretary, DHHS can approve such research after consultation with experts and receiving public comments.

Further restrictions are that recruitment should be fair and not influenced by the prison's administration or any promise of leniency during parole proceedings. How one defines "minimal risk" for prisoners is a tricky issue, because the prison environment is in many ways more risky than the outside world. Prisoners encounter different risks during their daily lives than nonprisoners. Therefore, some argue that the standards of risks "normally encountered in daily lives" should be the same as those for everyone else in the world outside of prison.

MISCONDUCT IN CLINICAL RESEARCH AND CLINICAL TRIALS

As discussed in chapter 5 on scientific misconduct, all clinical research supported by the federal government must follow the federal policy on scientific misconduct. Therefore, the policy applies to all federal agencies. Each agency provides an oversight for compliance with the scientific misconduct policy, including when human subjects are involved. The U.S. Public Health Service provides much support for clinical research. Scientific misconduct within the context of clinical research provides a unique challenge to agencies because it involves human subjects. The Office of Research Integrity (ORI) has issued specific draft Guidelines for Assessing Possible Research Misconduct in Clinical Research and Clinical Trials, which attempt to adapt the scientific misconduct policy to clinical research. The ORI emphasizes that the guidelines are to be used as a supplement to the ORI's model for responding to allegations of research misconduct.

In brief, the guidelines require that any investigation into misconduct in clinical research and trials should follow these elements:

1. Coordination of human subject protections with the IRB
2. Informing physicians and patients when significant public health issues are involved

3. Informing the Data and Safety Monitoring Board
4. Informing the affected journals
5. Coordination of the investigation with Office for Human Research Protection and FDA, if appropriate

The investigation should include the assessment of discrepancy of the data submitted to federal agency, publications, or other forms, from the original clinical data in the medical records.

Under the Freedom of Information Act, Shamoo (2001) obtained the institutional incident reports for NIH-supported research that contain adverse events, including deaths, for the years 1990–2000. Only eight deaths and 386 adverse events were reported throughout the 10 years, even though tens of millions of human subjects took part in these experiments. This likely represents an underreporting of adverse events in this large population. This high level of underreporting casts doubts as to the integrity of some clinical data.

QUESTIONS FOR DISCUSSION

1. Is the media paying too much, just enough, or too little attention to questionable research with human subjects? Why do you think that is so?
2. Do you think freedom of inquiry should surpass other values? Why?
3. What risks would you and members of your family take for public good? Why?
4. In your opinion, should there be a difference between informed consent for volunteering as a human subject and informed consent for medical treatment? What would those differences be, if any? Why?
5. Do you think IRBs are doing a good job of protecting human subjects? Can they? How would you improve the system, if you believe improvement is needed?
6. How would you design a system to ensure enrollment of mentally ill individuals into research studies while protecting them from harm? Why?

CASE FOR DISCUSSION

Case 1

An announcement in the newspaper and radio encourages people to enroll in research protocols to test a new anti-flu medication. The announcement emphasizes that subjects will receive a free physical exam, free health care for 60 days, and $400 compensation. The new drug is very promising in either stopping the full-blown symptoms of the flu or preventing it altogether. The protocol has already been approved by an IRB.

- What questions would you ask if you were a potential subject?
- Should the IRB have approved the protocol? Why?

Case 2

A hospital associated with a research university has a policy that every new employee should give a blood sample. The employee is told that the blood sample will be frozen for a long time. The hospital's purpose in collecting the blood sample is to reduce their liability in case anyone contracts HIV. From the frozen sample they can determine whether the patient had the HIV virus prior to employment. This will reduce the hospital's liability. A few years later, a researcher at the hospital is developing an HIV diagnostic instrument directly from the blood. The instrument, if it works, would advance HIV screening. The researcher wants to use the samples without any names attached to it. He just wants to test different samples from different people. The researcher designed the protocol such that once the samples are obtained, no one would know which sample belonged to which person.

- What concerns would you have if this was your blood sample?
- What should the IRB do?
- What should the informed consent form contain?

Case 3

Many clinical faculty members at research universities receive 20–90% of their salary from research grants and contracts, a large percentage of which consist of clinical trials sponsored by pharmaceutical companies.

- Do you see potential problems with this arrangement?
- Can you suggest some solutions?
- Should a university engage in routine clinical trials?

Case 4

Subjects for a research study will be recruited from private pain treatment clinics and the medical school's pain service. Preliminary studies have shown that the drug thalidomide may provide some relief for migraine headaches, arthritis, and neuropathy conditions. Because thalidomide's harmful effects on fetuses are well known, women of childbearing age will be excluded from this study.

- Are there social/scientific benefits from the study?
- If you are a member of the IRB, what questions would you ask?
- What should the risk/benefit analysis include?

Case 5

A company is developing a safer pesticide for use on a variety of crops, including tomatoes, corn, apples, green beans, and grapes. The company plans to use healthy subjects (its employees) to test the pesticide for toxic effects. Subjects will be paid $500 and will be monitored carefully for three days. They will report toxic effects, such as dizziness, nausea, headache, fatigue, shortness of breath, anxiety, and so forth. If the pesticide proves to be safe, it may replace many existing pesticides commonly used on crops.

- What are the risks to subjects?
- What are the benefits to subjects?
- Would you put any conditions on the protocol before going forward? What would they be?
- Do you see any conflicts of interest? Can they influence the outcome of the study?

Case 6

The aim of a study is to better understand condom use among adolescents and the psychosocial factors that increase or decrease condom use. The study is a survey of adolescent attitudes and beliefs about sexuality. It will include many different questions about sexuality as well as questions about alcohol and drug use, violence, musical tastes, and religion. The subjects will not be told the exact purpose of the study when they take the survey, but they will be told the results of the study. Subjects will be recruited from three local high schools. Personal identifiers will be removed. High school health education teachers will help administer the survey. Taking the survey will suffice as proof of consent. Subjects may refuse to take the survey without penalty. Parents will be notified about the study and may refuse to allow their children to participate.

- In what specific category of risk (discussed above) would you place this protocol and why?
- How would you protect the privacy of subjects?
- Why should the parents be involved?
- Should there be any concern for the community?

Case 7

Subjects with Alzheimer's disease will be recruited from 10 nursing homes in the area. Subjects or their legally appointed representatives will give consent. Subjects will provide a blood sample for genetic testing. Personal identifiers will be removed from the samples, although researchers will retain the ability to link samples to subjects. Researchers will develop a DNA database and attempt to find common genes associated with the disease, including variants of the APOE gene. Researchers will also compare the database with a database drawn from a matched set of patients without the disease.

- Do you have any concerns and, if so, what are they?
- If the patient was your father or mother, would you encourage your parent to enroll?

Case 8

A full professor/researcher at a major research university is a member of the National Academy of Science. In her research protocol, she describes briefly how she proposes to remove 100 schizophrenia patients from their medications for four weeks while outpatients. The protocol calls for randomly selecting 50 as controls, and thus these 50 will receive placebo for the duration of the experiments (60 days), and the other 50 will receive a promising new drug that presumably will have many fewer side effects. A colleague at a different department at the university raises some concerns during IRB deliberations.

- What you think the IRB member's concerns were?
- What are the risks/benefits of this protocol? Do the benefits outweigh the risks? Why?
- How would you deal with these concerns?
- Should the protocol proceed?

Case 9

An informed consent form describes a research protocol briefly. The protocol involves the washout of 60 patients from their current antidepressive drug. The research protocol dwells on potential worsening of the patients' condition if they are removed from their current medication but does not cite literature discussing that the washout may worsen prognosis in the future. The informed consent form makes the passing reference, "You may experience some symptoms of depression." The forms do mention alternative medications.

- What are the risks and benefits? Do the benefits outweigh the risks? Why?
- How much should the informed consent form reflect the protocol? How much should it reflect the literature?
- What do you think of potentially scaring patients away from participation?

Case 10

Six schizophrenia patients experienced medication washout for four weeks. The experimental protocol calls for subjecting three patients to a chemical that will induce, in part, symptoms of schizophrenia such as psychosis. The other three patients will be the control group and will remain without medication for the duration of the protocol (one week). All six will undergo repeated PET scans. These experiments are needed to study the mechanism of psychosis and what types of receptors are involved.

- Do these experiments violate the Nuremberg Code?
- Do these experiments violate U.S. federal regulations?
- What additional and unique safeguards, if any, would you undertake for such experiments?

Case 11

A research protocol calls for using 80 healthy young children to test a new vaccine. The new vaccine's safety has been tested, and all indications are that it is a fairly safe vaccine, and probably safer than the current vaccine for the same deadly disease. Half of the children will receive a placebo, and half will receive the new vaccine. All 80 children were screened to make sure that they have not yet received any vaccine for this disease. Informed consent forms were very detailed on risks and benefits. However, the forms did not mention that those receiving the new vaccine will not be able to receive the old vaccine.

- Should the informed consent forms have mentioned the fact that the children can no longer obtain the old vaccine?
- Was the description of risks and benefits appropriate?
- Would you allow your children to enroll?

Case 12

A nontenured assistant professor at a medium-sized university is a member of her university's IRB. One of the human subject protocols the IRB is reviewing is from a world-renowned professor at another department at her university. This world-renowned professor is a member of the promotion and tenure committee. The assistant professor's package for promotion to tenured associate professor will go to the committee in six months. The assistant professor has a great deal of concern about the proposed protocol. She feels that the risks are watered down and the benefits or potential benefits are exaggerated.

- What should the assistant professor do? What you would do?
- How should the university handle the problem?

Case 13

One hundred children, aged 6–12 years, from poor Hispanic American communities were recruited into a research protocol. They were offered a $25 gift certificate to Toys 'R Us. The parents of these children were given $125 to cover transportation costs plus the inconvenience of taking their kids to the hospital for a whole day. The children were identified as siblings of individuals incarcerated for violent crimes. The children have committed no crimes and have no illness. The university researcher obtained the information regarding the siblings through sealed court records, without the parents' or the courts' permission. The protocol calls for giving the youngsters fenfluramine (a diet drug). If the children were predisposed to violence, they may show a large increase in serotonin due to fenfluramine. Samples of spinal fluids (by spinal taps) will be collected every 3 hours for 12 hours. Blood levels of serotonin will be monitored continuously through a vein catheter. Informed consent forms were signed by parents, who in some cases were unable to read or write. There was no notation of which parents were not able to read. Research on youth violent behavior is crucial to help those children with violent tendencies before they become criminals.

- If you were an IRB member, would you approve the protocol?
- What kind of questions should IRB members ask?
- How could you design this protocol and the informed consent forms to make certain the IRB will approve it?

Case 14

A research proposal and its informed consent forms were submitted to an IRB of an independent nonprofit research facility in San Francisco. The protocol deals with 300 drug addicts, of whom 20% are also suspected of having HIV. The protocol is a survey of social habits of these addicts. The surveyor will follow the addicts around in their daily routine for one week to register their food intake, drugs used, sexual habits, and so forth. The researcher considered the study to be a minimal risk study and said so on the proposal submitted to the IRB.

- What should the IRB do?
- What should the informed consent form contain?
- Should confidentiality of information be dealt with in the informed consent form?
- Is this research of minimal risk? Why?

10

The Use of Animals in Research

> This chapter discusses the use of animals in research. It provides a brief history of animal research and examines the ethical arguments for and against animal experimentation. The chapter discusses the animal rights views of Peter Singer and Tom Regan and considers some morally significant differences between animals and humans. It also discusses some principles for the ethical treatment of animal in research, such as the "three Rs"—reduction, replacement, and refinement—as well as animal research regulations.

Experimentation on (nonhuman) animals is one of the most controversial issues in research ethics. Like the abortion debate, the issue has been hotly contested and often violent. Animal rights activists have freed laboratory animals and destroyed research records, materials, equipment, and buildings to protest what they consider immoral uses of animals (Koenig 1999). Animal welfare organizations have not condoned violence, but they have taken strong stands against specific types of animal research. Researchers, on the other hand, have rallied around the cause of animal research and have developed professional organizations, such as the National Association for Biomedical Research and the Foundation for Biomedical Research, to promote the humane use of animals in research. Given the highly polarized nature of this debate, one wonders whether there can be any hope of some consensus on the issue (DeGrazia 1991).

Estimates of the number of animals used in research vary from 17 to 70 million animals per year (LaFollette and Shanks 1996). Advances in technology have made it possible to eliminate some uses of animals in research and replace animal models with other testing procedures, such as tissue cultures and computer simulations (Barnard and Kaufman 1997). Researchers are also finding ways to obtain valid results using fewer animals. Additionally, universities are using fewer live animals in educating graduate and undergraduate students. The number of animal experimental procedures conducted in the United Kingdom declined from 5.2 million in 1978 to 3 million in 1998. However, this trend may reverse as researchers increase the number of animals used in transgenic research (Stokstad 1999).

Approximately 40% of animals used in research are used in basic or applied research, 26% are used in drug development, and 20% are used in safety testing. The remaining 14% are used for educational or other scientific purposes (Pence 1995). Most of what we know about basic animal physiology, anatomy, biochemistry, embryology, development, genetics, cytology, neurology, immunology, cardiology, and endocrinology has been gained through experiments on animals. Animals are commonly used in applied research to test new medical therapies, such as drugs, vaccines, medical procedures, or medical devices. Indeed, U.S. Food and Drug Administration (FDA) regulations require that new drugs and medical devices be tested in animal populations before they are tested in human populations (Bennett 1994). Animals are also used in environmental studies to determine the toxic or carcinogenic effects of compounds that are released into the environment, such as pesticides, herbicides, or pollutants. They are also used in agricultural research in the development of hybrid breeds, clones, or transgenic species, and in cosmetic research to test the toxicity of mascara, shampoo, hair dye, lipstick, and other products. Transgenic animals are playing an increasingly important role in research: researchers have developed varieties of transgenic mice that contain genes for specific diseases, such as diabetes, obesity, cancer, and Parkinson's disease. Transgenic animals are playing an increasingly important role in agriculture as well: researchers have developed sheep that produce human hormones in their milk, and they are attempting to develop pigs that will produce organs suitable for transplantation into human beings (Wilmut 1997, Marshall 2000c).

Although people have spoken on behalf of animals for many years, a book by the philosopher Peter Singer, titled *Animal Liberation* (1975 [1990]), spurred and buttressed the modern animal rights movement. But before examining Singer's views on animals, we provide a brief history of the animal rights movement.

HISTORICAL PERSPECTIVE

For many years, scientists who used animals in research were influenced by the views of the seventeenth-century French philosopher René Descartes (1596–1650), who argued that animals are like machines and that their behaviors result from instincts, reflexes, and other internal mechanisms that do not involve consciousness or rationality (Descartes [1970]). Descartes' view probably had a significant influence in the early vivisection practices: seventeenth- and eighteenth-century vivisectionists nailed dogs to boards and cut them open without anesthesia or analgesia. They interpreted their howls and cries as mere noises produced by a machine (LaFollette and Shanks 1996). Pain-relieving measures were not used in animals before the discovery of anesthesia in 1846 (Sideris et al. 1999). In the twentieth century, the behaviorists held that we could know nothing about the inner workings of the mind, although we can study behavior; because it is not possible to know whether an animal can think or feel, they did not pay sufficient attention to animal pain or suffering (Rollin 1989).

These attitudes toward animals began to change in the 1800s, as philosophers Jeremey Bentham (1748–1832) and John Stuart Mill (1806–1873) advanced the notion that animals can suffer and thus deserve moral consideration. Their views provided a philosophical and moral basis for the nineteenth-century's animal welfare movement. From the mid-1800s until the early twentieth century, there was a strong antivivisection movement in England and the United States. Leaders of this movement opposed the use of animals in experiments and opposed all forms of cruelty to animals. The American Society for the Prevention of Cruelty to Animals (ASPCA) was formed in 1866, and local societies for the prevention of cruelty to animals soon followed. The American Humane Organization, founded in 1874, opposed the use of animals in experiments as well as inhumane experiments on human beings. Many of the leaders of this movement, such as Caroline White and Mary Lovell, were women with strong religious and moral convictions. The antivivisection movement also received support from the Women's Christian Temperance Movement, the Department of Mercy, and *Life* magazine. There were two main arguments that antivivisectionists made against animal experiments. First, they argued that these experiments cause unnecessary and unjustifiable suffering to animals. Second, they argued that our attitudes toward animals could influence how we treat human beings: cruelty to animals can lead to cruelty to human beings. In this light, the antivivisection movement also drew connections between exploiting animals in research and exploiting human beings and helped draw attention to unethical experiments on children, mentally ill people, poor people, African Americans, and prisoners (Lederer 1995).

In Britain, animal rights activists helped pass the "Martin Act" in 1822 entitled "Act to Prevent Cruel and Improper Treatment of Cattle." A few years later the Royal Society for the Prevention of Cruelty to Animals (RSPCA) was founded. In 1829, New York State passed a law to protect domestic animals such as horses, oxen, and other cattle. By the end of the nineteenth century, Britain passed stricter animal protections laws. Feminist and animal activist Frances Power Cobbe became more active in opposing vivisection. Late in the 1800s, all experiments with animals in Britain required a yearly license. During the same period Darwin's theories on evolution tended to inextricably link human beings to animals. This linkage heightened sensitivity to subjecting animals to pain. The animal rights movement in England remained dormant until the 1960s. In 1972, Richard Ryder, Ronald Lee, and Clifford Goodman founded the Animal Liberation Front in England.

In the United Sates, the National Academy of Sciences and the American Medical Association formed a coalition to push for legislation in the late 1890s to disarm vivisectionists and promote medical progress. The animal rights movement was practically nonexistent in the United States until the 1960s and the advent of the civil rights movement. This was followed by Peter Singer's book *Animal Liberation* (1975 [1990]). In the 1980s, a new force came to existence, People for the Ethical Treatment of Animals (PETA), which was founded by two strident activists, Alex Pacheco and Ingrid Newkirk (Sideris et al. 1999). PETA has since engaged in numerous high-profile activities to highlight the plight of animals in certain experiments. Although PETA has not condoned the use of violence, many people have alleged that the organization has used unethical and illegal means to reach its goals (Oliver 1999).

THE ARGUMENT FOR USING ANIMALS IN RESEARCH

Why do scientists use animals in research? The main argument can be understood in starkly utilitarian terms (Cohen 1986, Botting and Morrison 1997): animal research produces important basic and applied knowledge that promotes human health and welfare. Proponents of animal research also note that animal research can be justified on the grounds that it also improves the health and welfare of animals, but this point plays a minor role in the overall argument. The argument is utilitarian because it holds that the ends (promoting human health and welfare) justify the means (animal research). Those who criticize this argument argue either (1) that the ends do not justify the means or (2) that the means are not effective at achieving the aims. The first type of critique raises moral objections to animal research; the second raises scientific or technical objections to animal research. Below we examine both of these critiques as well as replies to them.

Moral Critiques of Using Animals in Research

To understand moral arguments against using animals in research, it is useful to draw an analogy with human research. Two of the guiding principles in human subjects research are beneficence and respect for persons (National Commission 1979). We can use humans in our research provided that we take steps to promote and respect their inherent moral worth. The phrase "human guinea pig" literally means treating a research subject (or person) like an animal, that is, treating the research subject as something that can be sacrificed for a greater good (Jonas 1980). Moral objections to animal research include the argument that research protections pertaining to human beings should be extended to animals: we should take steps to promote and respect the moral worth of animals (LaFollette and Shanks 1996). If we are not morally justified in performing an experiment on a human, then we should also not perform that experiment on an animal. Animals, like human beings, have inherent moral worth and should not be sacrificed for a greater good. This claim is supported in two very different ways, a utilitarian argument, defended by Peter Singer (1975 [1990]), and a rights-based argument, defended by Tom Regan (1983).

According to Singer, the central question in our treatment of animals is whether they deserve moral consideration. But Singer does not believe that all organisms deserve moral consideration: for example, he would not claim that bacteria deserve moral consideration. Merely being a living creature is not a sufficient reason for special moral treatment. On the other hand, Singer thinks that the question of whether animals can reason or communicate is not the only relevant issue in deciding whether they deserve moral consideration—what matters is that animals have the ability to suffer. Singer cites the seventeenth-century philosopher Jeremy Bentham on this point. In discussing the moral status of black slaves, Bentham argued that the color of their skin was irrelevant to determining their moral status. And he extended this argument to animals: the most important question in determining the moral status of a being is not whether the being can think, talk, or reason, but whether it can suffer (Bentham 1789 [1988]). According to Singer, many animals can suffer and therefore they pass the key test for determining whether they deserve moral consideration. This view implies that human beings have a moral obligation to refrain from causing animals to suffer.

Most people would likely accept most of this argument: it is certainly wrong to inflict *needless* suffering on animals, and one should take steps to minimize animal suffering. But most people would say that animal suffering could be justified to promote important causes, such as improving human health and welfare. Animals have some moral worth, but human beings have a higher moral status or worth (Cohen 1986, Frey 1994). Thus, we should consider animal suffering in deciding how to treat animals, but we should give far more weight to human suffering.

However, Singer does not believe that we should give more weight to human suffering. According to Singer, all beings that deserve moral consideration deserve equal moral consideration. Thus, we should give equal weight to human and animal suffering. Our refusal to give equal consideration to animals is a form of bias that Singer calls "speciesism." Singer equates speciesism with racism and sexism because these "isms" discriminate morally between different classes of beings based on irrelevant characteristics. Just as skin color and gender are not relevant to a person's moral standing, species membership is also not relevant. According to Singer: "Speciesism . . . is a prejudice or attitude of bias toward the interests of members of one's own species. It should be obvious that the fundamental objections to racism and sexism made by Thomas Jefferson and Sojourner Truth apply equally to speciesism" (Singer 1975 [1990], p. 7).

Singer's view does not prohibit animal experiments on species not considered to have moral worth, including plankton, worms, and many other lower species. Nor does it imply that experiments on animals with moral worth can *never* be morally justified. Because Singer is a utilitarian, he believes that animal experiments could be justified if the experiments promote the greatest good for the greatest number of beings that deserve moral consideration—humans and animals. However, his view implies that most of the animal experiments that are performed today should be stopped, and that we should consider performing experiments on human beings that lack rationality or consciousness, such as severely retarded infants or adults, instead of performing those experiments on animals.

In responding to Singer's view, many writers have attempted to refute the charge of speciesism. According to Cohen (1986), Frey (1994), Caplan (1983), Carruthers (1992), and others, there are morally significant differences between humans and animals. Some of these include:

- Rationality: the ability to reason and solve problems
- Communication: the ability to communicate information
- Self-consciousness: the awareness of one's self in one's environment; the awareness of one's own beliefs, emotions, desires, and attitudes

- Self-determination: the ability to make deliberate choices in controlling one's own behavior
- Consciousness: the awareness of sensations, including the capacity to feel pain

According to these critics, many of the higher animals used in research lack rationality, communication, self-consciousness, self-determination, and possibly even consciousness. For these reasons, the moral worth of a single human being is far greater than the moral worth of, for example, a thousand laboratory mice. Thus, we are justified in causing 1,000 laboratory mice to suffer in order to prevent or diminish the suffering of a single human being. According to Cohen (1986), the charge of speciesism is unsound and morally offensive because, although there are no morally significant differences among races, there are morally significant differences between humans and other species.

We return later to the question of important moral differences between animals and human beings. Note at this point, however, that such blanket assertions as "humans and animals are morally the same" or "humans and animals are morally different" are likely to be misleading, because one must consider the specific species in question before comparing that species with *Homo sapiens*. For example, chimpanzees and human beings have more in common (morally) than do mosquitoes and human beings.

Note also that Singer's use of the term "suffering" is somewhat naive and simplistic. It would appear that Singer uses the term "suffer" as a substitute for "feel pain," but suffering is not merely the same the same thing as feeling pain (Cassell 1991). There are many different types of suffering: unrelieved and uncontrollable pain; discomfort, as well as other unpleasant symptoms, such as nausea, dizziness, and shortness of breath; disability; and emotional distress. However, all of these types of suffering involve much more than consciousness: they also involve self-consciousness, or the awareness that one is aware of something. For a creature to experience unrelieved pain, the creature must be aware that it is in pain and that the pain is not going away.

If we think of suffering in this fashion, then it may not be at all obvious that animals suffer, because we do not know the extent to which animals are self-conscious. Although one might argue that it is also difficult to prove that animals feel pain, most people find this easier to accept (based on behavioral and neurological similarities) than the claim that animals are self-conscious. However, once again, a great deal depends on what species of animal we have in mind. Monkeys, dogs, and cats probably have enough self-consciousness to experience suffering. But what about fish, frogs, and mice? Perhaps Singer has chosen the wrong word to describe animal experiences. If he had said that the key point is that animals can feel pain, rather than suffering, then perhaps his claims would be less contentious (Rollin 1989).

Tom Regan, like Singer, also believes that animals have moral status. But Regan, unlike Singer, argues that animals have rights. This seems like an outrageous claim to those who believe that only moral agents can have moral rights—a moral agent is someone who participates in the moral community: he or she can follow moral rules, make moral choices, and discuss moral issues. Rights and responsibilities go hand in hand: one cannot have a moral right unless one can also accept moral responsibilities. Because animals are incapable of following moral rules, making moral choices, or discussing moral issues, they are not moral agents. Thus, they are not members of the moral community and have no moral rights (Fox and DeMarco 1990).

To make sense of the idea that animals have rights, Regan (1983) draws a distinction between moral *agents* and moral *patients*. Regan argues that moral communities include members who have moral rights but not moral responsibilities, such as young children, mentally retarded adults, and permanently comatose adults. We grant moral rights to these people because they still have interests even if they do not have responsibilities. Moral patients do not have all the rights accorded to moral agents. For instance, children do not have the right to vote, the right to enter a contract, or the right to marry, but they do have some basic rights, such as the right to life, the right to health, and so on.

Animals, according to Regan (1983), are moral patients because they have inherent value. By this he means that animals are capable of valuing their own experiences and their own lives. They can prefer pleasure to pain, freedom to captivity, and life to death. They have perception, memory, and a sense of their own past and future. Since animals have inherent value, one should treat them just like other beings that have inherent value, because inherent value does not come in degrees. Indeed, it would be a form of speciesism to insist that humans have more inherent value than do animals. Thus, animals should be accorded the same rights that we grant to other moral patients, such as children. According to Regan, and many other writers, the purpose of rights is to serve as moral "trump cards" to protect and promote individual interests. For example, when we say that a person has a right to vote, we imply that this right should not be taken away in order to promote a greater good. Animal rights also function as moral trumps cards that forbid us from sacrificing animals for some "greater good." In particular, we should not use animals in experiments that are not designed to promote their interests. Because more than 99% of animal experiments yield no benefits for the experimental subject, almost all animal experiments are immoral (Regan 1983). The only kind of animal experiment that could be justified would be an experiment that is designed to benefit the animal or promote its interests. Here we can draw an analogy with the ethics of experimentation on children: according to most research ethics regulations and policies, we should conduct research on children that is more than minimal risk only if the benefits to the subjects outweigh the risks. Research on children should promote that subject's best interests (Glantz 1998).

Many different writers have criticized Regan's view. Some of the critiques address the theoretical underpinnings of his position and argue that he has not adequately explained how animals can have rights (Carruthers 1992). First, one might ask whether the claim that animals *really* value their own experiences and their own lives has any plausibility. The word "value" connotes more than having a preference, want, or desire: to value something, one must make a judgment about the worth of that thing. Wanting a drink of water is not the same thing as a valuing a drink of water: a person who values a drink of water also makes a judgment that the water is good in some respect, for example, good for quenching thirst. It is not at all clear that animals have the cognitive capacity to make judgments about value even if they have desires or preferences.

Second, according to most accounts of rights, rights promote or protect interests (Feinberg 1973). An interest, on this view, is a something that one *needs* to promote one's overall well-being. For example, people need food, shelter, freedom, companionship, freedom from pain, and many other things that promote well-being. Regan's view implies that animals also have various interests, such as interests in living, in freedom of movement, in food and water, and in freedom from pain. But how can we make sense of the interests of animals? If we are not careful, we may find ourselves accepting the idea that plants have interests, if we maintain that animals have interests. Plants need water, sunlight, and soil to grow and flourish. But do plants have interests? This view seems patently absurd. So, there must be some difference between an interest and a *biological* need. One might argue that interests are different from biological needs in several ways. First, beings with interests are aware of those interests. Second, beings with interests can communicate those interests. Although a plant may need water, it is not aware of this need, nor can it communicate it (as far as we know). Although laboratory mice may be aware of their biological needs in some sense, they cannot communicate those needs.

Finally, other writers have objected to the practical problems with making sense of animal rights (LaFollette and Shanks 1996). One problem would be how we should resolve conflicts of rights among animals. For example, if a lion and a zebra both have a right to life, should we stop the lion from killing the zebra in order to protect the zebra's rights? How do we weigh the rights of a beaver to make a dam against the rights of those animals who will have their homes flooded if the beaver makes a dam? If we accept the idea that animals have rights, and that these rights are held equally, then there are no satisfactory solutions to these types of problems. To solve these issues, we would need to have some way of assigning value to various rights claims, for example, that the lion's right to food is more important than the zebra's right to life. But this opens the door to assigning greater value to the rights of human beings, which is a move that Regan wishes to avoid. If we say that animals and human beings both have rights but that human rights are more important, then we can also justify animal experimentation on the grounds that human rights to health and welfare outweigh animal rights to life, freedom from pain, and so on.

Although we think that Singer's and Regan's critiques of animal research have some serious flaws, they offer society and the research community some important lessons about our treatment of animals. In particular, these critiques allow one to see more clearly the importance of developing an account of the moral status of animals that is sensitive to both the similarities and differences between humans and animals (LaFollette and Shanks 1996). Singer and Regan, incidentally, do recognize that there are moral differences between humans and animals (Regan and Singer, 1989). Singer (1975 [1990], 1985) holds that it is worse to kill a normal human adult with rational life than to kill a mouse, and Regan (1983) admits that if one must choose between saving the life of a human and saving the life of an animal, greater harm will occur if one does not save the human. But these concessions offer little comfort to those who place much greater value on human life than on animal life.

On the other hand, it is important to remember that for many years many researchers held very little respect or consideration for animal pain or suffering. Some, such as the Cartesians and the behaviorists described above, adopted this stance based on their judgment that animals are unthinking, unfeeling, and nonconscious beings, much like robots (Rollin 1992). We believe that the most sensible view lies somewhere between the extreme positions staked out by Singer and Regan on the one hand, and the Cartesians and behaviorists on the other. Most people, including most researchers, believe that we have moral duties toward animals and that we should respect and promote the welfare of animals (Bulger 1987). For example, most researchers favor extending the Animal Welfare Act to laboratory animals, including rats and mice (Plous and Herzog 2000). However, many people, including researchers, also recognize the importance of animal research (Botting and Morrision 1997). The only way to make sense of the competing claims is to adopt the view that animals have moral status (or moral value) but that human beings have a greater value (Frey 1980). There are degrees of moral value, and not all species have the same moral worth. To understand this kind of view, we now discuss why human beings have moral worth and why differences between humans and animals imply differences in moral worth. We believe that the value of a species depends on its degree of similarity to the human species: species that closely resemble humans, such as chimpanzees, have greater moral worth than do species with little in common with humans, such as cockroaches.

So what makes human life valuable? To answer this question, we first need to draw a distinction between intrinsic and extrinsic value. Something is intrinsically valuable if it is valuable for its own sake; something is extrinsically valuable if it is valuable for the sake of something else. Human life is both intrinsically and extrinsically valuable. For example, a person may have value as a soldier in a war, as another laborer in a factory, as a source of organs for transplantation, and so on. There are many things in society that we view as extrinsically valuable, such as money, real estate, commodities, and so on. But human life has more than extrinsic value; it also has intrinsic value. So what makes human life intrinsically valuable? We do not think there is a single answer to this question. Instead, we offer a list of characteristics that people frequently mention when defending the value of human life:

- Free will: the ability to make decisions and freely act on them
- Rationality: the ability to solve problems and make judgments and inferences; the ability to develop abstract ideas and theories
- Creativity: the ability to come up with new ideas, behaviors, solutions, and expressions

- Emotion/Feeling: the ability to experience anger, fear, joy, sadness, jealousy, and other emotions; the ability to experience moral emotions, such as sympathy and empathy; the ability to feel pleasure or pain
- Spirituality: the ability to form a concept of higher power or being; the need to find meaning in life and a connection to the whole universe
- Morality: the ability to choose between right and wrong; the ability to experience moral emotions
- Personality: the ability to form and act upon various traits of character, such as honesty, courage, kindness, humor, modesty, sincerity, loyalty, and integrity
- Communication: the ability to communicate thoughts through language; the ability to understand language
- Self-consciousness: the awareness of being aware; the awareness of one's self in one's environment; the awareness of the past and anticipation of the future; the awareness of one's own thoughts, feelings, judgments, personality traits, and decisions
- Consciousness: awareness of sensory stimulation

Items in this list should not be surprising to most readers; since ancient times, philosophers and theologians have discussed these features of human life. (This list also has some relevance to question about the status of the human fetus; see chapter 11.)

If we apply this analysis to animals, we can say that animal life also has extrinsic value: animals are valuable sources of food, clothing, labor, amusement, companionship, and so on. But assigning animals extrinsic value provides very little in the way of any moral restriction of our conduct toward animals. One might appeal to the extrinsic value of animals in many different ways to justify restrictions on our conduct toward animals. For example, one might argue

- that it is wrong to torture a cat because people find this to be degrading or offensive
- that it is wrong to kill dolphins because people like dolphins
- that it is wrong to kill lions because people think lions are beautiful
- that it is wrong to exterminate prairie dogs because they play a vital role in the ecosystem of the Great Plains of North America
- that it is wrong to cause an animal species to become extinct because the species is an important source of biodiversity
- that it is wrong to harm an animal because a person who harms an animal is more likely to harm a human being

These arguments, while important, are highly contingent, relativistic, and tentative because they depend on human wants, beliefs, and desires or features of the ecology. For instance, if no one liked dolphins, then it might be acceptable to kill dolphins; if prairie dogs did not play a vital role in the ecology, then it might be acceptable to exterminate them; if people were not offended by

someone who tortures a cat, then it might be acceptable to torture a cat, and
so on. For these reasons as well as others, it is important to show that animals
have intrinsic value, not just extrinsic value (Taylor 1986). Thus, it is wrong to
torture a cat because this act harms a valuable life, not just because people find
it offensive.

So how might one *prove* that animals have intrinsic value? How does one
prove that anything has intrinsic value, for that matter? We suggest that the
process of assigning intrinsic value to something is not entirely rational, in
that one does not arrive at judgments of intrinsic value based solely on empirical evidence or logical argument. In ethics and morality, judgments of intrinsic value are basic premises (or assumptions or axioms). Over 2300 years ago
Aristotle argued that one cannot "prove" basic premises; one accepts basic
premises and then makes arguments on the basis of those premises (McKeon
1947). Since that time, other philosophers have argued that it is not possible
to conclusively "prove" that one should accept basic principles of deductive
logic such as modus ponens, basic principles of inductive logic such as Bayes'
Theorem, or basic axioms of Euclidean geometry such as the parallel postulate
(Quine 1969, Putnam 1981).

So how does one come to accept basic premises? Arguments can be helpful,
but experience is also important. For example, consider how one develops an
appreciation for a piece of classical music, such as Mozart's *Eine Kleine Nacht-
musik*. You might start to like this piece after someone convinces you by means
of an argument that this is good music. Someone might argue that the music
is well ordered, creative, intelligent, expressive, lively, and so on. But you will
probably only come to appreciate this piece after listening to it. You experience the value or worth of the music after becoming familiar with the music.
Some might even describe this psychological phenomenon as a "conversion"
experience or a Gestalt shift: you simply come to "see" the value of the music
much as you come to "see" that a picture of a witch is also a picture of a young
woman. We suggest that the same psychological mechanisms apply to coming to appreciate the intrinsic value of animals: arguments can play a role in
helping us to accept the value of animals, but we also must have some experience with those animals in order to fully appreciate their value. For instance,
if you have never had a pet pig, then an argument may convince you of the
worth of the pig, but you will not truly appreciate the worth of the pig until
you have come to know the pig, much in the same way that one would come
to know the worth of Mozart's music.

Although we admit that it is not possible to *conclusively prove* that animals
have intrinsic value, we do believe that *arguments by analogy* can play a role in
helping people come to appreciate the value of animals. We assume, therefore,
that people already accept the claim that human beings have intrinsic value. To
show that animals also have intrinsic value, one may construct an argument by
analogy with human beings: animals have value insofar as they are like human
beings. As the analogy increases in strength, the value of animals should also increase (LaFollette and Shanks 1996). An argument by analogy does not conclusively establish basic premises about moral worth, but it can help people be-

come more willing to accept those premises. To develop the analogy between humans and animals, one must consider the above list of characteristics of human life and ask whether animals are like us in relevant ways.

Many of these questions are very difficult questions to answer and require a great deal of scientific investigation and research. After many years of treating questions about animal cognition and emotion as "unscientific," we are just now beginning to understand in greater detail important aspects of animal consciousness, experience, emotion, self-consciousness, and communication (Bonner 1980, Rollin 1989, Griffin 1992, De Waal 1996). Evidence that can help us answer these questions can come from the study of animal behavior, evolution, genetics, physiology, neurology, or endocrinology. Because different animal species have different behavioral, physiological, neurological, genetic, and biochemical traits as well as different evolutionary histories, it is likely that some species will be more like humans than other species. For example, given what we know about chimpanzees and mice, we have a strong argument that chimpanzees are more like humans than are mice. Thus, chimpanzees have greater moral worth than do mice. One can make similar comparisons for other species, such as dogs, cats, elephants, dolphins, monkeys, birds, and so on.

Ethical Animal Experimentation and Scientific Validity

How does this argument, that the more like humans a species is, the more moral worth its members have, apply to experimentation on animals? Before deciding whether to conduct an experiment on animal, we must decide whether it is morally acceptable to use the animal in the experiment, given the purpose of the study, the experimental design, the methods used, and the species of the animal. If we decide that the animal has some moral value and that the experiment would harm the animal in some way (e.g., by causing pain, suffering, disability, or death), then we must argue that the experiment can be ethically justified, given the expected benefits. What this view implies is that researchers can conduct experiments on animals, provided that they provide a sufficient moral justification for the experiments (LaFollette and Shanks 1996). Because many different animal species may have some degree of moral value, the moral burden of proof rests with researchers who plan to conduct experiments on animals; researchers do not simply have a moral "free ticket" or "blank check" regarding animal experimentation. Moreover, because animal species may differ with respect to their moral worth, an experiment can be morally acceptable on one species but not be morally acceptable in a different species. For example, it may be morally acceptable to create a transgenic mouse that is prone to various forms of cancer (i.e., an oncomouse), but it may not be morally acceptable to create an "oncochimp" or an "oncomonkey," because chimpanzees and monkeys have more moral value than do mice by virtue of their higher degree of similarity to human beings.

Because animal species have some degree of intrinsic value, our view also provides justification for a policy that resembles the three "Rs" of animal research defended by Russell and Birch (1959):

- Replacement: When it is possible to answer a research question without using an animal, replace the animal use methodology with a methodology that does not use animals. When it is possible to answer a scientific question using a morally "lower" species of animal, replace the "higher" species with a lower one.
- Reduction: When it is possible to answer a research question using a smaller number of animals, reduce the number of animals used.
- Refinement: Wherever possible, refine research methods, techniques, concepts, and tools to reduce the need for animals in research and to reduce harms to animals, such as pain, suffering, disability, and death.

The three Rs can be justified on the grounds that they minimize harm to animals and promote animal welfare within the context of animal experimentation. Of course, these three Rs make sense only if one believes that the research protocols are likely to yield results with scientific, medical, or social value. Thus, a fourth R should also apply to animal research:

- Relevance: Research protocols that use animals should address questions that have some scientific, medical, or social relevance; all risks/arms to animals need to be balanced against benefits to humans and animals.

Finally, a fifth R is also important (and plays a key role in U.S. animal research regulations):

- Redundancy avoidance: Avoid redundancy in animal research whenever possible—make sure to do a thorough literature search to ensure that the experiment has not already been done. If it has already been done, provide a good justification for repeating the work. Avoiding redundancy is important to avoid using animals unnecessarily and to save research resources.

This approach to the ethics of animal experimentation suggests that researchers also need to address the five Rs relating to the scientific validity of every research protocol they propose, because these issues can affect the ethical soundness of the research. This idea is conceptually similar to examining scientific validity of human experimentation: good experimental design is a moral requirement for human subjects research because a poorly designed experiment may not yield generalizable knowledge and may therefore impose unnecessary risks on human subjects (Levine 1988). Some of the scientific issues that researchers need to address are as follows:

(1) The scientific need to do the experiment at all: If the experiment has already been done, it may or may not be worth repeating. Although it is often important to repeat new experimental findings, unnecessary repetition should be avoided (redundancy avoidance).

(2) The appropriateness of the animal model: Animal research protocols specify the species used to answer a research questions. These protocols should therefore provide a rationale for the particular species chosen; they should de-

scribe how the experiment would provide evidence that is relevant to the research question. For example, if one is interested in learning about the conduction of nerve signals along axons, then the squid may be a good animal model because it has giant axons that are easy to study. Moreover, knowledge about squid axons may be generalized to other species. If one wants to know whether a specific chemical is likely to be toxic or carcinogenic in humans, then it is important to use an animal species that is metabolically similar to the human species. For many years, researchers have more or less assumed that toxicity studies in mice can be generalized to humans, but this assumption is now being questioned (LaFollette and Shanks 1996). For example, researchers at one time thought that saccharin can cause bladder cancer in humans based on studies in which mice were fed huge doses of the saccharin and then formed tumors in their bladders. However, we know that laboratory mice have a mechanism of waste elimination that is different from the human mechanism. When mice eliminate saccharin, they build up uric acid crystals in their bladders. Human beings, on the other hand, do not form these crystals. Thus, conclusions about the carcinogenic effects of saccharin in laboratory mice probably do not apply to human beings.

(3) The number of animals used: The principle of reduction implies that researchers should reduce the number of animals used, whenever this does not affect their ability to obtain useful data, but researchers must also make sure that they use enough animals to obtain statistically significant data and results. Otherwise, the experiment causes unjustifiable harm to the animal subjects. Here, good statistical design and ethical practice go hand in hand (see the discussion of statistics in chapter 2).

(4) Efforts to promote animal welfare and reduce animal harm: Because animal research should promote animal welfare and minimize animal harm wherever possible, researchers need to take measures to minimize pain, suffering, disability, and death. Researchers must consider the appropriate use of analgesia and anesthesia; humane forms of euthanasia, when this is required for pathological findings; appropriate and sterile surgical procedures; disease control; and living conditions, such as nutrition, living space, and exercise. The United States and many other countries have many regulations addressing these issues (discussed below). However, although regulations govern this important aspect of research, we want to stress that these regulations have a sound moral justification; they are not needless rules or "red tape" (LaFollette and Shanks 1996).

(5) Alternatives to the animal model: As mentioned above, the principle of replacement implies that researchers should find alternatives to animal models, wherever possible. In the last few decades, scientists have made greater strides in developing alternatives to animal models, such as tissue cultures and computer simulations (Office of Technology Assessment 1986, LaFollette and Shanks 1996, Stokstad 1999). We encourage further developments in this direction. However, it is unlikely that researchers will be able to completely eliminate the need for animal subjects, because many complex physiological, behavioral, and developmental phenomena can be understood only within the

context of a whole organism. For example, to understand how a vaccine protects an organism against infection, one must eventually use the vaccine in whole organisms. Inferences about the vaccine from tissue cultures or computer models simply will not provide relevant knowledge about whole organisms. Most research questions related to animal behavior, such as research on Parkinson's disease, obesity, aggression, and addiction, will probably require whole organisms.

REGULATIONS

Here we briefly review some of the regulations that govern research on animals in the United States. Many of these regulations embody the ethical and scientific considerations mentioned earlier in this chapter. The two main laws that govern animal research in the United States are the 1966 Animal Welfare Act (AWA), since revised several times (1970, 1976, 1985), and the U.S. Public Health Service (PHS) *Policy on the Humane Care and Use of Laboratory Animals* (PHS 2000b; see also VandenBerg et al. 1999). The PHS policy applies only to animal research conducted using PHS funds, but the AWA applies to all animal research. In addition, many research institutions and professional societies have their own guidelines for the humane care and use of animals in research (Bennett 1994). There are also private organizations, such as the American Association for the Accreditation of Laboratory Animal Care (AAALAC), that accredit research institutions. Institutions can legally conduct animal research without AAALAC accreditation, but accreditation stills plays an important role in shaping research practices.

The PHS policy applies to all vertebrate animals used in research supported by USPHS funds. The National Institutes of Health (NIH) is one of the units of the PHS, and the largest in supporting research with animals. The PHS policy requires compliance with AWA and the National Research Council (NRC) *Guide for the Care and Use of Laboratory Animals* (1996). The Office for Protection from Research Risks (OPRR) is the NIH office responsible for monitoring recipients of USPHS funds for compliance with the regulations. Compliance with the OPRR takes the form of a written assurance of compliance by the research institution. OPRR can inspect animal care facilities "for cause."

The AWA, originally titled the "Laboratory Animal Welfare Act," promulgates rules that apply the commercialization and use of animals, including the use animals in research. Animals originally covered by the AWA included (nonhuman) primates, dogs, cats, guinea pigs, hamsters, and rabbits (Bennett 1994). In 1970 the AWA was expanded to cover all warm-blooded animals, but in 1976 the Secretary of Agriculture excluded rats, mice, birds, farm animals, and horses from being covered under the AWA. The U.S. Department of Agriculture (USDA) oversees compliance with AWA. In 2000 the USDA announced a plan, later suspended, to once again include rats, mice, and birds under the AWA (Malakoff 2000). Although some researchers have objected to including rats, mice, and birds under the AWA, polls suggest that many researchers welcome this change (Plous and Herzog 2000).

Both the AWA and the USPHS policies stipulate rules and guidelines for the humane care and use of animals in research. These regulations address a variety of issues, including living conditions, such as cage sizes, food, and exercise; efforts to reduce pain and discomfort, including analgesia and anesthesia; surgical procedures, including antiseptic procedures and euthanasia methods; veterinary care and disease prevention and control; procurement and transportation; and the qualifications, health, and safety of personnel. The NRC's *Guide for the Care and Use of Laboratory Animals* spells out many of the standards for animal experimentation contained in AWA and PHS regulations. The NRC established the Institute for Laboratory Animal Research to study, prepare, and distribute documents on the care and use of animals in the research community. The AAALAC also considers the NRC guide when deciding whether to accredit an institution. All researchers and students are advised to consult the NRC guide when preparing animal experimentation protocols and proposals (Bennett 1994, VandenBerg et al. 1999).

The AWA and USPHS regulations also address institutional responsibilities for ensuring and promoting the humane care and use of animals in research. These regulations require that institutions that conduct animal research to establish an institutional animal care and use committee (IACUC) to review and approve animal research protocols and to monitor animal research. IACUCs are also charged with educating researchers about scientific and ethical aspects of animal research and relevant regulations. IACUC members should include a veterinarian, a scientist, and a community representative. Many IACUCs also include an ethicist or a lawyer. IACUCs have the authority to stop any animal research protocol that does not meet the standards set forth in relevant policies. IACUCs also conduct inspections of laboratories on a biannual basis. IACUCs function much like institutional review boards (IRBs) in that both of these research committees are charged with ensuring institutional compliance with relevant regulations and with protecting research subjects.

QUESTIONS FOR DISCUSSION

1. How can we know whether an animal can feel pain or suffer?
2. What is the difference between the ability to feel pain and the ability to suffer? Do you agree with this distinction? Why or why not?
3. Do you agree with Singer that speciesism is like racism? Do you think speciesism can be justified? Why or why not?
4. What is the moral status of nonhuman animals? Do they have rights? Should we promote their welfare?
5. What criteria should we use to decide whether a being has moral status, that is, whether it is a member of the moral community?
6. Are there some types of animal experiments that you regard as unethical? Why?
7. Do you think that animal research always has important benefits for human beings? Are there some types of research that are not very beneficial?

8. Do you think animal research is overregulated, underregulated, or is regulated just about the right amount?
9. Are there some ways in which we take better care of animals in research than we do humans?

CASE STUDIES

Case 1

A graduate student, while conducting an experiment for her mentor on repairing spinal chord injuries in rats, severs the spinal chord, allows the rat to heal, determines the degree of paralysis, and then injects neural stem cells into the site. She will use 25 rats in her protocol. In one of the experiments, one of the rats dies after surgery, and her mentor replaces the rat. She asks him what he planned to do in response to this death, and he says nothing. She prods him a bit further, and he says that he knows why the rat died—he gave the rat too much anesthetic—and he doesn't think the death will have any effect on the experiment's results. He also does not want the IACUC to know about the death.

- How should the graduate student respond?
- What should the IACUC do if it finds out about this incident?

Case 2

A researcher is planning to test a new analgesic medication in dogs. The medication may prove useful in relieving pain associated with severe burns. To conduct the experiment, he will use two groups of 12 dogs each, an experimental group and a control group. Both groups will receive a burn on the back. Both will receive treatment for the burn, but only one group will receive the medication under study. He will also attempt to measure their degree of pain and discomfort by touching the burn to evoke a response, such as behavioral clues, heart rate, and blood pressure.

- Would you approve of this experiment? Why or why not?

Case 3

The army is developing a new lightweight helmet for soldiers. It plans to test the helmet first on animals with heads similar to the human head, including chimpanzees. In the tests, the animals wearing the helmets will be subjected to head trauma, including gunshots and blows with an iron pipe. After the trauma, the researchers will examine the helmet and the animal to determine the extent of damage. Animals will receive CT scans and will be followed for several months after the event. If animals require surgery to repair an injury, they will receive it. The animals will also receive appropriate analgesia during the experiments and may be euthanized, if necessary.

- Is this experiment ethical? Why or why not?

Case 4

A cosmetics company is developing a new hair dye for eyebrows. Currently, there are no hair dyes for eyebrows that are safe for human use, because these dyes can cause blindness. In testing the new dye, the company will use rabbits. It will drop dye into the rabbits' eyes and measure the degree of injury. Rabbits will receive treatment for eye injuries as well as appropriate anesthesia and analgesia. When the study is complete, the rabbits will be euthanized for pathologic analysis.

- Should the company be allowed to do this experiment? Why or why not?

Case 5

Researchers are developing an HIV vaccine and would like to test it on (non-human) primates before they test it on humans. Because HIV does not cause AIDS in primates, the researchers are planning to test their vaccines using two different viruses, a mutated form of HIV that can cause AIDS symptoms in primates, and a simian immunodeficiency virus (SIV), similar to HIV, that can cause simian AIDS. The researchers plan to develop vaccines to both viruses and inject these vaccines into the primates. They will inject live viruses into one group of primates and give a control group live viruses but no vaccinations. They will provide appropriate veterinary care to all subjects and will euthanize all subjects at the end of the study treatment for pathologic studies.

- Do you believe this experiment is ethical? Why or why not?

Case 6

Surgeons are developing a robotic device for performing heart surgery. The device, if successful, would be a safer and more reliable way to perform heart surgery than current human techniques. One of the main benefits of the robotic system is that it minimizes unstable movements. It is also expected to reduce the risk of infection. In developing the device, the surgeons are planning to test it on dogs, cats, and pigs. They also plan to use animals to teach surgeons how to use the device. For each animal, the protocol will include a surgical procedure followed by a postoperative recovery period, followed by euthanasia and pathologic analysis. One of the research protocols also involves using the device for emergency surgery to respond to heart trauma, such as gunshot or knife wounds. For this protocol, animals will be shot or stabbed and prepared for surgery. All animals will be given appropriate analgesia and anesthesia.

- Would you approve of this protocol? Why or why not?

Case 7

A researcher is studying aggression in rats. She is experimenting with a variety of environmental and hormonal influences on aggression in order to study the relationship between aggression and overcrowding, stress, food deprivation, and levels of sex hormones. In some of her experiments, she will be place rats in crowded cages; in others she will deprive them of food; in others, she will give them high doses of testosterone. She will attempt to minimize pain and discomfort to the rats, but they are likely to fight and injure each other.

- Would you allow the researcher to do this experiment? Why or why not?

Case 8

Researchers at a company are developing a new insect repellant as an alternative to their current products. They plan to assess its toxic effects on animals. Among other tests, they plan to use the "lethal dose 50%" (LD_{50}), in which they will expose 100 mice to the amount of chemical required to kill 50% of the subjects. Other tests will expose groups of 100 subjects to lower doses of the chemical to observe other effects, such as seizures, anemia, organ failure, and malnutrition. The rats will be given the chemical in several different ways, including orally and intravenously. They will also have the chemical applied to their skin and eyes. All rats will be euthanized for pathologic analysis.

- Is this experimental ethical?

Case 9

Researchers are developing an animal model for a rare genetic disorder known as osteogenesis imperfecta. Children born with this disorder have a genetic mutation that prevents them from forming strong bones. Neonates usually have many broken bones at birth and usually die within 6 months, or within a year at most. They usually also have severe brain damage, organ damage, and a variety of infections. Researchers plan to develop a transgenic mouse with a genetic defect that results in a condition similar to osteogenesis imperfecta. They will study the etiology of the disease in mice as well as a variety of treatment modalities.

- Do you have an ethical problem with this experiment?

Case 10

A researcher is conducting experiments with transgenic oncomice on tumor suppression. In his experiments, he allows the mice to develop cancerous tumors, and he then treats them with different gene therapy vectors designed to inhibit cell cancer growth. Two graduate students and two lab technicians work with him on his project. Last week, one of his graduate students informed the IACUC chair that several mice had developed tumors that impeded their free movement in the cages. The tumors were growing around their front legs, and on their chests. The graduate student also reported that the researcher has been out of town consulting with biotech companies and has not been paying close attention to work being conducted in his lab.

- How should the IACUC handle this problem?

11

Genetics and Human Reproduction

This chapter provides background and an overview of genetics and human reproduction, including its scientific, social, and historical context. The chapter mentions ethical issues that arise in different areas of research related to genetics and human reproduction, including genetic testing and screening, genetic counseling, prenatal genetic testing, preimplantation genetic testing, surrogate pregnancy, reproductive cloning, somatic gene therapy, stem cell research, and genetic engineering of plants, animals, and humans. It also outlines some traditional critiques of attempts to control or manipulate human genetics and reproduction.

This chapter and chapter 12 address topics that are quite different from those covered in the rest of the book. Chapters 2 through 10 address ethical problems and issues that arise within the process of research itself, and do not discuss in any significant depth issues that arise because of the effects of research on society or the social context of research. Many issues, such as concerns about authorship, plagiarism, data management, publication, and peer review, have important impacts on the integrity of research but often have little direct impact on society. Other issues, such as intellectual property and the use of animal and human subjects, raise important issues for researchers and for society. This chapter and the next address topics that arise when scientists consider the social impact of research and its social context. This chapter considers ethical issues in genetics and human reproduction. (Much of the material covered in this chapter will be familiar to students of the biological sciences, and we apologize in advance for any material that seems introductory. However, many students of physics, chemistry, psychology, the humanities, and other disciplines are not familiar with some of the basic facts pertaining to genetics and human reproduction. Moreover, it is impossible to understand the ethical and political issues without having a firm grasp of the relevant scientific, historical, and social facts.)

THE DARWINIAN REVOLUTION

Charles Darwin's (1809–1882) theory of evolution by natural selection was one of the most significant scientific developments in the nineteenth century. The publication of Darwin's book *The Origin of Species* (1859) had profound effects on the biological and social sciences as well as philosophy, politics, literature, and religion. Before this time, most scientists believed that all species, including human beings, did not change or evolve over time. Species were regarded as fixed forms or archetypes created and made by God (or Nature), and human beings were regarded as fundamentally different from animals because humans and animals have different essences, or defining features. This "essentialist" approach had been developed by Aristotle and was articulated by such esteemed scientists as Carl Linnaeus, George Cuvier, and Louis Agassiz. Before Darwin developed his theory, scientists such as Lamark had defended the idea of evolution. Moreover, the Enlightenment idea of "progress" had a significant influence on the science and philosophy of the era.

Darwin germinated his theory during his five-year voyage as the ship's naturalist on the *H.M.S. Beagle*, but he did not publish his ideas for two decades to ensure that he could develop a clear, cogent, and well-documented argument for evolution. Darwin synthesized an abundance of evidence that species evolve, from a variety of sources, including island biogeography, the fossil record, and selective breeding. His theory provided an explanation of this evidence under a common principle: organisms within a common population that are better able to survive and reproduce than their competitors in a given environment will transmit their characteristics to the next generation. Over time, those characteristics (or phenotypes) that confer an adaptive advantage to their possessors will persist and spread through the population: the "fittest" will survive.

Darwin also argued that all living things, including human beings, are descended from common ancestors. The argument for common descent generated more controversy than any other aspect of his theory because it challenged religious claims that human beings have a special place in the creation (Mayr 1982). It implied that man is not different from the other animals. Indeed, Darwin argued that cognitive, emotive, social, and moral traits found in man had evolved from "lower" animals.

SOCIAL IMPLICATIONS OF COMMON DESCENT

The idea of "common descent" from animals has had profound implications for ethics, philosophy, and religion (Dennett 1995). The initial reaction from many religious groups was to vilify Darwin's theory and regard it as sacreligious because it removed man from the center of God's creation and made him just an animal. In 1927, the famous John Scopes "Monkey Trial" pitted creationists against evolutionists in battle over teaching Darwin's ideas in the public schools. This battle continues today, as evidenced by the debate in Kansas about teaching evolution in public schools (Dennett 1995, Dalton 1999). Additionally, philosophers and ethicists have been examining Darwin's theory in light of moral theories and principles. As discussed in chapter 10, most moral theories and principles hold that human beings are more valuable than animals, and this idea implies what Peter Singer calls "speciesism." How can we make sense of the worth we place on human beings once we realize that we are descended from animals and in fact share 98% of our DNA with chimpanzees?

Another idea that had a profound effect on science and politics was improving our species through selective breeding. People began to realize that the same principles of selective breeding that apply to plants and animals might also apply to the human population. This led to the idea of eugenics, or controlled breeding of the human population to promote "desirable" or eliminate "undesirable" characteristics. Founders of the eugenics movement include Francis Galton, who argued for selective breeding in human beings, and Herbert Spencer, who defended the "struggle for existence" as a principle of social policy known as social Darwinism. According to this idea, society should allow its weakest members to perish and should encourage the survival of its strongest members. This idea was used to justify laissez faire capitalism as an approach to social and economic policy, that is, capitalism with little government regulation and no social safety net. In the 1890s, the German philosopher Friedrich Nietzsche incorporated some ideas of Darwinism into his writings. Nietzsche described existence as "will to power" and envisioned the emergence of an *ubermensch* (superman) who would be superior to normal human beings. Nietzsche's writings influenced many writers, philosophers, and politicians, among them Adolph Hitler (1889–1945).

During the early twentieth century, many states in the United States and countries in Europe adopted eugenics laws and policies, including immigration quotas based on race and ethnicity and mandatory sterilization laws for the "feeble-minded." In the United States, the Supreme Court upheld mandatory sterilization laws in *Buck v. Bell* (1927). Nazi Germany extended eugenics ideas even further, with mandatory sterilization for people with schizophrenia, blindness, alcoholism, feeble-mindedness, and physical deformities. The Nazis also sterilized people of Jewish ancestry and enacted laws forbidding Aryans to breed with Jews, to promote "racial purity." They eventually exterminated millions of Jews and other "impure" or "inferior" people in the name of cleansing the Fatherland (Kevles 1995).

MENDELIAN GENETICS

Although Darwin's theory of evolution is one of the most impressive works in the history of science, it lacked a satisfactory explanation or mechanism of inheritance. According to a theory popular during Darwin's time, known as the blending theory, different traits or characters blended during reproduction. Thus, if one bred a tall pea plant with a short pea plant, the resulting offspring should be average-sized pea plants. The problem with this theory is that breeding experiments often do not result in the blending of traits. Moreover, the theory could not account for the variety of traits one finds within species, because variety should decrease over time as different traits blend together. The Austrian monk Gregor Mendel (1822–1884) provided a solution to this problem with his theory of inheritance. According to Mendel, different characters (traits or phenotypes) are caused by different factors (genes or genotypes), which can be inherited. The combination of these factors determines the types of traits one observes in breeding experiments. For any given phenotype, there are two factors, one from each parent. These factors randomly assort during reproduction to produce different combinations. Moreover, some of these factors "dominate" other factors; for example, a tall plant and a short plant might produce tall and short plants in the next generation but not "average" or blended plants. An organism that has two identical copies of a factor is homozygous for that factor, whereas an organism with two different copies is heterozygous.

Mendel developed his laws of inheritance during his famous breeding experiments involving peas. Unfortunately, most scientists, including Darwin, ignored his work, which was not appreciated or discovered until the early 1900s, when DeVries, Correns, Hunt, Morgan, Hardy, Weinberg, Fisher, and others developed the discipline known as Mendelian genetics (Mayr 1982). As a side note on scientific honesty, some commentators have argued that Mendel may have "fudged" his results because the ratios he claims to have observed are "too good to be true." R.A. Fisher, an eminent biologist and statistician, analyzed Mendel's results and argued that they do not contain the types of random statistical variations one finds in genuine scientific data. Today, the Office of Research Integrity uses similar methods to prove that data have been fabricated (Broad and Wade 1982 [1993]).

CELLS, TISSUES, EMBRYOS, AND ORGANISMS

In the 1900s, this new science of genetics became integrated into the established sciences of cytology, embryology, pathology, immunology, and physiology. During the 1800s, biologists and pathologists such as Schwann, Schleiden, Weissman, Roux, Huxley, Pasteur, and Koch had developed the cell theory. Thus, by the end of the century scientists knew that all living things (except viruses) are made of cells; that cells are organized into tissues, which form organs and organ systems; that the physiological and behavioral traits and functions of multicellular organisms, including digestion, movement, growth, and reproduction, are made possible by activities occurring at the cellular level; that many diseases are caused by cellular pathogens, such as bacteria; and that cells have various parts, such as a membrane, mitochondria, the cytoplasm, Golgi bodies, and the nucleus. Biologists knew that the nucleus somehow transmits genetic information, but it took several decades to explain how this occurs.

From 1900 to the 1920s, cytologists and embryologists identified structures in the nucleus known as chromosomes, which carry genetic information. They studied different processes of cell replication known as mitosis and meiosis. In diploid organisms (i.e., organisms with two sets of chromosomes, such as most plants and animals), somatic cells (cells in the body) replicate using mitosis, a process whereby the chromosomes line up and divide, and then the cell separates to form two daughter cells, each with their own nuclei and cytoplasm. Diploid organisms use meiosis to produce haploid cells (cells with one set of chromosomes). These haploid cells are known as gametes, and the tissues that produce haploid cells are known as germ tissues. Together these constitute germ cells or the germ line. During sexual reproduction, male and female gametes (sperm and ova) fuse together to form a fertilized egg (or zygote), which becomes an embryo. The cells of the developing embryo undergo many millions of mitotic divisions as the embryo develops and differentiates.

In vertebrate animal species, shortly after fertilization the embryo becomes a hollow ball of cells, or blastocyst, which flattens out and divides into different layers of cells, the ectoderm, mesoderm, and endoderm. Cells from these different layers become different tissues. For example, ectodermal cells differentiate into the epidermis, hair, and nerves; endodermal cells become the liver, pancreas, bladder, and lining of the gut; and mesodermal cells become muscle, bone, cartilage, and blood (Ville 1977).

DNA, RNA, AND PROTEINS

By the 1930s, biologists had a solid understanding of cell structures and functions and the mechanisms of reproduction and development, but they still lacked precise knowledge of how chromosomes divide and how they transmit genetic information, and how they influence the activities of cells, tissues, and entire organisms. The fields of biochemistry and molecular biology began to emerge as biologists began to study organic molecules, such as proteins, lipids, hydrocarbons, hormones, vitamins, and nucleic acids. Biochemists also began to understand the chemical processes that occur in cells, such as aerobic and anaerobic metabolism, photosynthesis, chemical transport, and signaling.

By the 1940s and early 1950s, biologist began to learn more about the nucleic acids, deoxyribonucleic acid (DNA) and ribonucleic acid (RNA), and their role in transmitting genetic information. Although biologists knew that chromosomes contain DNA and proteins, they were still not sure whether or how chromosomes encode genetic information or how they are able to divide. Watson and Crick's discovery of the structure of DNA in 1953 provided the key to understanding heredity as well as cell regulation (Mayr 1982). Using data from chemical analysis, x-ray crystallography, and models of chemical bonding, Watson and Crick showed that DNA is a very long molecule composed of pairs of only four deoxyribonucleotides (or nucleotides) in two complementary strands that take a helical shape. The four nucleotides are deoxyguanosine monophosphate (G), deoxycytidine monophosphate (C), deoxyadenosine monophosphate (A), and thymidine monophosphate (T): A always pairs with T, and G with C. A strand of DNA consists of some combination of these basic units. For almost all organisms, hereditary information resides in combinations and permutations of G, C, A, and T. So, for example, the strand of nucleotides AATTCG would pair with the complementary strand TTAAGC. This "base pairing" provides the key to understanding how DNA can replicate itself: DNA replicates when an enzyme (DNA polymerase) causes the two complementary strands of DNA to unwind and separate. With a protein, other nucleotides nearby bond with their respective pairs, forming two new complementary strands.

Ribosomes in the cell translate the genetic information contained in DNA ("read the code") to manufacture proteins. Proteins are compounds that regulate cell function and growth and form basic cellular structures. For instance, all enzymes, receptors, hormones, and antigens are composed of proteins. Proteins provide the structural foundation for muscles, bone, hair, cartilage, nerves, membrane channels, chromosomes, ribosomes, and mitochondria. Proteins are long chemical structures composed of 20 amino acids. It takes three nucleotides to make one codon, which codes a single amino acid. Different combinations of nucleotides may code the same amino acid.

During the 1950s, scientists discovered the relation between DNA, RNA, and proteins known as the central dogma of molecular biology: DNA codes RNA, and RNA codes proteins. More precisely, this happens when a segment of DNA known as a promoter triggers the enzyme RNA polymerase, which starts a process where a segment of DNA is transcribed into messenger ribonucleic acid (mRNA). The DNA that constitutes the genes is double stranded, but the strands separate so that mRNA can form. The mRNA consists of sequences of nucleotides complementary to those of DNA: A becomes uracil (U), C becomes G, T becomes A, and G becomes C. After this initial transcription of DNA, two other types of RNA, transfer RNA (tRNA) and ribosomal RNA (rRNA), translate the message encoded in mRNA to form proteins. The entire machinery for protein synthesis from RNA resides in the ribosomes, which read the RNA and string together and process proteins. The process ends when another sequence of DNA, known as a terminator, triggers an enzyme that stops DNA transcription. Therefore, the sequence of events is as follows (the central dogma): DNA is transcribed into mRNA, and in turn mRNA is translated into proteins. Proteins have different structural properties, including the primary structure (the sequence of amino acids) as well as secondary, tertiary, and quaternary structures that are attached, which form the three-dimensional shape of the protein (Beaudet et al. 1995, Kitcher 1997).

A gene can be defined as the DNA sequence needed to code for the primary structure of a protein, which would include the region of DNA that codes for amino acids, as well as other sequences, such as promoters and terminators, that regulate protein synthesis. Not all of the genes in a cell function at the same time in the cell's life. Different genes are activated or deactivated at different times. For example, homeobox genes are important in development but may not function during adulthood. Some genes, known as "terminator" genes, play a key role in initiating the process of cell death, or apoptosis.

The human genome has an estimated 35,000 genes or approximately three billion base pairs (Claverie 2001, Beaudet et al. 1995). DNA consists of two regions: coding sequence (exons) and a non-coding sequence (introns), or so-called "junk DNA." Introns are cleaved off by an enzyme prior to duplicating the mRNA. Thus, the complementary DNA (cDNA) contains exon regions only; 90% of DNA consists of introns, but their precise functional role remains unknown. Introns known as single nucleotide polymorphisms (SNPs) vary from organism to organism and across species, and they are useful in reconstructing molecular evolution and phylogenies and in identifying individual human beings—DNA fingerprinting (Roberts 1992, Kitcher 1997). Almost all (99%) of the DNA in a cell resides in the nucleus (nDNA), but mitochondria also have their own DNA (mtDNA), which replicates, codes for proteins, and can be inherited through the maternal line. mtDNA plays an important role in coding proteins that carry out mitchondrial functions, such as oxidative phosphorylation and other metabolic processes.

A single gene may consist of a few hundred to a thousand base pairs, and a chromosome may contain thousands of genes. During a cell's resting stage (when it is not dividing), the chromosomes resemble long strings loosely contained in the nucleus. At the beginning of cell division, the DNA replicates, the chromosomes divide, and the long strings become a tightly wound structure. Chromosomes have proteins known as centromeres in their middle and telomeres at each end. Centromeres hold chromosome pairs together and attach to spindle fibers during cell division. The fibers are anchored to centrioles, which pull chromosome pairs to opposite sides of the nucleus during mitosis. Telomeres help keep chromosomes from unraveling. Each human cell contains 46 chromosomes, consisting of 22 pairs of nonsex chromosomes (or autosomes) from each parent and one sex chromosome from each parent. The ova and sperm are the only cells that each contain 23 chromosomes only (Beaudet et al. 1995).

MUTATIONS AND GENETIC DISEASES

DNA replication is not a perfect process. Many different changes in DNA known as mutations can occur before, during, or after replication. Random events, viruses, exposure to chemicals, radiation, or errors in the different steps of DNA transcription and translation cause mutations. Some common mutations include deletions, where DNA sequences are deleted; insertions, where an extra sequence is inserted; and transpositions, where sequences are transposed. Even a point mutation (i.e., deleting or inserting a single nucleotide) can lead to problems reading the DNA known as frame shifts. Thousands of different point mutations are associated with the disease cystic fibrosis. Larger mutations occur in diseases such as Down's syndrome, where individuals have a whole extra chromosome, and fragile X syndrome and Huntington's disease, where a codon multiplies itself in the genome over successive generations (Beaudet et al. 1995).

Cells attempt to correct mutations and have mechanisms for "proofreading" and repairing DNA. Although the word "mutation" connotes something bad or pathological, mutations produce the random variation that is crucial to the process of evolution. Indeed, it is likely that millions of years ago a variety of mutations allowed human beings to evolve from primate ancestors. Many mutations are neutral—they have no significant effect on evolution, survival, or reproduction. However, many other mutations cause abnormal conditions known as genetic diseases. A disease state arises when the product of the genetic code (i.e., the protein, which could include enzymes and non-enzyme proteins needed for structure and function of the cell) is not functioning at the needed level. The error in the genetic code could occur at the DNA or RNA levels. However, diseases can also occur not at the genetic code level but at the level of protein modification after the protein has been synthesized (posttranslational errors). For example, phenylalanine is coded in DNA as AAA and in mRNA as UUU, which becomes phenylalanine on translation. Therefore, any error in AAA or UUU will translate into a different amino acid in the protein and thus potentially create a dysfunctional protein. In sickle cell anemia, for example, patients have a mutation that causes the improper formation of hemoglobin, a protein that allows red blood cells to carry oxygen (Kitcher 1997). Mutations on mtDNA can cause metabolic disorders, such as mitochondrial encephalomyopathy with lactic acidosis and stroke (MELAS).

The frequency of mutations in somatic or germline cells depends on a complex array of factors. Some base pairs and some amino acids are more vulnerable to mutations than are others. Some mutations are inherited, and some are not; Duchenne dystrophy is both inherited and spontaneous. New mutations usually are not inherited unless they occur spontaneously in the germ cells. When mutations occur only in germ cells, then the offspring will inherit the phenotype (the apparent characteristics). However, other mutations can still cause diseases such as cancer. According to the "two-hit" theory of cancer, a cancer arises when both alleles of a gene develop a mutation (An allele is a gene at a locus on a chromosome with different DNA sequences.) If individuals inherit one mutated allele, they may develop cancer if the other allele develops a mutation as a result of chemical exposure, radiation, or some other cause.

There are about 6,000 loci (or points of mutation) in humans, and about 4,500 of these are known to cause diseases (Beaudet et al. 1995). In other words, of the 35,000 genes in humans, so far in evolution about 4,500 genetic mutations can cause diseases. At present, we have identified 2,500 of these genes. If we think of a genetic disease specifically as a condition, such as sickle cell anemia, which is caused by a heritable mutation, then nearly 10% of the human population has a genetic disease. However, genes can produce predispositions to develop disease even when they do not cause diseases. For example, BRCA1 and BRCA2 mutations give people a genetic predisposition to develop breast cancer: women with these mutations have an 80% lifetime risk of developing breast cancer, compared with 10% risk for women who lack the mutation. Taking this perspective into account, an estimated 60% of the human population has diseases with a significant genetic influence. Geneticists also use the term "penetrance" to describe genetic pathology: a gene is 100% penetrant if every person with the gene will develop the disease. For example, Huntington's disease is almost 100% penetrant, although it is exceedingly rare. Variability describes the opposite type of causal relationship: a disease is highly variable if it has many different causes other than genetic ones. For instance, breast cancer is highly variable in that only about 10% of breast cancers are caused by genetic mutations, and an even smaller number of these are caused by BRCA mutations. Down's syndrome (trisomy 21), on the other hand, has low variability in that it has no other known causes besides the mutation that produces three copies of the chromosome 21.

Genetic diseases are classified into four types based on the site of mutations: chromosomal disorders; monogenic disorders, where the disorder is a single gene mutation; multifactorial disorders, where the disease is due to several different single gene or chromosomal mutations; and mitochondrial disorders (discussed above). Monogenic disorders occur in about 10 per 1000 births, or 1% (Beaudet et al. 1995). Examples include familial hypercholesterolemia (1 in 500), Huntington's disease (1 in 2,500), and Marfan syndrome (1 in 20,000).

A disorder is said to be Mendelian if it follows Mendel's laws of inheritance and involves a single base-pair mutation and a single protein. Mendelian disorders include autosomal dominant disorders, such as Huntington's disease, in which the individual needs only one copy of the gene to be affected; autosomal recessive disorders, in which an individual must have both copies to be affected; and X-linked disorders, in which the gene is linked to the X chromosome. Examples of autosomal recessive diseases include sickle cell anemia (1 in 655 U.S. African Americans), cystic fibrosis (1 in 2,500), and phenylketonuria (1 in 12,000). Examples of X-linked diseases include Duchenne muscular dystrophy (1 in 3,000 males), hemophilia A (1 in 10,000 males), and fragile X mental retardation (varies, 1 in 700–2,000 males; Beaudet et al. 1995). Because many diseases are autosomal recessive disorders, it is estimated that each person on average carries five genes that cause diseases (Kitcher 1997). Carriers (heterozygotes) are not affected because that they still have an allele (one copy of the gene) that functions well enough to make the required protein in the required amount.

In an autosomal dominant disorder, a person who has a single defective allele will be unable to manufacture the normal protein in the normal amount. In X-linked disorders, only males contract the disorder because the mutation occurs on the X chromosome and males lack an extra X chromosome carrying the allele needed to make the protein. Therefore, any mutations in the X of the male will result in the disease, whereas the female has XX gene, which reduces her odds of contracting the disease. Females are carriers of X-linked disorders.

GENETIC DETERMINISM

Since Mendel's time, geneticists have attempted to understand the causal relationship between genotypes (or genetic characteristics) and phenotypes (or biological, psychological, and social traits). At various times, scientists and popular writers have asserted or proposed a simplified approach to this difficult issue known as genetic determinism, i.e. the view that genotypes causally determine or explain phenotypes (Dennett 1995). In the 1970s, Harvard biologist E.O. Wilson took the work on kin selection by Robert Trivers and others and launched the field of sociobiology, which attempts to provide genetic and evolutionary explanations of social behavior, including human behavior. For example, a sociobiological explanation of why a bee will sacrifice itself for the good of the hive (biological altruism) is that the bee is promoting the inclusive fitness of its genes because its sisters carry copies of its genes. Since that time, biologists have developed genetic and evolutionary explanations of asocial behavior, intelligence, emotion, and cognition. Darwin himself speculated about the evolutionary and genetic causes of human behavior and intelligence.

Although sociobiology and related fields are legitimate domains of inquiry, and they have generated many useful explanations and models, critics have argued that sociobiology is a form of genetic determinism. Modern societies tend to overemphasize genetics and genetic explanations, and daily press reports relate research on genes "for" obesity, sexual preferences, various forms of cancer, humor, risk taking, and even religion (Nelkin and Lindee 1995). Aside from scientific problems, discussed below, genetic determinism has troubling social and ethical implications. Many of the important practices that guide human conduct, such as ethics, law, and religion, assume that people have free will, that is, that they can freely choose their behavior. But if our behaviors are caused by genetic factors, how can we have free will? Without a satisfactory accounting of the precise effects that genetics may have on behavior, genetic determinism can undermine responsibility. People with a "gene" for alcoholism could argue that they should not be held responsible for their excessive drinking. Genetics might be used an excuse for criminal behavior as well. Genetic determinism also has troubling implications for racial and ethnic prejudice and bias insofar as people have asserted that specific traits, such as intelligence or creativity, are associated with racial or ethnic characteristics. The belief in genetic determinism helped to fuel the eugenics movement. More recently, publication of *The Bell Curve*, a controversial book on race and intelligence (Herrnstein and Murray 1994), reopened issues of eugenics and genetic determinism.

It is unfortunate that simplistic explanations of human behavior and intelligence pervade our society, but researchers can and should do their best to dispel myths and misinterpretations through education. Even relatively simple traits, such as height or weight, are not entirely caused by genetic factors. A pea plant will not grow tall without water, and a person will not become an alcoholic if they never drink alcohol. The more realistic view of the issue is that phenotypes result from several different causal factors, including genetics, development, the environment within the organism, the environment external to the organism, and physical and chemical constraints. Determining the causal role of these different factors is a difficult task. One could classify traits according to the degree to which they are genetically caused, ranging from virtually 100% genetic to almost 0% genetic.

Shamoo (1997a) describes a simple model that one can use to understand genetic causation. Picture an organism as four spheres, each one within the other in a concentric arrangement. The inner sphere represents genetic causes with a single Mendelian locus, where identical twins have 100% concordance for the trait; for example, such traits as eye color and such diseases as sickle cell anemia fall in this sphere. The second concentric layer represents the genetic disorders or traits with multiple loci, such as some types of cancer, where the concordance for identical twins is less than 100%. The third layer of the concentric spheres represents disorders that occur posttranslationally (i.e., after DNA is translated to RNA and then to proteins), where proteins and other materials are involved. The fourth layer represents those biochemical reactions that are interactive with the environment, such as height, weight, intelligence, and so on. Factors such as aging, major life events, gender, and growth and development could influence directly the outer two layers of this sphere. Factors such as toxicants, drugs, and alcohol abuse also affect the outer two layers and may affect the inner two layers (i.e., genetic factors). However, factors such as nutrition, infections, and radiation could affect the entire sphere, including the inner monogenic single-locus spheres. The two outer layers can be influenced by environmental factors such as psychosocial factors, family, society, and religion, whereas drug therapy can influence (i.e., ameliorate) the *symptoms* of disorders from all four layers, but only gene therapy can influence, ameliorate, and alter all four spheres, including the genetic ones.

Numerous diseases have complex and multifactorial origins. This is especially true in diseases of the brain that affect behavior. Schizophrenia is a good example. Despite the complex nature of schizophrenia, genetics plays an important role. Among identical twins, the proband concordance—the expression of genetic traits in a group (not a pair) of twins—is 48%, reflecting a genetic contribution to the heredity of the illness (Kendler and Diehl 1993). But it also reveals the strong contributions of other factors in the manifestation of the illness. Bipolar disorders and affective disorders have a stronger presence of genetic contributions. The concordance among identical twins is 65% for affective disorders, 80% in bipolar disorders, and 59% in unipolar disorders (Nurnberger et al. 1994).

Although genetics plays an important role in causing disease states and "normal" traits, it should be clear from this discussion that other factors, such as the environment and development, also play important roles. Moreover, only a small portion of known diseases and "normal" traits result from a single, Mendelian locus; most traits result from a variety of different causal factors (Kitcher 1997, Holtzman 1989). Thus, it would be serious mistake to focus too much on genetic factors in science, medicine, and social policy because this may encourage us to ignore important nongenetic causes, such as social, economic, and cultural factors (Holtzman 1989).

GENETIC ENGINEERING

In the early 1970s, molecular biologists developed techniques for transferring genes from one organism to another as well as across species. These techniques, known as recombinant DNA, use vehicles, or vectors, to transfer genes into cells, for example, bacteria, through small vesicles known as plasmids. A plasmid contains a piece of DNA enclosed in a membrane. When the plasma attaches to the surface of the bacteria, the DNA enters the cell and is recombined in the genome. The additional gene can be inherited and can also function in the cell to make a protein. Vectors developed since the early 1970s include viruses, lysosomes, lipids, artificial chromosomes, and DNA alone. Charkrabarty's bacteria (see chapter 6) resulted from transferring a gene into bacteria that coded for a protein that allowed it to metabolize crude oil.

There are many different reasons for transferring DNA into cells. First, because cells that receive the gene will make copies of the gene and its associated protein, gene transfer enables researchers to clone (or copy) genes and proteins. Other processes, such as the polymerase chain reaction, can be used to manufacture thousands of copies of genes or proteins. Second, gene transfer is useful in developing genetically modified organisms (GMOs), because genes that are transferred to germ cells will be present in the adult and can be inherited. Gene transfer techniques have been used to transfer genes to plants, such as tomatoes, corn, and rice, as well as sheep, mice, and rhesus monkeys. No one has yet transferred genes to germ cells in human beings, although the same techniques are used in somatic gene therapy, which treats genetic conditions by transferring normal genes to the somatic cells of patients to allow them to make the required protein.

Gene transfer experiments have caused a great deal of excitement as well as concern among both scientists and the general public. In the early 1970s, many people became concerned about genetic accidents that might occur if GMOs or genetically engineered "superbugs" escaped from a laboratory. Michael Crichton's book *The Andromeda Strain* (1971) and Kit Pedler and Gerry Davis's book *Mutant 59: The Plastic Eaters* (1972) depict such an event. Other science fiction writers have speculated about biological warfare and the future evolution of the human race. In February 1975, over 140 concerned scientists from all over the world held a historic meeting at Asilomar, California, to discuss the benefits and risks of recombinant DNA and genetic engineering. They recommend that scientists proceed with the experiments with appropriate regulations and safeguards to minimize the risks from biohazards. Their recommendations led to the formation of the Recombinant DNA Advisory Committee (RAC), which oversees gene transfer protocols falling under regulations of the National Institutes of Health (NIH) or the Food and Drug Administration (FDA). In 1990, French Anderson performed the first gene therapy experiment in a human subject. Though gene therapy holds much promise, it still faces several technical hurdles related to transferring genes to cells in such a way that they function normally in protein synthesis (Walters and Palmers 1997).

Ever since gene transfer experiments began, they have faced some outspoken critics, such as Jeremy Rifkin (1998). For example, during the 1990s, a controversy erupted in Europe over genetically modified (GM) foods and crops, which led to some countries banning these products. People have expressed concerns about the risks to their health and safety posed by GM foods and crops. Others are concerned about environmental hazards or about commercial control over agriculture. Critics have raised similar objections to GM animals. To the extent that these concerns have a legitimate basis, they should be based on sound scientific evidence. In a sense, GMOs are not different from the plants and animals that we have produced through selective breeding for thousands of years. So one might argue that the risks are negligible or at least no greater than risks that we already accept. On the other hand, critics argue that gene transfer experiments can produce novel combinations of genes, such as tomatoes with fish genes. Critics also point out the GM plants and animals let loose in the wild, like a nonnative species, can upset the ecological balance. In any case, since these issues concern empirical questions relating to risks and hazards, they require further study (Reiss and Straughan 1996, Rollin 1995).

ASSISTED REPRODUCTION

During the 1970s, scientists and clinicians made significant advances in assisted reproduction technology (ART). Artificial insemination had been available for decades, but on July 25, 1978, Louise Brown became the first child conceived via *in vitro* fertilization (IVF). In this procedure, doctors give women hormones to cause ovulation, and then they use a needle to extract eggs from their ovaries. The eggs can be fertilized in a petri dish and implanted in the womb or stored for future use. Because couples almost never use all of the embryos created in IVF, thousands of unused embryos are destroyed each year, which itself raises ethical issues for people who regard embryos as having some moral value or status. In some instances, divorcing couples have fought battles for "ownership" or "custody" of the embryos. At the time that Louise Brown was born, the risk and benefits of IVF were not well documented. Although the procedure had been tried in animals, it had not been tried in humans. The procedure was performed under the guise of "therapy" and therefore was able to sidestep the questions, delays, and red tape that would have been involved in a research protocol. Fortunately, Louise Brown was born healthy, and over 100,000 "test-tube babies" have been born since then. The procedure is now considered "routine," although at one time people were concerned that it could cause defects. The procedures developed for IVF also have made it possible for women to donate their oocytes (or eggs) for use in reproduction. These procedures involve some discomfort and risks, and egg donors often receive a fee for their services. Many commentators are concerned about the emerging market for human eggs and question whether human reproductive materials should be treated as commodities (Andrews 2000, McGee 1997).

In the 1980s, surrogate pregnancy became popular. In this arrangement, the mother who carries the child, the birth mother, agrees to give the child up for adoption and may or may not be the child's biological (or genetic) mother. Under one type of arrangement, a surrogate may agree to carry a child for a couple and undergo artificial insemination with the man's sperm. In this instance, the woman who does not carry the child then adopts the child, along with the man, once the child is born. In another type of arrangement, the couple may use IVF to conceive an embryo, which can be transferred into the womb of a surrogate. Although some surrogate mothers do this for purely altruistic reasons, many act as surrogates for a fee. As a result of surrogate pregnancy, IVF, and sperm and egg donorship, it is now possible for a child to have five different parents: the biological mother, the gestational mother, the adopting mother, the biological father, and the adopting father (Andrews 2000).

During the 1970s and 1980s, researchers and clinicians also developed a variety of prenatal genetic tests (PGTs), such as amniocentesis and choronic villi sampling, that test for genetic conditions *in utero*. For example, either test can determine whether a fetus has Down's syndrome. If a fetus has a genetic disease, a couple may choose to abort the fetus in order to avoid giving birth to a child with a genetic disease. Selective abortion raises a variety of ethical issues relating to the morality of abortion and the definition of a genetic "defect" or "disease." Even if one assumes that abortion should be available to prevent the birth of a child with a serious genetic condition, the question arises as to what should count as "serious" (Parens and Asch 2000). Should a couple be able to abort a fetus because it will be a female, a male, have Down's syndrome, or be short or deaf? Currently, PGTs do not cover many genetic conditions. In the future, however, it will be possible to isolate fetal cells in the mother's blood and test those cells for many conditions. During the late 1990s, researchers also developed tests that can be used before an embryo is transferred to the womb. In preimplantation genetic diagnosis (PIGD), researchers can remove a cell from an embryo at the eight-cell stage and perform a genetic test on that cell without harming the embryo. For instance, if a man and woman both carry sickle cell anemia, to avoid a 25% chance of having a child with this disease, they can choose PIGD and implant an embryo that does not have the sickle cell gene (Andrews 2000).

Long before researchers developed prenatal or preimplantation genetic tests, couples took genetic tests to decide whether to have children. A couple anxious about their risks of having a child with cystic fibrosis (CF), for instance, can take a genetic test for CF mutations. Because CF is an autosomal recessive disorder, if both partners carry the CF gene, they have a 25% chance of having a child with CF. If only one partner has the gene, they may have a child who is a carrier, but they will not have a child who is affected. Today couples who are concerned about passing on genetic diseases are usually offered genetic counseling after they take genetic tests. To promote patient autonomy and chance, genetic counselors have adopted a position known as "nondirective" counseling: counselors provide patients with information about risks, benefits, and options, and they may offer advice, but they allow patients to make their own choices. Thus, a genetic counselor could tell a couple that they have a 50% chance of having a child with Huntington's disease but should not tell the couple to not have children (McGee 1997).

Unlike many other areas of medical practice or research, ART in the United States developed with very little regulation or oversight. Some commentators argue that additional regulations are necessary to protect children, parents, and society. One troubling aspect of ART procedures is that they are often performed as "therapy" rather than "research," which avoids the regulation and oversight that accompanies medical research. As a result, there continue to be concerns about the health and safety of patients and future children. One health and safety issue that has become a sticking point is the high incidence of multiple births, such as sextuplets, septuplets, and higher (ISLAT Working Group 1998). To ensure a successful pregnancy, ART practitioners usually transfer several embryos to the womb. Also, some women who take fertility drugs for ART do not heed warnings from their physicians and become pregnant with four or more fetuses. In these cases, many obstetricians recommend selective abortion to reduce the number of fetuses in the womb to improve the health of the other unborn children and the mother. But many women refuse selective abortion on moral grounds.

Many critics of ART are also concerned about its impacts on the traditional family structure (Callahan 1998, Kass 1985). Lesbian couples and single mothers can use artificial insemination to have children. Male homosexuals can use surrogate mothers to have children. A woman's sister, mother, daughter, or cousin could be the surrogate mother for her child. A family could have children with a variety of biological, social, and gestational parents, and other variations are possible. Some claim that children who are born into to these nontraditional families may suffer irreparable psychosocial harms. According to the critics, ART will harm society as well as undermining the traditional family. Proponents of ART, on the other hand, point out that these procedures benefit parents and the children who would not have been born without ART (Robertson 1994). A life in a nontraditional family is far superior to no life at all, one might argue. Besides, it is futile to insist that all families conform to some "traditional" norm in this era of working mothers, divorce rates as high as 50%, adoptions, grandparents raising children, gay couples, single-parent households, and so on. A family, one might argue, exists as long as there is love among human beings living together. Moreover, reproduction is an important human right that should not be restricted unless it causes harms to other people. As long as ART procedures are safe and effective, couples should have access to them. Apart from the safety issues, ART could result in separating the human activity of sex from reproduction. This may have some adverse outcomes, especially if society does not provide a period of dialogue and transition.

Other critics object to the idea of "designer babies" inherent in attempts to control human reproduction, because many of these techniques attempt to help parents give birth to children who are free from genetic diseases or conditions. Although most tests conducted so far focus on conditions such as Down's syndrome or Huntington's disease, which most people recognize as genetic disorders or diseases, it will one day be possible to select children for other characteristics, such as height, resistance to disease, longevity, eye color, and perhaps even intelligence. A number of commentators find this pursuit of human "perfection" deeply troubling and compare it to the eugenics programs of the Nazis (Kass 1985). Others are concerned that parents will impose excessive expectations and demands on their children. If you want to have a child who is the next Mozart, how will you react if the child lacks musical ability or has musical ability but dislikes music? (Andrews 2000). If a surrogate mother gives birth to a child with a defect that develops *in utero*, what will happen if the contracting parents refuse to adopt the child on the grounds that it is "damaged goods"? Finally, disability advocates are concerned that many ART techniques could increase discrimination against the disabled and send a "hurtful" message to people with disabilities (Parens and Asch 2000). How will society view people with disabilities if many couples are attempting to abort fetuses with disabilities? Will people with disabilities be viewed as mistakes?

One key conceptual issue that plays a large role in all debates about preventing genetic diseases, disabilities, or disorders is defining the concepts of health and disease. "Health" can be defined as the absence of disease. But what is a disease? From a biological point a view, a disease can be defined as a deviation from normal functioning that results in harm to the organism. Because this definition still allows for a great deal of variation within a biological range of normalcy, social, economic, and cultural factors often influence the distinction between "normal" and "abnormal" in clinical medicine. For example, 4' 6" would be considered a normal height for Pygmies, but it would be abnormal in the United States. A person diagnosed with dyslexia in the United States might not be considered to have any disorder in a nonliterate society. Philosophers, scientists, and clinicians continue to debate these issues (Humbr and Almeder 1997).

Finally, as we mentioned above, some critics object to the commercial aspects of ART (Andrews and Nelkin 2001), such as the selling of reproductive products, such as sperm or eggs, or reproductive services, such as serving as a surrogate mother or an adoption agent. Critics argue that many of the financial arrangements in ART can lead to exploitation of women (or parents) and may be equivalent to "baby selling." Commodification issues reinforce concerns about "designer babies" mentioned above, because parents may come to view their children as products that can be designed, perfected, bought, and sold.

THE ABORTION DEBATE

The abortion issue plays a crucial role in most of the ethical questions surrounding human reproduction and genetics. This issue has sharply divided U.S. citizens ever since the monumental *Roe v. Wade* (1973) decision by the Supreme Court. This decision overturned anti-abortion laws adopted by various states and granted women a constitutional right to abortion based on the right to privacy. The right to privacy ensures that U.S. citizens have dominion over a sphere of private decisions, such as reproduction, family life, and privacy in the home, child rearing, and refusal of medical treatment. It is mentioned in the Constitution, but judges and legal scholars have found a basis for this right in the first, fourth, ninth, and fourteenth amendments. This right is not absolute, however, because states can restrict privacy rights in order to prevent harm to people or to protect state interests.

In the Court's ruling in *Roe v. Wade*, the majority held that a woman's right to an abortion could only be restricted in order to protect her health or to promote the state's interests in human life. The Court did not state that the fetus has a legal right to life, but it carved out the "trimester" system, effectively giving the fetus some legal status in the third trimester. According to its ruling, abortions should be available to women on demand in the first trimester of pregnancy, with few restrictions. In the second trimester, the state can impose additional restrictions on abortion in order to safeguard the health of the mother. In the third trimester, the state's interests in promoting human life become paramount, and abortions should be allowed only in exceptional circumstances. The third trimester represented an important legal demarcation, according to the Court, because fetuses are considered to be viable by this time. One problem with this position is that medical technology continues to change the time of viability—the ability to live outside the mother's womb. Currently, in the United States fetuses born at 22–23 weeks of gestation are considered viable. In theory, abortions are legal at any time during pregnancy, even though the state can impose various restrictions. Ever since this important ruling, various states have enacted laws that attempt to whittle away abortion rights, such as requiring parental consent for minors to have abortions, a 48-hour waiting period for all abortions, and mandatory counseling about the psychological risks of abortion.

Leaving aside medical and legal issues for a moment, the key moral issue in abortion is the status of the fetus. Abortion opponents (the "pro-life" view) regard the fetus as a human being from the moment of conception, with at least some moral rights, including the right not to be killed. Abortion, according to this view, is equivalent to murder. Abortion proponents (the "pro-choice" view) regard the fetus as having some moral status as a "potential" human being, but they do not consider the fetus to be an actual human being with moral rights. Abortion may be irresponsible or wasteful, but it is not murder, according to this view. In the United States, the abortion debate affects political elections and key decisions in government. Pro-life and pro-choice advocates often stage protests, and some resort to intimidation and violence. We do not take a stand on the moral status of the fetus in this book, but we do suggest that this moral issue is similar to questions one might raise about the rights of animals (see chapter 10). A coherent moral position would be one that comes to terms with the moral status of various entities, such as embryos, fetuses, animals, plants, ecosystems, and so on.

The abortion issue also has far-reaching effects on debates about genetics and human reproduction. For example, the main reason for conducting prenatal genetic testing is to obtain knowledge that could lead to an abortion. Those who oppose abortion therefore have problems with prenatal genetic testing. In IVF, unused frozen embryos are destroyed. But those who view the fetus (or embryo) as a human being may oppose IVF because it involves the creation and destruction of embryos. Abortion opponents also oppose the use of fetal tissue in research because they believe that this may encourage people to have abortions and because using fetal tissue shows a lack of respect for the fetus. As discussed below, the abortion issue has also affected debates about cloning and stem cell research.

THE HUMAN GENOME PROJECT

In mid 1980s, the U.S. Department of Energy (DOE) initiated a discussion about sequencing the entire human genome (Green et al. 1995). These discussions, which were initiated and led by the visionary DOE scientist Charles DeLisi, were in part initiated by the need to identify mutations due to radiation among atomic bomb survivors. Another impetus for the DOE to make such a suggestion was the agency's experience in carrying out large projects successfully. Congress mandated that both the NIH and the DOE administer this large project, with the NIH taking the leadership role. In 1988, the Office of Human Genome Research was created within NIH, and the Nobel Laureate James Watson was installed as its first director. The project began in early 1990. Since 1990, the United States has contributed over $20 billion to the Human Genome Project (HGP), which was completed in February 2001, well ahead of schedule. A big reason the HGP was completed ahead of schedule is that in the mid 1990s, private corporations, such as Celera Genomics (see chapter 8) also took an interest in the sequencing the human genome. Celera developed new techniques, such as the "shot-gun" approach, and employed automated sequencing machines and supercomputers. Although there have been many tensions between public and private efforts over the years, Celera and the National Human Genome Research Institute (NHGRI) collaborated on this project and published separate versions of the genome in *Science* and in *Nature* (Pennisi 2001).

The HGP was divided into several segments, including the creation of the human genome map; what model of genome map should be used; ethical, legal, and social impact of the project; and the development of technology to carry out the project. The HGP analyzed the DNA from several human beings (or libraries) of European descent. Although human beings have about 99% of their DNA in common, the HGP needs to include additional studies relating to genetic diversity to ensure that scientists and clinicians have an adequate basis for understanding health and disease in the entire human population.

The HGP has already had profound implications for a variety of disciplines, including clinical genetics, oncology, pathology, immunology, and pharmacology, and has helped create new disciplines, such as pharmacogenomics, proteomics, and gene therapy (Fox 1999). The HGP will help scientists understand the genetic basis of health and disease, as well as various forms of diagnosis, treatment, and therapy. For example, genetic information can play a key role in drug discovery insofar as sequence data can be used to manufacture proteins. Many important drugs are themselves proteins or affect proteins in the body. Proteomics, the study of protein structure and function, is an important spinoff of the HGP. Moreover, that biochemical differences between individuals affect their responses to drugs has been known for a number of years. A particular drug may help some individuals lower their blood pressure but may cause an adverse reaction in others. Because genetics plays an important role in how different individuals respond to drugs, by studying genetic differences among people scientists can tailor drugs and prescription regimens to an individual's genetic profile. Pharmacogenomics, the study of how genes affect pharmacology, is another promising science arising from the HGP. Although the HGP has provided scientists with a wealth of information about basic sequence data, it will still take decades to understand how the different genes are translated and transcribed into proteins and how they function in cell regulation. Although supercomputers and large information databases will make deciphering the human genome easier, it may take another century to understand what it means.

PRIVACY AND DISCRIMINATION

One reason why the government set aside 5% of the HGP's funding for an ethical, legal, and social issues program is that scientists and policy analysts recognized that the project would raise a variety of moral and political issues, chief among them the issue of genetic privacy. As discussed above, genetic information can be useful in diagnosing diseases and in predicting disease predispositions. In the future, DNA tests could also be used to predict personality traits, intelligence, and longevity. Thus, genetic information comprises highly sensitive, medical data. These data can be very useful to patients and their doctors, but third parties, such as insurers or employers may also want this information to use it in decision making. A health insurer might want to use genetic information to rate a person's genetic risk. The insurer might use the information to deny insurance coverage to a risky patient or to raise the patient's rates. Employers could use genetic information in order to manage occupational safety hazards or to ensure a healthy workforce. For instance, a factory could test workers for a gene that increases their risk of developing cancer as a result of exposure to some workplace toxins. The employer could use this information in its employment decisions. An employer might also decide to not hire a person who tests positive for Huntington's disease on the grounds that they do not want to invest training and development costs in an employee who will only be able to work until his 40s. And these are just a few of the many situations that could lead to genetic discrimination (Annas and Elias 1992, Rothstein 1997, Juengst 1998).

In addition to genetic discrimination against specific individuals, many writers have expressed concerns about the stigmatization of specific racial or ethnic groups, due to their association with genetic conditions or diseases. For example, sickle cell anemia is much more common in African Americans than in the rest of the U.S. population. We also now know that cystic fibrosis, Tay-Sachs disease, and certain types of hereditary breast cancer (see below) are more common among Ashkenazi Jews. What is ironic about this situation is that we would not have discovered these facts if these populations had refused to participate in genetic studies. Thus, participation in genetic research can lead to benefit for a population as result of genetic knowledge, as well as harm related to discrimination or stigmatization (Fletcher 1989, Clayton 2001).

As a result of these concerns about genetic discrimination, many states have enacted laws against certain types of genetic discrimination, although these laws have not been tested, and there is no federal law on genetic discrimination. However, the Americans with Disabilities Act as well as the Civil Rights Act provide U.S. citizens with some protection against some types of genetic discrimination under federal law (Rothenberg et al. 1997). One way to handle concerns about genetic discrimination is to protect the privacy of genetic information, because people cannot use information for discrimination if they do not have access to it. All states have laws protecting the privacy of medical records, and if genetic information is regarded as part of the medical record, then it can be protected under existing medical records laws. However, these laws do not forbid third parties from asking people to grant them access to their medical (and genetic) records. If a person signs a form giving their insurer access to their medical record, then the insurer does not violate their privacy or confidentiality by examining the record. A federal privacy initiative was passed in 1996 as part of the Health Insurance Portability and Accountability Act (HIPAA). HIPAA prohibits health insurers from using genetic information in making insurance coverage decisions. The act also states that genetic disorders cannot be viewed as preexisting conditions for insurance purposes. However, the health care industry argues that it will cause a great deal of inconvenience and will be too costly to implement.

Although opposition to genetic discrimination is very high among health consumers and clinicians, insurers continue to argue that they should be able to use genetic information in making decisions or they will go out of business because of a problem known as "adverse selection." For example, suppose a patient knows that he has a genetic condition, such as Huntington's disease, and he therefore decides to buy extra life and health insurance so that he will have adequate coverage. He incurs great costs for the insurance companies that cover him. If they do not have access to his genetic information, then they cannot use that information, even though he can. One might argue that this asymmetry is unfair in that the insurer signs a contract while lacking important knowledge and that in the long run it will reduce the insurer's ability to manage the risk pool, a key economic assumption in insurance (Actuarial Foundation 1998).

Several other issues in human genetics are controversial because they raise concerns about privacy and discrimination. These issues include developing DNA databases for epidemiological research, using DNA markers (or "DNA fingerprints") in the criminal justice system, the use of human tissue in medical research, genetic testing to determine paternity, and family genetic testing (see below).

GENETIC TESTING AND SCREENING

Genetic screening programs have existed in the United States since 1963, when Massachusetts developed a screening program for phenylketonuria (PKU). PKU is a rare but treatable disorder in which the body lacks an enzyme for metabolizing the amino acid phenylalanine. If children have this condition and ingest phenylalanine, they can develop severe mental retardation. The treatment for PKU is fairly simple: eliminate phenylalanine from the diet. Because PKU is a treatable genetic disorder and the PKU test is reliable, effective, and inexpensive, all 50 states now require PKU screening for infants. Other common screening tests include tests for other metabolic disorders, such as galactosemia and sickle cell anemia. Although genetic screening programs have been fairly successful and popular, critics have raised various objections, including problems with the reliability and accuracy of tests (false-positive and false-negative rates), the cost-effectiveness of tests (are they worth it?), as well as concerns about genetic discrimination (Rothstein 1997, Clayton 2001).

In addition to genetic screening programs, many individuals are now opting for genetic testing to allow them to make important health care decisions. For example, BRCA1 and BRCA2 mutations are more common among Ashkenazi Jews (1% frequency) compared with the general population (0.1% frequency). Women with these mutations have an 80–90% lifetime risk of developing breast cancer and a 44% chance of developing ovarian cancer before age 70. Women in the general population have a 10% lifetime risk of developing breast cancer. About 5–10% of all breast cancers are due to hereditary syndromes, and about 70% of these are due to BRCA1 or BRCA2 mutations. If a woman is an Ashkenazi Jew, she may want to be tested for BRCA1/2 mutations. If the results are negative, she benefits from having some reduced anxiety. Although she could still get breast cancer, her risk is probably lower than 80–90%. If she tests positive for the mutations, she may decide to take steps to try to prevent breast cancer, such as more frequent mammographies, tamoxofin therapy, or even prophylactic breast removal (Clayton 2001).

Because many genetic conditions, such as Huntington's disease, are not currently treatable, and other genetic disease, such as cancer, are multifactorial and highly variable, and still other disease, such as Alzheimer's, have a low degree of penetrance, patients and clinicians often face difficult choices when it comes to genetic tests. Many patients may decide that they would rather not know the results of a genetic test. It is estimated that 20% of the population will develop Alzheimer's dementia by the age of 80. What will a patient gain by taking a test that, if positive, will increase their risk from 20% to 40%, especially given that we now have no effective treatment for this disease? Genetic tests on children also pose difficult questions, because it may not be obvious whether a test is in a child's best interests. If a child's grandmother has Huntington's disease, should the child be tested or can a test wait until the child is no longer a legal minor? What if a mature minor wants to be tested for BRCA1/2 mutations but the parents object?

Dilemmas also arise in genetic testing because genetic conditions are inherently family conditions—often more than one member of a family carries defective genes. Thus, the risks of discrimination may impact not just the person taking the test, but possibly the entire family. For example, if several women in a family test positive for BRCA1 or BRCA2, then the whole family may become stigmatized. Confidentiality issues also arise in family genetic testing. For example, a person who tests positive for a genetic condition, such as BRCA1/2, may not want to tell her sisters. Most people would agree that her confidentiality and privacy should be respected. On the other hand, one might argue that there is an obligation to break confidentiality in order to inform the woman's sisters that they may want to be tested. Or if a man tests positive for Huntington's disease but does not want to tell his fiancé about his condition, one might argue for breaking his confidentiality in order to relay important information to his future wife.

On the other hand, some members of a family may prefer to maintain their right not to know the results of genetic tests or their own genetic condition. Because information from a genetic test on a single individual can often give us reliable information about other family members, the "right not to know" may conflict with someone else's "right to know." For example, if a daughter tests positive for Huntington's disease and her father tests negative, we can know that her mother has the disease without testing her mother. Her mother may not want to know, but she may have this choice denied. Although we do not advocate breaking confidentiality in genetic testing and we think that it is important to respect a person's right not to know, we recognize that there are differing opinions about how to handle these ethical dilemmas related to genetic testing (Rothstein 1997).

GENE THERAPY

In an important paper on the ethics of gene therapy, Walters (1986) made two influential distinctions. The first distinction is between somatic gene therapy (SGT) and germline gene therapy (GLGT). The goal of SGT is to transfer genes to somatic cells; and the goal of GLGT is to transfer genes to germ cells, such as gonadal tissue, gametes, or embryos. Because therapies designed to affect somatic cells may inadvertently affect germ cells, SGT poses a small risk of accidental GLGT (Walters 1989, Holtug 1997, Walters and Palmer 1997). The second distinction made by Walters was between genetic therapy and genetic enhancement: genetic therapy aims to treat or prevent diseases in human beings, whereas the goal of enhancement is to change, improve or enhance human beings.

In early discussions of gene therapy, Anderson (1989) argued that it was ethically acceptable to attempt SGT in human beings on a limited basis, but he and other writers held that other interventions, such as GLGT, were ethically questionable. Controversies about gene therapy continue today. The main ethical argument for proceeding with SGT was that it was conceptually similar to existing forms of therapy, such as chemotherapy, radiation therapy, or surgery. The rationale for all of these procedures is the same: therapy can be justified on the grounds that the benefits of therapy outweigh the risks for an individual (existing) patient. Many therapies, such as cancer treatments, have a high degree of risk, but these risks can be justified if they offer important benefits, such as the only hope for a cure for a terminal disease. If SGT passes the risk/benefit test, then it can be used in human beings. (This argument assumes, of course, that we can distinguish between "therapy" and "enhancement," discussed below.)

The first SGT experiment took place in 1990 to treat a child with adenosine deaminase deficiency. Since then, there have been a variety of other SGT procedures to treat conditions such as glycogen storage disease type Ia;

α_1-antitrypsin deficiency, familial hypercholesterolemia, cystic fibrosis, Duchene muscular dystrophy, Huntington's disease, and breast cancer (Beaudet et al. 1995, Walters and Palmer 1997). The general idea behind SGT is to use a vector, such as a plasmid or a virus, to deliver a gene to a cell that lacks a normal copy of the gene. For this procedure to be effective, one needs to deliver the gene to the cell and to ensure that the gene functions properly in the cell (i.e., it is expressed as a protein in the right way, at the right time, in the right amount). Although SGT has had some successes, it still suffers from technical difficulties. The body often develops a powerful immune response to the vectors used in gene therapy as well as to foreign genes. So the human immune system often destroys foreign transgenes (genes that are transferred from one organism to another). Even when transgenes penetrate the body's defenses, they may not integrate into the genome or function in the cell. Although SGT has suffered some technical setbacks and has yet to deliver on the promises made in the early 1990s, it is a young science that will take some time to develop (Resnik 2001d).

GLGT has been much more controversial than SGT. The idea behind GLGT is to transfer genes to germline cells in order to correct harmful mutations and prevent the development of a genetic disease or condition. As already discussed, other methods of reproductive control, such as genetic testing and counseling, PGT, or PIGD, have been used to prevent genetic diseases. These methods are safer than GLGT and do not involve making changes to the germline. GLGT would make the most sense for situations in which parents cannot use these methods to give birth to healthy children who are 50% genetically related to each partner. Some cases might include the following:

- A woman has a mitochondrial disease, such as MELAS. Because mitochondria are transferred from one generation to the next via the cytoplasm in the ova, they are inherited through the maternal line. The only way for a woman with a mitochondrial disease to give birth to a child who is 50% (actually more like 49.5%) genetically related to her is to (a) transfer normal mitochondria into an embryo produced by her or (b) transfer a nucleus from one of her embryos into an egg with its nucleus removed. The first procedure has already been performed — the child is reported to be healthy — but some would consider this a form of GLGT because it involves transfer of mtDNA to germline cells (AAAS 2000).
- A couple are both homozygous for an autosomal recessive disorder, such as sickle cell anemia. Because neither the man nor the woman has the normal gene, the only way to produce an offspring related to each of them by 50% and with the normal gene is to perform GLGT.
- For a woman or a man homozygous for an autosomal dominant defect, such as Huntington's disease, all of their children, including heterozygotes, will express the gene.
- A woman homozygous for an X-linked recessive defect, such as hemophilia B, wishes to have a male child. Assuming that the woman is

fertile, she could give birth to a healthy male only with the aid of GLGT. (For a review of other scenarios, see Resnik and Langer, 2001).

As far as we know, GLGT involving the transfer of nuclear DNA has not been performed on human beings, although it has been performed successfully on animals for many years—the procedures would be identical to those used to produce transgenic mice, sheep, pigs, and monkeys.

The arguments for performing GLGT in a human being are to benefit the future child by preventing a genetic disease in that child, to benefit the parents by allowing them to have a child free from a genetic disease, to respect parental procreative rights, and to benefit society by reducing the economic and social burdens of genetic disease. Although these arguments have some cogency and make some sense in the abstract, there are still many technical problems with GLGT that make it too risky to perform in a human being. The first problem is that GLGT is simply too dangerous at this point in time. The procedure entails immediate dangers, such as risks to the patient (child) and risks to the mother, as well as long-term threats, such as risks to future generations and to the gene pool (Resnik et al. 1999). As discussed above, one small mutation can lead to a harmful genetic condition. GLGT could induce artificial mutations with devastating effects. If a gene randomly inserts into the genome, then it could cause a major frame-shift mutation or it could disrupt genes that are functioning normally. Even if a gene is inserted into the gene in the right place, it still might not be expressed at the right time and in the right amount. Problems could arise if the gene is overexpressed or underexpressed, or if it is expressed at the wrong time, such as early in embryonic development. Many genes are expressed in development but not later in life and vice versa. Risks to the mother are not as severe as the risks to the child, but they are real nonetheless. For example, the child might grow too big for the womb or suppress the mother's immune system. Because genetic changes induced by GLGT can be inherited, there are also risks to future generations, some of which may not manifest themselves for many years. It is possible that a child produced by GLGT would be healthy but that its offspring would have a genetic disease. Finally, it is also possible that the human gene pool could be adversely affected if we use procedures such as GLGT (or other forms of genetic control) to reduce the genetic diversity of the gene pool. Although our species is not in any immediate danger of extinction as a result of disease or predators, genetic diversity is important in the survival of any biological species, including human beings.

Although these arguments constitute the main ethical problem with GLGT, they do not raise any objections to the procedure in principle, because they would lose their force as soon as GLGT becomes safe and effective. One might argue that that day will never occur, because we will always lack sufficient knowledge or wisdom to successfully alter the human genome (Rifkin 1983). On the other hand, as late as 1950 many people believed it was impossible to send a rocket to the moon. Given the rapid pace of progress in biomedical science and biotechnology, we expect that GLGT will be technically possible in less than a decade and perhaps even "safe" in less than two decades. If GLGT can be made as safe and effective as other currently accepted ART technologies, such as IVF, would it be acceptable? Some critics have argued that we should never perform GLGT, even if it proves to be safe and effective. Their arguments claim that GLGT is wrong as a matter of principle. Some of these arguments are as follows [see Resnik et al. (1999) for further discussion]:

1. GLGT is "playing God" or interfering with the natural order. Genetic engineers are modern-day Dr. Frankensteins.
2. GLGT will take us down a slippery slope toward genetic enhancement.
3. GLGT will result in unjust distributions of genetic resources or genetic "haves" and "have-nots."

In addition, some arguments made against other types of ART, noted above, also apply to GLGT:

4. GLGT is a dangerous pursuit of human perfection.
5. GLGT will impose oppressive expectations and demands on future children.
6. GLGT will increase genetic discrimination.
7. GLGT will have adverse impacts on disabled people.

In response to item 1 in this list, many would argue that scientists and doctors already "play God" and interfere with the natural order. Virtually all of modern medicine is an attempt to "play God" and overcome or modify nature, but few would argue that we should do away with modern medicine. Indeed, one might argue that God gave us a brain so that we could use it to develop science and technology to reduce suffering, disease, famine, and poverty and to improve the human condition. One might also argue that human beings, including human science and technology, are simply a part of nature. What we do cannot really interfere with nature if it is in some deep sense "natural." What this objection seems to boil down to is not that "playing God" or "interfering with nature" is inherently wrong, but that we must use our science and technology wisely and appropriately.

In response to item 2, it does seem that GLGT as well as SGT will probably take us on a slippery slope toward genetic enhancement. Many of the drugs developed for therapeutic purposes, such as anabolic steroids, amphetamines, Ritalin, Viagra, and Prozac, can be used to enhance performance. Surgical techniques used to treat facial wounds or cancer can also be used to enhance the body through cosmetic surgery. Thus, the distinction between therapy and enhancement is a key problem not only in genetics but also in all of medicine (Parens 1999). Although this seems like a fundamental distinction, its importance and cogency become less clear when one examines borderline cases. For example, male pattern baldness is a normal trait. Would there be anything wrong in developing an SGT cure for baldness? If we accept drugs to treat baldness why not also accept gene therapy for baldness? Or consider genes designed to enhance human health. If we had a gene that conferred immunity to HIV, and if it were possible to use GLGT to produce a child that is immune to HIV, would this procedure constitute enhancement? Would it be wrong? Or consider aging. Aging, as we know, is normal. But what about genetic therapies (somatic or germline) designed prolong the human life span or counteract the effects of aging? Again, would these therapies be enhancement? Would they be wrong?

It will not be easy to answer these questions because they are closely connected to the concepts of health and disease discussed above. Most people would view "therapies" as technologies designed to treat or prevent diseases and would view "enhancements" as technologies designed to meet other goals. As we discussed above, ongoing controversies concern the definition of "disease," and there are some good reasons for thinking that this concept has normative as well as social, economic, and cultural dimensions. Moreover, the goals of "health promotion" or "disease prevention" lie in the murky ground between "therapy" and "enhancement" because effective health promotion or disease prevention techniques, such as vaccination or rigorous exercise, often enhance the body beyond normal functioning. Finally, one needs to address, at a fundamental level, what it is that is wrong about enhancement. Are enhancements wrong because they give people an unfair advantage? Are they wrong because they are unnatural? Are they wrong because they are dangerous? Are they wrong because they lead to or reinforce social injustices? Or are they not wrong at all? [For further discussion, see Parens (1999).]

We do not address item 3, the issue of haves and have-nots. For further discussions on this matter, see Resnik et al. (1999).

HUMAN CLONING

A clone, in biotechnology, is understood to be an exact copy of a molecule, such as DNA or a protein, or an exact copy of a cell or an organism. For many years, botanists and agronomists have been able to clone plants from cuttings. For example, a jade plant grown from a leaf will have almost exactly the same genome as its parent (there may be some slight genetic variations due to mutations). For years scientists have also been able to clone mammals, such as cows (Rollin 1995). It is possible to split an early embryo or take a cell from it without damaging the offspring. This procedure, known as "twinning" or "embryo splitting," has been used successfully for many years to produce cows and other livestock. Indeed, identical human twins are natural clones.

Before 1996, however, scientists had not produced a mammalian clone from an adult cell. Philosophers and scientists had discussed this possibility, and science fiction writers had written about it. For example, Aldous Huxley's book *Brave New World* (1932) depicts a fascist state that uses cloning and other technologies to produce distinct castes; the movie *The Boys from Brazil* (1978) is about scientists who clone Hitler, and the movie *Jurassic Park* (1993) depicts the cloning of dinosaurs. However, cloning of this sort did not become a reality until the birth of Dolly, the world's most famous sheep.

On February 23, 1997, Ian Wilmut and his colleagues at the Roslin Institute announced that they had produced Dolly, who was actually born on July 5, 1996. The story soon made headlines around the world as the media rushed to report the event. On the following day, U.S. President Clinton asked the National Bioethics Advisory Commission (NBAC) to review the legal and ethical implications of this new development. A few days later, President Clinton banned the use of federal funds for cloning a human being (NBAC 1997). Several European countries have followed suit. Congress considered but ultimately rejected a ban on human cloning. So far, the biomedical community is observing a voluntary moratorium on human cloning, although a few individuals have said they would try to clone a human being for money.

Wilmut and his colleagues created Dolly by taking a nucleus from a mammary cell from a sheep and transferring it into an egg that had been stripped of its nucleus. They then stimulated the egg with an electric charge to induce normal embryonic development, and transferred the developing embryo into the womb of a sheep. Thus, Dolly is an identical twin of the sheep that donated the nucleus. It took 277 failed attempts to produce Dolly. Most of these failures occurred before implantation, but many others occurred after implantation; the embryos either failed to implant or were aborted (Pence 1998). This was a new milestone in reproductive biology because the enucleated egg was "reprogrammed" with the full genetic complement from an adult sheep to go through the life cycle again. Prior to this feat, scientists were able to speculate that cloning would be feasible from embryonic cells but not from adult cells because adult (differentiated) cells have lost their ability to develop into a new organism.

In 1993, two reproductive biologists were able to produce embryonic clones by splitting human embryos. This event also prompted a great deal of media attention and public debate and prompted the National Advisory Board on Ethics in Reproduction to hold a workshop to hear from embryologists, ethicists, reproductive biologists, public policy experts, legal scholars, journalists, and government officials (Cohen 1994). In 1993 as in 1997, reasonable people disagreed about the ethics of human cloning (Macklin 1994, Annas 1994).

The arguments for cloning are similar to the arguments for developing GGLT as well as other reproductive technologies: cloning could be justified on the grounds that (1) it benefits children who would not exist without the procedure, (2) it benefits infertile couples or other people who want to reproduce, (3) it respects the right to procreation, and (4) it benefits society if it is used to reduce the economic and social burden of genetic disease. The strongest case for reproductive cloning would be for a couple who lack fertile gametes because of exposure to radiation or chemicals. Others have argued that cloning allows homosexual couples to have genetically related children or that cloning might be useful in preventing genetic diseases (Pence 1998). Some people have suggested that it might be appropriate to clone a child with leukemia in order to produce a bone marrow donor, or to clone a "replacement" for a dead child.

On the other hand, many people have raised objections to reproductive cloning. The strongest objection raised so far is that cloning is too risky. This procedure has not been tested on human beings, and we do not know whether it is safe or effective. Although scientists have produced many mammalian clones, these offspring have had some physical problems. Others have pointed out the possible psychological harms to the clone. Would clones regard themselves as freaks? As objects produced or manufactured to fulfill their parents' goals? Although the psychological risks are real, it is important to note that most children born via ART techniques have faced these risks and as far as we know, they have not proven to be significant. When the first test-tube baby was born, many people speculated that she would regard herself as a freak, but we have no evidence that this has happened or is a problem. However, the physiological risks of cloning are far greater than the risks of IVF, because IVF does not involve nuclear transfer. In a sense, cloning can even be regarded as a type of germline therapy (or enhancement) because it involves manipulation of the germline (American Association for the Advancement of Science 2000).

Many of the objections to cloning are similar to objections to other ART procedures, such as GLGT:

1. Cloning will have adverse impacts on the family structure, birth, death, and marriage (Shamoo 1997b).
2. Cloning threatens social or religious values.
3. Cloning is "playing God."
4. Cloning threatens the human gene pool.
5. Cloning leads to the commodification or commercialization of people.

We do not explore all of these arguments in detail, but refer to the NBAC (1997) and Pence (1999). These arguments, to some, are not very convincing, and they have been addressed above. But consider two other arguments against cloning:

6. Cloning will lead to various abuses by dictators, millionaires, and others.
7. Cloning will threaten the individuality or uniqueness of the clone.

Item 6 is an argument against any type of technology, including genetic testing, gene therapy, surgery, and chemotherapy. As such, the argument is trivial and naive. Because any technology can be abused by anyone with bad motives, the key is to regulate and control technologies to prevent abuses.

Item 7 is a common, though ill-informed objection. In popular accounts of cloning, some people have assumed that the clones will be exactly alike. Of course a person's individuality would be threatened if you could produce an exact copy, but this cannot occur. Even identical twins, who are natural clones, have different personalities. Twins also have anatomical differences. For example, twins do not have the same fingerprints, and they may have different birthmarks. We know that twins are able to form their own identities, and they do not consider themselves "copies." We should expect that a clone would also develop his or her own personality and sense of self (McGee 1997, Pence 1998). On the other hand, recognizing that clones would be unique people does not take away from the fact that genetics would play a key role in influencing the behavior of the clone. Because we know that heredity plays an important role in mental illness, intelligence, and personality, we would expect that clones would be very similar to each other. However, because genes do not determine behavior, each clone would still have his or her own "will" and "ego" (see the discussion of genetic determinism, above).

STEM CELL RESEARCH

Although it is beyond the scope of this textbook to delve into all ethical aspects of the use of stem cells, we describe here some basic concepts and the controversial issues they bring up in stem cell research. Above we described how the body forms different layers of tissue during development that differentiate into various tissue types as the single cell of an early embryo develops into an adult organism. Cells that can differentiate into various cell types are called stem cells and include embryonic stem (ES) cells and adult stem cells. Because ES cells can become a new organism or can differentiate into any tissue type, they are said to be "totipotent." Adult stem cells, on the other hand, because they cannot (as far as we know) become any type of tissue, are said to be "pluripotent." For example, bone marrow stem cells can become red blood cells, T-lymphocytes, or B-lymphocytes, but not muscle or bone cells. Nerve stem cells can also become different types of nerve tissue. Stem cell research attempts to engineer tissues from the body's stem cells to replace defective, damaged, or aging tissues. In 1998, scientists were able to grow human ES cells indefinitely. Since then, researchers have conducted stem cell experiments on mammals and have had some success in repairing spinal chord injuries in mice.

Because scientists cannot use federal funds to conduct research on embryos, private corporations, most notably the Geron Corporation, have funded ES cell research. Geron, in anticipation of potential ethical concerns, appointed its own ethics advisory board (Lebacqz et al. 1999). The Clinton administration sought to loosen the interpretation of the ban on embryo research to allow the government to sponsor research on the use of ES cells once they were available, but not on the derivation of those cells; it is unclear how the Bush administration will react to this idea. President G. W. Bush had made the decision to allow use only of about 60 existing cell lines, and not the production of embryonic cell lines specifically made for the purpose of use for stem cells.

Most of the stem cell procedures proposed to date would use the ES cells from embryos created by couples in fertility clinics. In the United States, thousands of embryos are discarded each year because IVF couples cannot use all of their embryos. A couple may create 300 embryos in an attempt give birth to one child. Another approach to stem cell research proposes that researchers create embryos for scientific and medical purposes. This approach, known as therapeutic cloning, or somatic cell nuclear transfer (SCNT), involves transferring the nucleus from a cell in a person's body into an enucleated egg. The

ES cells from this new embryo would match the tissue in the person's body, thus avoiding the potential tissue rejection problems that could arise in stem cell therapy (Solter and Gearhart 1999).

The potential of stem cell research is enormous, because so many diseases result from tissue damage. Stem cell research could lead to advances in treating paralysis, diabetes, heart disease, pancreatitis, Parkinson's disease, liver disease, arthritis, and many other conditions. The main objection to this promising research has to do with the source of ES cells. ES cells can be obtained from aborted embryos, embryos remaining after infertility treatments (IVF), embryos created solely for research by IVF techniques, and from SCNT techniques (i.e., therapeutic cloning). To obtain ES cells, therefore, one must either create embryos that will be used, manipulated, or destroyed, or one must obtain embryos leftover from infertility treatments.

But here is where the abortion debate resurfaces, because these techniques would involve treating embryos as mere things or objects and would not give embryos the respect they deserve, according to some critics. If one views embryos as human beings with dignity and rights, then one should refrain from ES cell research, because this would be equivalent to using human beings in an experiment without their consent, murdering human beings, and so on. Using embryos from abortions is problematic, according to critics, because this practice can encourage abortions. The NBAC (1999) report on this topic recommends that embryos merit respect as a form of life but that they do not merit the same respect as adult human beings. The NBAC made several recommendations, among them, separating the abortion decision from the procedure to use fetal tissues, and that there should be no payment for fetal tissues.

QUESTIONS FOR DISCUSSION

1. Should we try to "improve" the human race? Why or why not?
2. Couples often seek to produce children that are free from genetic diseases, and some seek to produce children with enhanced traits. Is there a moral difference between these "eugenics" decisions made by couples and those made by the state?
3. Some people have developed sperm banks of famous men scientists. In theory, one could also develop egg banks for famous women scientists. Would you contribute to such banks? Would you use them?
4. Are there limits to the future of genetic engineering technology? Should there be a societal imposition of limits? If so, what would they be?
5. If your wife were pregnant and both of you knew the fetus would survive with an IQ of 10, how would you feel about selective abortion? Would you use it?
6. What if in the scenario in item 5, you were offered prenatal gene therapy to have a normal child? Would you use it or select abortion? Why? What about somatic gene enhancement to ensure a high IQ for the baby? Why or why not?

7. Your sister had genetic testing for a dozen diseases. She is a writer and is writing a popular book to talk about her results. What do you think she should do regarding your rights, if anything? Would you interfere with her book publication? Why or why not?

8. Three major events in our lives are interwoven into our social fabric: birth, marriage, and death. Do you think cloning could change the social context of these three events? Why? How?

CASES FOR DISCUSSION

Case 1: Prenatal Genetic Testing

A couple who are both Ashkenazi Jews are concerned about Tay Sachs disease; they both have relatives who were born with the disease. Their physician refers them to a genetic counselor. They take a preconception genetic test and discover that they are both carriers. They have a 25% chance of having a baby with Tay Sachs. Their options include (a) don't reproduce and adopt instead, (b) reproduce with no technological assistance, (c) reproduce with technological assistance. If they pick option c, they can use IVF and PIGD to select an embryo without the disease; the others would be discarded. If they don't want to use IVF/PIGD, they can conceive, conduct a prenatal genetic test to detect Tay Sachs, and abort the baby if the test is positive. They may also use the sperm or eggs from someone who does not carry the gene. This would result in a child who is only half genetically related.

- What should this couple do?
- How should the genetic counselor advise them? To promote autonomy and avoid eugenics policies, most genetic counselors subscribe to nondirective counseling: give the couple information and options, but don't tell them what to do. Consider in this case (a) best interests of future child, (b) rights of the couple, and (c) effects on society.
- Would it be irresponsible for this couple to procreate naturally, knowing that they have a 25% chance of having a child with Tay Sachs? Would it make a difference if the disease is Huntington's (50% chance if one parent has the gene)? Hemophilia (50% chance if one parent has the gene)?

Case 2: Selective Abortion to Prevent a Disease

A 39-year-old woman gets the results of amniocentesis and discovers that her fetus has Down's syndrome. She is in her eighteenth week of pregnancy. She already has three children, ages 1, 3, and 5.

- Should she have an abortion?
- Suppose she discovers that her fetus has Tay Sachs. Should she have an abortion?

Case 3: Selective Abortion for Gender Selection

You are the Ob-Gyn for Mrs. Jones. Mr. and Mrs. Jones have three boys, and they very much want to have a girl. They do not particularly want to have another child if it is a boy, and they have told you this much. "I've got enough boys around the house!" says Mrs. Jones. They have even mentioned that they might consider aborting a male child. They are very eager to learn more about determining the sex of the child. During an ultrasound scan at 16 weeks gestation, you learn that the child is a male. Mr. and Mrs. Jones also see something that looks like a penis and they ask you what it is.

- Should you tell them the sex of the child?
- How would you tell them?

Case 4: PIGD for a Tissue Match

A couple has a 4-year-old daughter with Fanconi's anemia, a rare genetic disease, who needs a bone marrow transplant or else she will die. If the couple have another child, this child may or may not be a possible tissue match, and he or she may or may not have the disease. To ensure that they have a child that is a tissue match and does not have the disease, the couple plans to use IVF and egg-cell nuclear transfer (ECNT) to select an embryo to be implanted.

- Should society allow this procedure?

Case 5: PIGD for a Deaf Child

A deaf couple comes to a fertility specialist with an unusual request. They have had previous genetic testing/counseling and they have discovered that the wife is genetically deaf, and the husband is deaf as a result of a childhood disease. They are both members of a deaf community and speak American Sign Language (ASL). They want to have a child but do not think they could accept a nondeaf child. They would like to have a deaf child. To accomplish this, they would like the fertility specialist to use PIGD to select an embryo that is homozygous for the deafness gene.

- Should society (i.e., represented by their government) allow them to do so?

Case 6: ECNT for MELAS

A woman has mitochondrial encephalomyopathy with acidosis and stroke (MELAS), a mitochondrial genetic disease that is inherited through the egg cytoplasm, not the nucleus. She would like to have a baby that is genetically related to both her and her husband. Their Ob-Gyn, who is a fertility expert, says that he can use ECNT to create an embryo that would not have the disease. Its nuclear DNA (nDNA) would come from the couple, but its mitochondrial DNA (mtDNA) would come from an oocyte donor.

- Should she and her doctor be allowed to use this procedure? Why or why not?

Case 7: Cloning

A childless couple are sterile as a result of radiation exposure during their work at a nuclear weapons plant. Neither the man nor the women can produce gametes. They want very much to have children. They approach a fertility specialist, who says that he could perform a cloning procedure similar to a protocol used to create Dolly. He would use a donor oocyte and transfer a nucleus from one of the couple's somatic cells. If they would like, they could have a daughter and a son. He says the procedure has now been well tested in animals and is quite safe.

- Should they have access to this procedure? Why or why not?

Case 8: TGR for Genetic Disease

A couple who both have an autosomal recessive disorder are seeking assistance in reproduction (they are heterozygous for the gene). Their fertility specialist informs them that any children they produce with their gametes will have their disease. Using a donor sperm or egg, IVF, and PIGD, they could have a child who is 50% genetically related. He mentions that targeted gene replacement (TGR) might be appropriate in their case. According to his protocol, the couple would produce some embryos, he would remove some embryonic stem (ES) cells and use TGR to produce ES cells that have the normal gene but not the defective gene. He would obtain a copy of the functioning gene from ES cells produced by another couple. He would then transfer the nuclei from altered ES cells into several of the woman's enucleated oocytes, allow these oocytes to become embryos, test the embryos, and then implant an embryo with the normal gene. The couple would also have the option of selective abortion if anything went wrong. The procedure has been tested in animals but not humans.

- Should the couple be allowed to attempt this procedure? Why or why not?

Case 9: Artificial Chromosomes

A biotech company has developed an artificial chromosome for transferring genes to animals. The chromosomes can carry a variety of genes. In humans, they could carry genes designed to confer immunity to communicable diseases, including HIV, or protection against cancer via tumor suppression. Animal studies have shown that these chromosomes do not interfere with normal gene expression.

- Should they ever be used in human beings? Why or why not?

Case 10: Sterilization

WW is a severely retarded, 22-year-old man with fragile X syndrome. He is also sexually active. He lives at home with his parents; his father is his guardian. His parents would like to have him sterilized so that he and they will not have to be responsible for any children. They believe it would be in his best interests, their best interests, and society's best interests for him to be sterilized.

- Should society allow the procedure to go forward? Why or why not?

Case 11: Confused Parentage

Baby Z has six parents: a sperm donor father and an adoptive father, as well as two egg donor mothers, a surrogate mother, and an adoptive mother.

- Is this a problem? Why or why not?

Case 12: Huntington's Testing

A prominent member of the Smith family, Henry Smith, age 55, has developed Huntington's disease. He has told family members about his condition and has encouraged them to be tested. He has two sons, John (35) and Robert (32), and a daughter, Nancy (28). John took the test and tested positive for Huntington's. He has three daughters, Melissa (13), Jessica (7), and Sarah (3). John and his wife Irene have decided to not have their daughters tested. They have not told Jessica or Sarah about the test, although Melissa found out and wants to be tested. Robert is planning to get married soon and does not want to be tested. Nancy tested negative for the disease. They are planning to contact other family members who could have the disease.

- What do you think is the problem here? The solution?

Case 13: BRCA1 and BRCA2 Mutations

Women with BRCA1 or BRCA2 mutations have an 80–90% probability of developing breast cancer and a 44% probability of developing ovarian cancer by age 70. Women without those genes have a 10% probability of developing breast cancer and less than 5% probability of developing ovarian cancer by age 70. About 1% of Ashkenazi Jews have these mutations, compared with 0.1% in the general population.

Of all breast cancers, 5–10% are due to hereditary cancer syndromes (two-thirds of these are due to BRCA1/2 mutations); 10% of ovarian cancers are due to hereditary syndromes. Males can carry these genes and get breast cancer. Men with BRCA1 or BRCA2 mutations have a 9% risk of developing breast cancer by age 70. The incidence of BRCA1/2-attributable cancer is higher in Europeans than in African Americans. There are 235 different BRCA1 mutations and 100 different BRCA2 mutations. Myriad Genetics will test for both of these types of mutations for $2,400; the Genetics and IVF Institute will test for a variant of the BRCA1 gene common among Ashkenazi Jews for $295.

Juliana has recently tested positive. She wants to make sure that her future children do not have these mutations and is planning to use PIGD to screen embryos. She will try to implant embryos that either do not have any of the mutations or have only a few mutations. After having children, she plans to have her breasts and ovaries removed.

- Do you agree with her decision? Why or why not?

Case 14: New Screening Program

It is the year 2005 and scientists have discovered a gene that confers an increased risk (25%) for attention deficit hyperactivity disorder (ADHD). A group of educators are proposing that the state enact a law requiring mandatory screening for this gene, because studies have shown that early intervention for ADHD can yield excellent results. If a child tests positive for the gene, parents can be educated about the condition and what steps to take to provide an appropriate environment for their child. The educators argue that this screening program will be very cost-effective, because about 5% of children have ADHD, the test is inexpensive, and the state can save a great deal of money on special education programs and medication through early intervention.

- How would you react to this for your children?

Case 15: Genetic Privacy

Leslie Green's mother, sister, and aunt have all developed breast cancer; her aunt died from the disease. Her mother appears to be "cancer free" after being in remission from all forms of cancer for 10 years, although her sister has developed ovarian cancer after having a mastectomy. The family recently learned about the BRCA1 and BRCA2 genes that have been linked to certain types of cancer. So far, her mother and sister have tested positive for the gene. The family recently exhumed the body of the aunt, and the aunt tested positive as well. Leslie is considering having a test for the BRCA1 and BRCA2 genes. She discusses this matter with her family physician. She is considering having her breasts and ovaries removed if she tests positive, as a way of preventing cancer. She is concerned, however, that her insurance rates will skyrocket (assume this is possible) if her insurance company discovers any test results (positive or negative). To keep her insurance company from finding out about the results, she wants to pay for the test out of her own pocket. She also wants these results kept secret.

- Should her doctor keep the test results secret?
- What should the doctor do if the insurance company asks whether Leslie has had genetic tests?
- Should the doctor keep two sets of records, the public record that the insurance company can review and a more private record?
- If Leslie tests positive, should she have her breasts removed?
- If she tests negative, should she inform her insurance company?

Case 16: Genetic Test for Mentally Retarded Man

HT is a 44-year-old white male hospitalized for impaction. He is mentally retarded and has physical deformities, which have been present since birth. He has one "normal/functional" limb, his right arm, and three abnormal ones (short, clubbed, stiff, drawn in). His family lives far away from town but wants to transfer his care to the outpatient service; they like the care he has received while a patient at the hospital. After examining the patient and seeing his niece, the attending physician begins to wonder whether HT has a genetic syndrome. A resident also comments that he has seen other members of the family (nieces, nephews, and siblings) who have a very similar appearance (face, skin, hair, body size, and build). HT is currently living with his niece. The plan of care is to stabilize his medications and send him home with a prescription for a laxative and recommend some physical therapy to help him with constipation. The team will also schedule a follow-up appointment in the outpatient clinic.

- Should the team bring up the issue of genetic tests for HT or possibly family members?
- What are the possible benefits and risks of these tests?

12

The Scientist in Society

This chapter discusses several important issues regarding scientists' role in society, including social responsibility, advocacy, expert testimony and expert opinion, public oversight of research, censorship of science, the clash between science and religion, and the public funding of research and development. The chapter also discusses the relationship between science and human values and provides a historical overview of the development of science and its impact on society.

THE ASCENSION OF SCIENCE

Most people find it difficult to comprehend that science was not always the complex, technical, intimidating, and powerful social institution that it now is. The term "science" was not even coined until the 1800s. Before this time, what we now call "science" was regarded as a type of natural philosophy. The full English title of one of the most important books in the history of science, Isaac Newton's (1642–1727) *Principia*, was "The Mathematical Principles of Natural Philosophy" (1687). Galileo Galilei's (1564–1642) two great books, *Dialogues Concerning the Two Chief World Systems* (1632) and *Dialogues Concerning the Two New Sciences* (1638 [1991]), were extended debates about natural philosophy written in the style of a Socratic dialogue. Some of the greatest scientists throughout history, such as Aristotle, Robert Boyle, Francis Bacon, René Descartes, Galileo, Newton, Charles Darwin, and Albert Einstein, also wrote on humanistic subjects, such as philosophy, theology, history, psychology, and politics.

In the modern world, a chasm has emerged between the "hard" sciences, such as chemistry, physics, and biology, and the "soft" sciences and humanistic disciplines, such as economics, sociology, psychology, history, philosophy, theology, literature, and law. C. P. Snow described this rift in an influential monograph, *The Two Cultures and the Scientific Revolution* (1964). According to Snow, the hard sciences deal with "objective" facts and use experimental methods, whereas the soft sciences and humanistic disciplines address "subjective" values and employ literary and philosophical methods. The two cultures have trouble communicating with each other, and there is a division of epistemological labor: scientists conduct research; humanists (and other members of society) address the value questions that arise in research. As a result of this split, many scientists have thought that they do not need to address the value implications of their work, and many humanists have felt that they do not need to understand the factual basis of public policy issues.

During this century, philosophers have written many books and articles about questions concerning the relations between "facts" and "values." Some have argued that this distinction is an oversimplification (Rudner 1953, Kuhn 1977, Putnam 1981, Longino 1990, Shrader-Frechette 1994). First, values play an important role in shaping scientific concepts, hypotheses, and explanations and in the decision to accept (or reject) scientific theories: science is not a value-free domain (Longino 1990). Consider, for example, research on human intelligence, which has been affected by social and political agendas and concerns ever since phrenologists and anthropologists in the 1800s attempted to show that some races were inherently less intelligent than others (Gould 1981). The very idea of "intelligence" is not purely objective but reflects value judgments relating to human cognitive abilities. Second, some have argued that values are not subjective. Although moral relativists point to the phenomenon of moral disagreement to argue that values are subjective or contextual, moral objectivists emphasize the phenomenon of moral agreement: although people disagree about specific issues, almost all of the world's cultures agree on some basic moral principles or values, such as respect for persons, beneficence, honesty, fairness, and so on. People agree with these basic values because these values reflect objective facts about human nature or human rationality, according to objectivists (Boyd 1988).

We do not need to rehearse these debates here, but we acknowledge them to give the reader a sense of these issues. Although we recognize the nuances and complexities in these debates, we agree with Snow's sociological observation that the distinction between facts and values plays an important role in Western societies. Moreover, the chasm between facts and values has serious consequences for the relationship between science and society. First, the idea that science is "value-free" has led many researchers to ignore the social, political, economic, legal, and ethical aspects of research. This attitude can undermine the integrity of research because it encourages scientists to pay insufficient attention to the responsible conduct of research (Resnik 1998a). For this reason, the study of responsible conduct in research must address scientists' obligations that extend beyond the laboratory setting, such as social responsibilities. As an aside, we are troubled that the Office of Research Integrity did not include a section on scientific responsibility in its recommended training, especially because much important work on the ethics of science explicitly discusses social responsibility (Bronowski 1956, American Association for the Advancement of Science 1980, National Academy of Sciences 1994, Whitbeck 1998, Bulger et al. 1993). On the other hand, one can understand why many scientists have adopted the view that science has nothing to do with ethics or values, because they have been taught since high school that science is "objective" and finds facts.

The idea that the humanities deal only in "value" questions has led many scholars and policy makers to pay insufficient attention to important factual and empirical issues relevant to policy questions. This attitude can undermine public policy because facts have an important bearing on the highly complex and technical issues of our era, such as global warming, strategic defense, genetically modified foods, energy use, alcoholism and drug abuse, and HIV/AIDS. On the other hand, one can understand why the public and politicians are wary of learning more about science and the relevant facts, because many people from a very early age have learned (from culture, peers, and the media) that science is "too complex," "inhumane," "arcane," or "impenetrable." Although our culture has made great progress in the last decade in science education in grade school, many people are ignorant of basic scientific ideas and findings and have an antipathy toward scientific thought (Nelkin 1995).

SCIENCE IN ANCIENT GREECE

To understand how the rift between science and values emerged in Western societies, and why this rift poses ethical dilemmas for scientists and for society, it is useful to examine the roots of science in ancient Greece (circa 600 BC to 100 AD). For several reasons, science historians claim that science began in ancient Greece, not Egypt, Babylon, China, or another ancient civilization (Cromer 1993). First, the Greeks attempted to develop natural explanations for natural phenomena. Second, they developed a way of thinking (or methodology) known as the critical or Socratic method. The Greeks, more so than previous civilizations, challenged existed assumptions and dogmas, argued back and forth, and debated about fundamental ideas. They valued intellectual honesty, integrity, openness, and free inquiry. Third, the Greeks developed abstract ideas and theories (Lloyd 1970, Cromer 1993). Finally, the Greeks also made careful observations and inductions and conducted experiments. Although many scholars view the Greeks, especially Plato, as excessively rational and philosophical, they were far more empirically minded than were other ancient civilizations, which often based their medical treatments on cosmologies, intuitions, or superstitious beliefs. Aristotle was a very careful observer and classified hundreds of species of plants and animals and types of minerals. He made several observations, such as the live birth of dogfish, which were not reconfirmed for over a thousand years. Hippocratic physicians kept detailed case histories of their patients and recorded signs, symptoms, healing, and death. The Greeks also made careful astronomical observations. By observing the shadow of the earth during a lunar eclipse, the Greeks came to believe that the earth is round (Burke 1995, Goldstein 1980, Cromer 1993).

In thinking about the role of science in Greek society, it is important to realize that the Greeks did not have a dramatic split between science (or natural philosophy) and other disciplines, such as philosophy, theology, politics, mathematics, rhetoric, logic, and literature. Most of the great Greek thinkers practiced, knew about, and learned about many different disciplines. For example, Aristotle's works included books on physics, biology, botany, zoology, meteorology, psychology, metaphysics, epistemology, ethics, politics, literature, drama, logic, and rhetoric. Our modern concept of a "liberal arts education" has its origins in Greek intellectual life. Moreover, the Greeks did not have the clear separation between a realm of facts and a realm of values that we find in modern society. For Plato, the highest type of knowledge was the form of the good. Because knowledge was objective, knowledge of goodness as well as justice was also objective. In Aristotle's cosmology, everything had a natural purpose or function that was determined by God. According to Aristotle, the function of the heart is to warm the blood, the function of the brain is to cool the blood, the function of the stomach is to digest food, and the function of man is to exhibit rationality in accordance with virtue. Human virtues are objective because they are based on natural functions, which are objective. The Greeks also did not view tools or artifacts as value-neutral, because every human-made object also had a purpose or function (Lloyd 1970).

If we skip about 1,300 years of history to the rebirth of culture in four-teenth century Europe, we find that Europeans began to reemphasize the im-portance of human reason, the beauty and dignity of the human body, and the wonder and glory of the natural world (Debus 1978). This transformation can be seen most clearly in European painting, which was highly stylized and un-realistic during the Middle Ages (1000–1200 AD) but became more expressive and realistic during the Renaissance or "rebirth" (1340–1450 AD). Medieval painters tended to focus on religious themes, such as the Crucifixion or birth of Christ; they drew angels and Christ larger than human beings, and they did not put much detail into the anatomical features of human beings. Renais-sance painters, on the other hand, made people with realistic faces. They drew shadows, blood, cuts, and wrinkles. They also addressed nonreligious themes, such as portraits of nobility or landscapes. Most important, European artists developed the techniques of perspective painting, which was a marriage of art, geometry, and optics (Goldstein 1980). The Europeans studied Greek and Roman art and architecture and hoped to recapture or even outdo ancient glory. Brunelleschi's famous cathedral in Venice and Michelangelo's statue of David combine the best of Renaissance science and art.

Renaissance European culture, like Greek culture, did not have a dramatic split between science and the arts. Students in universities studied a variety of subjects, and European scientists also had solid grasp of philosophy, history, politics, and art. The person who exemplified this fusion of science and art most clearly was Leonardo da Vinci (1452–1519), who drew very realistic pic-tures of the human body, plants, and birds in flight as well as portraits, such as the Mona Lisa. Da Vinci was also an inventor who designed a helicopter, an umbrella, and a submarine. Although da Vinci did not make important con-tributions to science during his time, his work exemplifies the intermixing of the worlds of science and the humanities characteristic of his era (Goldstein 1980).

THE SCIENTIFIC REVOLUTION

As discussed in chapter 4, the Protestant Reformation, led by Martin Luther, helped diffuse some of the church's authority in European society. Even so, the church and the state were by far the two dominant institutions until the Scientific Revolution (1500–1700 AD). The event that launched this revolu-tion was the publication of Nicholas Copernicus's (1473–1543) *The Revolutions of the Heavenly Spheres* (1543). In this work, Copernicus defended a heliocen-tric model of the solar system, which contradicted the Church's geocentric view. The theological significance of Copernicus's system is that it takes man out of his central place in the universe and makes the earth simply another planet revolving around one of many thousands of stars, the sun. In an important twist, a Lutheran cleric Osiander wrote a preface to the book claiming that Copernicus's system was only a convenient tool for making astronomical calculations; it should not be viewed as representing the world as it is. As a result of this introductory note, the Church did not object to the book, and the heliocentric theory did not win many converts (Burke 1995).

This accommodation did not last long. The controversial and arrogant Giordano Bruno (1548–1600), who followed the ancient Egyptian prophet Hermes and believed in alchemy and magic, traveled around Europe defending Copernicanism. Bruno also claimed that the universe was infinite and contained countless planets like the earth. Bruno was imprisoned by the Inquisition and burned at the stake for various heresies against the Church, such as practicing magic and denying the divinity of Christ. As a result, the Church began to turn against Copernicanism, because it was associated with heretical views. In the 1610, Galileo turned his telescope at the heavens and made observations that confirmed Copernicanism, such as moons orbiting Jupiter, rings around Saturn, mountains on the Moon, sunspots, and the phases of Venus. He also developed mathematical laws of free fall and motion based on controlled experiments, which challenged Aristotle's physics. In both of his *Dialogues*, Galileo defended Copernicanism, rejected Aristotelianism, and poked fun at superstitious beliefs as well as the Church. Although Galileo was not burned at the stake, he was punished for his heresies. He was confined to house arrest for the last nine years of his life. The Catholic Church placed his *Two Chief World Systems* on its index of prohibited books until 1835 and only formally admitted its wrongful treatment of Galileo in the 1990s (Burke 1995).

During the Scientific Revolution, many different fields of science emerged, and scientists also applied experimental and quantitative methods to existing disciplines, such as anatomy, physiology, medicine, and alchemy. The great anatomist Andreas Vesalius (1514–1564) defied religious prohibitions against dissecting human beings, reintroduced the practice of dissection, and developed accurate and beautiful drawings of the human body, which he published in his book *The Fabric of the Human Body* in 1543. The English physician William Harvey (1578–1657) conducted experiments on the circulation of blood in humans and animals. He proved that the function of the heart is to pump blood and showed how blood circulates throughout the body. Harvey also made accurate measurements of respiration, pulse, and blood pressure. Scientists developed new mathematical approaches to problem solving, such as calculus and probability theory, and formed professional associations and journals (Ronan 1982). In his book *The Skeptical Chemist*, Robert Boyle (1621–1691) attacked some of the mystical concepts and goals of alchemy, laid the foundations for the science of chemistry, and developed methods for chemical measurement and analysis (Debus 1978).

By the time Isaac Newton died in 1727, science had established itself as a powerful and important social institution distinct from the church and the state. In his *Principia* and other works, Newton described a world that was rational and knowable: the universe is a deterministic system that operates according to precise, mathematical laws. Newton developed laws of motion, gravitational attraction, and optics. Newton himself believed that these laws were created by God and written in the language of mathematics. Newton's view of the world began to have important influences not just on science but also on the broader culture. People began to view nature as rational, deterministic, and well ordered. They also began to believe that human beings can learn how nature operates if they conduct carefully controlled experiments to discover nature's laws. The general acceptance of Newton's ideas marked the beginning of a period in European history known as the Enlightenment, which is marked by a strong faith in science and technology and a belief in the power of human reason and the hope for material as well as moral progress. As an indication of how far science had come in 200 years, Newton was knighted for his scientific and political contributions (he served in Parliament and was master of the mint) and buried in Westminster Abbey (Ronan 1982).

SCIENCE VERSUS MORALITY AND RELIGION

These tremendous advances in science led Europeans to question the authority of religion and morality. Many different scientists and philosophers attempted to reconcile the new science with the old values and traditions. Francis Bacon (1561–1626) attacked religious and metaphysical dogmas and assumptions and defended an inductive and experimental approach to science. He argued that science should not concern itself with the search for teleological (purposive, goal-oriented) explanations but should focus on causal and mechanical explanations. Although Bacon defended scientific ideas and criticized the empirical claims made by the Bible, he also acknowledged the importance morality and religion. Bacon argued for a separation between science and metaphysics, and he argued that science should serve human goals (Cranston 1967).

In defending his views, Galileo argued that he was not saying the Bible is erroneous, because the Bible is not a scientific text. Galileo, and many other scientists who followed in his footsteps, argued that scientific theories and theological views do not clash because they address different domains: science is about nature and the physical world; religious books are about God, the soul, and the spiritual world (Burke 1995). Boyle, Galileo, and the English philosopher John Locke developed a distinction between primary qualities (or properties) of matter, such as length, width, and height, which are objective and measurable, and secondary qualities, such as colors, sounds, and feelings, which are subjective. Because primary qualities are thought to be "in the object," this distinction laid the groundwork for a modern distinction between "objective" and "subjective" (Hirst 1967).

We also find a split between science and human values in the work of René Descartes (1596–1650), who argued that the world consists of two types of substances, mental substances, such as God and the mind or soul, and physical substances, such as the human body and planets. The methods for studying the material world include observation, induction, and experimentation; the methods for studying the mental world include intuition and reason. The German philosopher Immanuel Kant (1724–1804) also sought to make room for religion and morality while providing a rational foundation for empirical science. Kant accomplished this reconciliation by making a distinction between observable features of the world (the phenomena) and unobservable features (the noumena). Science studies the phenomena, but morality and religion speculate about noumena. Even though it is not possible to prove the metaphysical claims of religion or morality in the same way that one can prove a theorem in mathematics or a hypothesis in physics, human beings must still make some metaphysical assumptions in order to sustain religion and morality. A century later, Charles Darwin himself would struggle with reconciling his theory of natural selection and his own religious beliefs.

THE MODERN WORLD

The period of time following the Enlightenment is what many scholars refer to as the modern period. As discussed in preceding chapters, during the industrial revolution science continued to grow in power and influence and drew closer to technology, business, and the military. As people began to realize the practical usefulness of science, science began to have important impacts way beyond the academic realm (Jacob 1997). Technological developments, such as the steam engine, factories, locomotives, machine tools, the telegraph, the cotton gin, crop rotation, the tractor, gas lights, electricity, electric lights, and the telephone, transformed the world by changing the way people live, eat, work, play, travel, and communicate. Society became more urban, mobile, literate, expansive, busy, complex, individualistic, materialistic, and wealthy (Jacob 1997).

Scientific ideas began having a broader impact on Western culture, as well (Jacob 1997). For example, people began to apply the scientific method to practical problems in business, finance, government, engineering, and public health. During the 1800s, the idea of a "social" science emerged as a way of using scientific methods to solve human problems. Science was also taught not only in universities but also in grade schools. The public began to read popularizations of scientific ideas as well as various encyclopedias. As discussed in chapter 11, many scientific ideas and theories, such as Darwinism, had a significant impact on Western culture. Other ideas that influenced common thinking included causation, equilibrium, force, acceleration, species, gas, boiling, and electricity.

By the 1800s, science and technology had grown so powerful and influential that they became targets of criticism. In 1808, Johannes Goethe published *Faust*, an epic poem about a man who sells his soul to the devil for scientific knowledge and technological control. In 1811, a group of English craftsmen known as Luddities objected to being replaced by tools and smashed machines in textile factories in protest. Amish communities in the United States attempted to resist the influence of modern science and technology. In 1844, Henry David Thoreau (1817–1862) spent a year in solitude at Walden Pond in Massachusetts. He kept a diary in which he reflected on nature, man, society, and technology. In his book *Walden* (1856), Thoreau denounced the busyness, crassness, and artificiality of modern life and argued for a return to a simpler, more natural, more spiritual way of life. Other romantic writers, such as Emerson, Hawthorne, Melville, Whitman, and Mary Shelley, echoed similar themes. In *Frankenstein* Shelley depicted a scientific experiment to create life gone awry and warned against tampering with nature. And Darwin's ideas about evolution and natural selection caused a great deal of controversy in science and in the public domain. Many religious and political leaders condemned his work as atheistic, heretical, and morally dangerous (see chapter 11).

Despite these protests, science and technology continued to grow in power and influence. The profound impact science had on business during the nineteenth century, led private research and development (R&D) investments, industrial laboratories, manufacturing, and the chemical industry. During this century, science also had an impact on humanistic disciplines, such as psychology, economics, sociology, anthropology, history, and philosophy. In each of these disciplines, many practitioners attempted to emulate the methods and techniques of the hard sciences in an attempt to attain respect or legitimacy. Sigmund Freud attempted to establish a scientific psychology, August Comte and Max Weber sought to develop a scientific sociology, and Karl Marx viewed himself as setting politics on a scientific foundation.

In the twentieth century, disciplines such as behaviorism and neurobiology applied experimental methods and rigorous concepts and principles to the study of human behavior. Researchers have also applied quantitative and experimental approaches to problems in economics and political science. In philosophy, an early twentieth-century movement known as logical positivism attempted to make philosophy into a rigorous discipline based on formal logic, probability theory, and set theory. Science has also had an impact on the broader culture through public education and the media. Since the nineteenth century, scientists had been depicted in literature, cinema, and television. For years reporters have also routinely covered scientific breakthroughs, problems, and events. Science literacy has become an integral part of K-12 education in Western nations so that children can become productive citizens and understand our complex world.

During the twentieth century, the governments of the world also began investing more heavily in R&D, especially in military R&D. World War I was the first major war in which science and technology played a key role. Both sides used new inventions such as tanks, dynamite, airplanes, steel battleships, machine guns, and mustard gas (Williams 1987). The strategic significance of military and nonmilitary R&D became obvious to politicians and the public in World War II. In this war, the United States, Great Britain, Germany, and Japan all invested heavily in R&D related to weapons and defense systems, such as rockets, jet airplanes, radar, sonar, and computers. Both sides used secret codes to communicate messages and mathematicians (cryptographers) to make and break codes (Williams 1987).

The most profound technical achievement of this war was the development and deployment of the atomic bomb. After the United States dropped the first bomb on Hiroshima, Japan, on August 6, 1945, the world could see the immense power, danger, and horror of modern science. In 1905 Albert Einstein proposed his special theory of relativity (known as $E = MC^2$) to explain the relationship between matter and energy in quantum mechanics. The equation implied that even a small amount of matter could be converted into an immense quantity of energy. During the 1930s, German scientists proposed the possibility of splitting large atoms, such as uranium, and developed models of nuclear fission. In 1939, Enrico Fermi, an Italian physicist who later immigrated to the United States and contributed to its war effort, conducted the first experiments proving that fission occurs, by bombarding uranium with neutrons.

In 1940, O. R. Frisch and R. E. Peierls, two refugee scientists from Nazi Germany, argued that the Allies needed to develop an atomic bomb to counteract Germany's nuclear weapons program; this led to the formation of a high-level scientific group known as MAUD, which recommended developing the bomb. Einstein also wrote a letter to President Roosevelt warning him about German efforts to build the bomb. Following the bombing of Pearl Harbor and the entry of the United States into the war in 1941, the Americans and British started a nuclear weapons program known as the Manhattan Project in June 1942. The British soon withdrew from the project for political reasons, but the United States invested $2 billion in the project. Most of the money was spent on building and operating a plant in Oak Ridge, Tennessee, to process uranium ore to obtain purified uranium-235. The government also established a laboratory and testing grounds in Los Alamos, New Mexico, which was directed by Robert Oppenheimer. The first atomic bomb, code named Trinity, exploded 60 miles south of Los Alamos on July 16, 1945 (Williams 1987).

Most of the scientists who worked on the development of the atomic bomb had political as well as scientific motives. All the scientists were aware of the Nazi threat, and most were glad to be able to do something to help the war effort. Once the project was started, many became excited about the idea of doing physics on a grand scale, and they were curious to see if the bomb would work. When the project was started, the United States was not winning the war, and the Germans seemed unbeatable. But by 1945, the Allies had defeated the Germans through more conventional means stemming from the invasion of Normandy, France. The Japanese, however, were determined to continue fighting, despite suffering thousands of civilian casualties in the fire bombing of Tokyo and other cities. At one point, some scientists had suggested that there was no need to drop the bomb on people because the Japanese would be impressed by a demonstration. As we know, this argument did not get very far, especially because many thought that it would take a full-scale invasion to force Japan to surrender. President Truman felt a strong duty to end the war as quickly as possible with minimal loss of American lives, so he made the decision to drop the bomb. Like a utilitarian (see chapter 1), Truman calculated that the ends (forcing Japan to surrender quickly) justified the means (dropping bombs on Hiroshima and Nagasaki).

After the war, many of the scientists who had played a role in the war effort felt a strong sense of guilt and moral revulsion over what had happened (Oppenheimer 1989, Heisenberg 1971). The incredible destruction wrought on the Japanese people became apparent to military personnel and physicians, who observed and recorded hundreds of thousands of deaths from radiation exposure, including cancers and birth defects, that took place for several years after the bombing, long after tens of thousands of victims had died during the bombing. Oppenheimer, one of the key physicists on the project, spoke eloquently of the need to never allow nuclear weapons to be used again and helped lead the "atoms for peace" movement. But soon the Soviets made and exploded their own bomb in 1949, and several years later the United States and Soviets both developed hydrogen bombs. Although these two opponents did not destroy the world during the ensuing Cold War, they came close several times, especially during the Cuban missile crisis in October 1963.

SCIENCE AND SOCIAL RESPONSIBILITY

One immediate impact of World War II on the scientific community was that scientists began to feel a sense of social responsibility. Without question, many scientists had a sense of social responsibility before the war, but afterward more scientists began to realize that science can be used for good or bad purposes and that there is a continuing need to use it wisely (Bronowski 1956, Lakoff 1979). Researchers could no longer ignore the social consequences of their work, once it became apparent to all that these consequences can be direct, immediate, and far-reaching. After World War II, many scientists took on the yoke of social responsibility and became involved in policy issues. As noted in chapter 1, Rachel Carson published *Silent Spring* (1961), which helped launch the environmentalist movement. Carson's book discusses the dangers of DDT and other pollutants for human beings and for the environment. In 1963, Barry Commoner published *Science and Survival*, a book with a similar theme. In 1966 Henry Beecher published a study in the *New England Journal of Medicine* on unethical studies in medical research (see chapter 9). The 1975 conference in Asilomar on recombinant DNA (see chapter 11) is another important example of scientists exercising social responsibility. In 1989, Roger Boisjoly followed his sense of social responsibility when he warned NASA about possible O-ring failure in the launch of the *Challenger* space shuttle (Whitbeck 1998).

Researchers have also formed organizations to address policy issues and social responsibility, such as the Union of Concerned Scientists, Doctors Without Borders, the Council for Responsible Genetics, Environmental Defense, the Natural Resources Defense Council, Worldwatch, Science for the People, the Center for Science in the Public Interest, the Skeptics Society, the World Resources Institute, and Student Pugwash. Moreover, many professional associations, such as the American Association for the Advancement of Science, the American Anthropological Association, the American Medical Association, the American Physical Society, the American Chemical Society, and the American Psychological Association, take stands on key policy issues or endorse social responsibility.

Although many researchers now recognize that they have social responsibilities, dilemmas can arise in deciding whether or how to exercise those responsibilities. First, many researchers have other obligations or duties that conflict with their obligations to society. As noted in chapter 1, researches also have obligations to be honest, open, and objective, to allocate credit fairly, to respect intellectual property, and to obey the law. For example, consider a researcher working for a pharmaceutical company who discovers that the company has done some preliminary work on a very beneficial drug, such as a treatment for HIV, that it does not want to develop until the patent expires on a similar drug. In a situation like this, the researcher is caught between obligations to society to help make this drug available as soon as possible and obligations to the company to not disclose confidential information. Similar conflicts can arise when researchers work for universities, the government, the military, or the criminal justice system. For example, consider a researcher who believes that a military project, such as a new airplane, has a design flaw that will hamper its effectiveness in battle. If her supervisors tell her to not worry about this problem, should she disclose this information to the public? In anthropology, researchers are often caught between obligations to be objective and open and the obligation to promote the best interests of the societies that they study (Resnik 1998b). If an anthropologist discovers some information that could harm the society that he is studying, should he publish it?

Second, social responsibility may also conflict with a researcher's personal interests or career ambitions, because sometimes speaking out on an issue or question can result in being fired, blackballed, or demoted by a company or institution. Even if none of these bad consequences happen, researchers may worry that their peers will perceive them to be "biased" or "political" if they get involved in efforts to influence social policy. Because researchers are taught that they should be objective, and society expects them to be objective, most researchers are wary of criticism that might damage their reputation for objectivity. Moreover, many researchers may want to be socially responsible but lack the time or effort to exercise their social responsibilities, due to the pressures of research and teaching. And some others may call that a cop-out. Like blowing the whistle on unethical or illegal conduct, acting to benefit society or prevent harm can be costly, risky, and taxing. Boisjoly, for example, exerted considerable effort studying the O-ring problem and trying to convince NASA to delay its launch of the *Challenger* until the weather was warmer (Whitbeck 1998).

Even when researchers decide to take some actions to meet their social responsibilities, questions can often arise relating to how they should go about exercising their responsibilities (Resnik 1998b, von Hippel 1991). Chapter 7 argues that researchers have ethical duties to be objective. Researchers should not fabricate, falsify, or misrepresent data or results. Although it is likely that they often fail to be completely objective, researchers should still strive to be objective. But how far do duties of objectivity extend? Should researchers always be objective, or can they sometimes advocate for a particular cause? Consider an environmental scientist who has strong beliefs about the importance of taking steps to reduce humanity's impact on global warming. How should he advocate for this position? Or consider a medical researcher who has strong opinions about the importance of protecting human subjects in research. How should she advocate for her views? Researchers, like other people, are also citizens who, like other people, have a right to voice opinions on policy questions. When should researchers be allowed to step out of their "lab coats" and into their regular cloths? This conflict between objectivity and advocacy can be as confusing for researchers as it is for the rest of the public, especially when one considers all the ways that researchers can influence policy:

1. Providing expert testimony in a court of law or to government committees
2. Providing expert opinions or advice for government agencies
3. Offering expertise to schools, hospitals, prison systems, accident investigators, and so on
4. Educating students, politicians, and the public about policy issues
5. Conducting research that benefits society or refusing to conduct research that may be harmful to society
6. Assessing the impacts (i.e., benefits and risks) of scientific research
7. Writing editorials in professional journals or popular publications
8. Lobbying Congress
9. Organizing political rallies or protests
10. Voting in elections

We believe that researchers should act as impartially as possible when they are required to provide expert testimony or opinion or to educate students or the public (1–4 above) because in these roles they are expected to be objective. A researcher who takes advantage of the privilege of being asked to be an expert by grinding a political axe, abuses this privilege and undermines the public's trust in science. The public has come to expect that when researchers are asked to serve as experts, they will do their best to act with competence, integrity, and impartiality. They expect the same for education: when members of the scientific community are asked to educate students or the public, they should provide up-to-date, balanced reviews of the material, not a biased account. On the other hand, when researchers are participating as citizens (7–10 above), and it is clear from the context that they are not acting as experts, then they are free to act as advocates.

Items 5 and 6 constitute a very important gray area in scientific responsibility. Because of their expertise, researchers are often uniquely qualified to assess the benefits and risks of research. However, risk assessment is not a purely objective activity (Shrader-Frechette 1994, Whitbeck 1998). First, following the discussion of human subjects research in chapter 9, risks are understood as the product of the probability and magnitude of harm. Although "probability" is (more or less) a scientific notion, "magnitude" is a value-laden concept, because it refers to the seriousness or severity of harms, which may be related to such notions as pain, discomfort, suffering, inconvenience, unhappiness, perceived injustice, debasing human values, or disability. Second, in making risk/benefit decisions, one must often decide whether to "gamble" or "play it safe," that is, whether to take a significant risk that could have a big payoff or whether to avoid the risk. Again, these decisions are based on values related to rational decision making (Resnik 1987). Consider, for example, the decisions made by the researchers who worked on developing the atomic bomb. At some point, each researcher who decided to work on the Manhattan Project probably decided that the benefits of the research outweighed the risks. So each researcher on the project acted in accordance with what he or she took to be his or her social responsibilities. Other risk/benefit decisions made by researchers, such as decisions related to human subjects research, animal research, drug approval, engineering design, environmental impacts, bioengineering, and product safety, involve some mix of "facts" and "values."

EXPERTISE VERSUS PUBLIC OVERSIGHT

The participation of scientists in public policy debates also raises importance dilemmas for society relating to authority and control (Dickson 1988, Jasanoff 1990, 1995). In most modern nations, scientists play a key role in governmental decisions by serving as experts witnesses, by providing expert opinions, or by providing education on the "facts" relevant to policy issues. Since the Scientific Revolution, scientists have provided political leaders with expert opinion on exploration, navigation, military affairs, sanitation, the census, and public health. During the twentieth century, Western nations became increasingly dependent on advice and opinion from experts to help their expanding bureaucracies regulate commerce, medicine, labor, transportation, agriculture, and communication (Westrum 1991). Today, expert scientists occupy key positions and provide important advice in various U.S. government agencies, such as the National Institutes of Health (NIH), the Centers for Disease Control and Prevention (CDC), the Food and Drug Administration (FDA), the Environmental Protection Agency (EPA), the Department of Energy (DOE), the Department of Agriculture (USDA), the Department of Health and Human Services (DHHS), the Department of Defense (DOD), the National Transportation Safety Board (NTSB), the Drug Enforcement Agency (DEA), the National Aeronautics and Space Administration (NASA), and the Federal Bureau of Investigation (FBI), to name but a few. The government also receives advice and opinion from semi-independent scientific organizations, such as the National Academy of Sciences (NAS) and the Institute of Medicine (IOM).

The use of experts in government is based on the idea of delegation of authority: although the power and authority ultimately resides with the citizens of a society, they (or their leaders) may choose to delegate some decision-making authority to promote effective decision making. To make efficient, well-informed, and reasonable decisions, governments must rely on experts. The FDA, for example, uses expert scientists and clinicians to help decide whether a new drug should be approved for human use. In making these decisions, the experts carefully examine the evidence from clinical trials with an eye toward benefits and risks. The NTSB uses experts to develop transportation safety standards and rules, to study the factors relevant to safety, and to investigate accidents to determine their causes.

Although the use of scientific experts benefits society greatly, it raises some fundamental political issues: How much authority should be delegated to experts? How much control should remain with the people? How can the public oversee and control experts? In the United States, the public oversees experts through the various branches of government. The legislative branch can oversee and control government agencies through legislation, and the executive branch can control agencies through executive orders. The courts can exert their authority by making judicial rulings on the legal impact of these decisions (Jasanoff 1990, 1995). All agencies must report their activities to the branch of government that oversees them. This type of oversight, though important, operates at a very general level. In the United States, the government sets policy that governs agencies, but it does not micromanage them. For example, legislative and the executive branches of government can both regulate the NIH by approving funding for various programs and establishing policies for the NIH. But members of Congress do not sit on NIH study sections or manage NIH grants.

Commentators have raised a variety of concerns about the use of experts in government decision making. Many bemoan the fact that society has become increasingly dependent on experts, and they would like to see more power and authority returned to the people (Dickson 1988). They argue that democracies are becoming nothing more than technocracies, that is, governments managed by bureaucrats and experts. The public should have more authority over governmental decisions, and experts should have less authority, according to the view. One issue where the public has demanded more input is the funding of medical research. Several years ago, the NIH established an Office of Alternative Medicine (OAM) in response to demands from the public for more research into alternative therapies. The NIH also recently established the National Center for Complementary and Alternative Medicine (NCCAM). Many biomedical researchers have opposed both of these moves on the grounds that these alternative therapies are little more than quackery and do not merit special funding. Researchers also objected to the public's meddling with the NIH's affairs. Those who support the OAM and NCCAM, on the other hand, claim that the medical establishment is biased against alternatives therapies (Boozang 1998, Stokstad 2000). For many years, the NIH has sought public input in setting funding priorities. The agency recently bowed to public pressure to overhaul its peer review system and has been experimenting with including members of the public on peer review panels. Researchers have also objected to public involvement in peer review (Agnew 1999b).

On the other hand, other commentators argue that the public should have less authority over government decisions due to its ignorance and incompetence. Uninformed people have no business making important decisions that affect public health, safety, national defense, and so on. These decisions should be left to the experts, with less meddling from public. The use of expert witnesses in the courtroom is one area where some commentators have argued that we need more, not less, expert authority (Angell 1997b). Several high-profile legal cases, such as the Dow Chemicals breast implant case, have involved legal and political controversies about the validity of expert testimony. Many writers have argued that the courts have been far too liberal in admitting expert testimony in that they have allowed people to testify who lack legitimate qualifications, valid data, or sound theories. In a key U.S. Supreme Court case, *Daubert v. Merrell Dow Pharmaceuticals* (1993), the Court ruled that judges must be the gatekeepers for admitting expert testimony and that they can use a variety of criteria for determining who qualifies as an expert. Prior to this case, judges could admit expert testimony only if it was based on generally accepted ideas, theories, or methods. The practical effect of the general acceptance standard was that it was often used to exclude "junk" or "fringe" science as well as novel or untested science from the courtroom. Some commentators have argued that the pendulum has swung too far in the other direction and that scientists should reassert some control over expert testimony in the courtroom. Some have suggested that scientists could establish panels or boards of independent experts to provide testimony or that they could certify or license experts (Huber 1991, Angell 1997b). In addition to the issue of expertise in the courtroom, commentators have made similar arguments regarding the approval of new drugs, claiming that the FDA should not bow to public demands to approve drugs.

Another argument against too much public involvement in science is that excessive governmental control can hamper the process of scientific discovery and innovation. Public involvement almost always involves more rules, regulations, and red tape, which can impede progress. Scientists should be allowed to be self-governing and should be free from excessive oversight. In his influential report to President Roosevelt, *Science: The Endless Frontier*, Vannevar Bush (1945 [1960]) defended the ideal of a self-governing scientific community free from excessive public oversight. This document laid out a social contract for science in which the government would fund R&D and researchers would take responsibility for ensuring the integrity and productivity of research (Guston 2000).

One can also use examples from history to argue against excessive government interference in R&D. Before the Nazi regime came to power in the 1930s, Germany had the best scientists and the best research programs in the world, but German science went rapidly downhill. At least three factors contributed to this demise. First, many German scientists with Jewish ancestry or who might be branded as Jewish sympathizers fled Germany to avoid persecution, torture, enslavement, or murder. Second, those who stayed in Germany faced a very difficult political situation, including the constant threat of persecution or forced resignation from university positions (Heisenberg 1971). Third, the Nazis started to redirect R&D funding toward the solution of more practical problems. They cut back on basic research and focused on research related to public health, nutrition, engineering, occupational safety, and the war effort (Proctor 1999). Although the Germans made great progress on specific areas of applied research, such as research on cancer, the overall effect of politicizing R&D was highly detrimental to science.

Indeed, throughout history, science has flourished in environments where researchers have been free from political or religious persecution. In the sixteenth and seventeenth centuries, the University of Padua in Italy became an important center for education and research because the climate in Padua was very tolerant. Many scientists, such as Galileo, studied at Padua to take advantage of the free, open, and welcoming environment (Butterfield 1957). Although public involvement in research is not the same thing as political or religious persecution, history shows us that movements to suppress, censor, or control research are often supported by or instigated by the public.

This question of public control of research raises the issue of "forbidden" knowledge. First, are there are types of experiments researchers should not be allowed to do? Second, are there any areas of inquiry researchers should not be allowed to explore? Earlier chapters have discussed many types of experiments on human and animal subjects that scientists should not be allowed to conduct because of moral concerns related to protecting human rights and dignity and animal welfare (see especially chapters 9 and 10). But we should be wary of placing any blanket restrictions on experimentation beyond those appropriate for conducting research on human or animal subjects. Other types of experiments should be evaluated on a case-by-case basis to assess their risks and benefits. For instance, some genetic engineering experiments may pose risks to human health or the environment. Others, such as nuclear tests or research on biological weapons, may be restricted for political reasons.

Throughout history, people have argued that some questions should not be raised or investigated scientifically. For example, the Catholic Church opposed dissections on the human body during Vesalius's day on the grounds that this would desecrate the body, which it viewed as the temple of soul. The Church also did not want Galileo to conduct research on Copernicanism. In Darwin's time, many people would rather not discuss the whole issue of evolution. In the twentieth century, some have argued that we never should have conducted research on nuclear fission, mind control drugs, assisted reproduction, genetic engineering, or animal cloning. Some wish that researchers had never opened "Pandora's Box" of knowledge in the first place.

Although it is always important to evaluate the benefits and risks of obtaining knowledge, we should hesitate to treat any area of inquiry as "forbidden." Human beings are like Pandora: we are naturally curious and rebel against authority. It is very difficult to keep knowledge forbidden for long, because someone, somewhere, usually will find out how to obtain it. At one time the design for an atomic weapon was a secret, but you can now download it from a web page. The only way society can control the proliferation of nuclear weapons is to control access to weapons-grade fissionable material. Even a ban on cloning human beings is likely to be ineffective in the long run, because some people are interested in conducting this experiment. We also do not believe that ignorance is bliss. It is better to expose the truth and learn how to deal with it, than to hide from the truth and pretend it can remain hidden. Although evaluating the risks and benefits of obtaining knowledge on a case-by-case basis, and regulating research to protect individuals and society, are important steps, making broad declarations that some questions are "too dangerous" to explore will accomplish little.

None of our comments in this chapter should be taken to imply that researchers should have a "free reign" or no public accountability. Rather, what society must do is develop appropriate and productive ways of regulating and controlling science (Guston 2000). Our comments should also not be taken to imply that society should delegate decision-making authority to scientists and other experts. Instead, society must find the proper balance of between expert and nonexpert (or public) decision making. The proper response to both of these problems related to the accountability of science may vary from case to case, depending on the nature of the research or the nature of the public decision. For example, research with direct, immediate, and clear impacts on individuals or society, such as research on human subjects, should have a great deal of regulation and oversight. On the other hand, research with only indirect, long-term, and unclear impacts, such as research on cosmology or quantum physics, should have much less regulation and oversight. When it comes to allowing experts to make decisions, some decisions, such as whether to lower or raise taxes, should be made by the public. Other decisions, such as how to manage a strategic or international crisis, should be made by experts. As an analogy, consider hiring a medical expert. Competent adults should be allowed to make medical decisions related to accepting or refusing treatment. But even an adult who consents to a treatment plan need not be involved in every decision affecting his or her treatment: the adult chooses to leave many of these decisions to medical experts.

FUNDING SCIENCE

World War II had a direct bearing on science's social status and economic and political power. Science emerged as an important and influential institution after the Scientific Revolution, but it did not become a dominant institution until after World War II. During the nineteenth century, science, religion, business, and the state fought for control in the societies of Europe and the United States, but after the war science's power increased dramatically as it displaced other institutions, such as the humanities, art, and religion, for control of society. Science got an economic boost from the government, which began increasing its investments in R&D through the 1970s, and business, which matched and then surpassed the government's investments in R&D (see chapter 8).

In 1995, the United States alone spent $170 billion on R&D, with the private sector contributing 60% of that total and the government 35% (Jaffe 1996). The United States spent about 2.5% of its gross domestic product (GDP) on research, and it is likely that the United States spent at least that amount in 2000 (Jaffe 1996). Projecting from these trends, a conservative estimate would be that in the year 2000, the United States spent over $200 billion on R&D. Other Western countries fund R&D at similar levels in relation to GDP (May 1997). In President G. W. Bush's 2002 budget request, total federal R&D amounted to $95.3 billion, with the biggest investments occurring in defense R&D (mostly DOD, $45.2 billion), NIH ($23.1 billion), NASA ($14.5 billion), and NSF ($4.4 billion; Malakoff 2001).

Since World War II, the question of the public funding of R&D has been debated many times. Although most people agree that the government should invest in R&D, the exact amount of that investment must be justified in relation to other types of government spending. R&D spending must compete with spending on education, health care, infrastructure, the military, social security, and so on. How can government investments in R&D be justified? Shouldn't other sectors of the economy, such as private corporations and private foundations, fund R&D? Although private investments in R&D account for 60% or more of the funding of science, the government also has a strong interest in funding R&D. During this century, scientists and politicians have developed several different rationales for public investments in R&D:

(a) R&D investments are important for national security and national defense. This argument played a key role in the U.S. investments in R&D during the Cold War (Guston 2000). After World War II, politicians realized the need to invest in science and technology. After the Soviets launched Sputnik in 1957, the U.S. beefed up its R&D investments to avoid falling behind. The massive investments in the space program during the 1960s and 1970s, which resulted in manned missions to the moon, can also be viewed in military terms in that superiority in outer space has strategic value. Although the argument justifies R&D spending on weapons systems, defense systems, military intelligence, and other military research, it is not clear that it justifies much investment in nonmilitary R&D, especially basic R&D. In response to this criticism, many commentators have argued that investments in basic R&D lead to important military applications and develop an overall knowledge base that has strategic value.

(b) R&D investments promote economic growth. With the end of the Cold War in the 1990s, politicians started relying on this argument for R&D funding more than the national defense argument. The Clinton administration argued that United States needed to continue investing in R&D to promote economic growth. Although many politicians and scientists find this argument convincing, some have begun to question this argument, claiming that increases in economic growth are based on many factors other than scientific and technological development (Shamoo 1989, Malakoff 2000b).

(c) R&D investments lead to practical applications. This is an argument made by Vannevar Bush in 1945 and by many commentators since then. Most people accept the idea that investments in applied research, such as medical and engineering research, lead to practical applications, such as new treatments and better bridges. But many have wondered whether investments in basic research have practical applications (Guston 2000). Many investments in basic research, such as research on black holes or planet formation, seem never to lead to any practical applications. On the other hand, one might argue that most basic research investments eventually lead to practical applications, even if we cannot imagine those applications when the research is being conducted. For example, basic research on the structure of DNA led to genetic engineering and gene therapy; basic research on quantum mechanics led to nuclear fission and transistors; basic research in Boolean logic led to the development of computers. Moreover, investments in basic R&D help build a knowledge base for any further practical applications. Even research in economics, history, and philosophy may lead to practical applications if it contributes to the overall base of human knowledge scientists need to develop ideas and test hypotheses.

(d) R&D investments are valuable for their own sake. Science is worth pursuing for its own sake, according to this argument. Knowledge itself has inherent value for individuals and society. Knowledge enlightens, satisfies, and edifies people. It is important to know why the dinosaurs went extinct, even if this knowledge does not lead to a new weapon or medicine or strengthen the economy. Any scholar or researcher will find this argument appealing, and many members of the general public are also convinced by it. The trouble with the argument is that, by itself, it does not distinguish science from other areas of inquiry that also have some inherent value, such as philosophy, literature, and history. Society is willing to spend billions on scientific R&D (as opposed to humanistic studies) because science pays dividends: science is valuable as a means to other social goals, such as military strength, economic development, public health, public safety, and so on.

(e) Science is too important to leave entirely in the hands of the private sector. This is an argument that has recently played a role in debate about funding biomedical research, especially controversial research, such as stem cell research. If an area of research has economic value, then companies will likely invest in it. If the government declines to invest in the area, then the research will remain in the private sector, under private control. As a result, results of the research may not be published in a timely fashion, if it at all. Private companies may also place restrictions on the use of research results, may demand excessive fees, and so on. Moreover, there is some danger that private research may be biased or erroneous, due to conflicts of interest or outright fraud. If there is no public research to offset or counterbalance the private research, this can affect the quality of research and threaten human health and safety (Resnik 1999a).

POLITICS AND RESEARCH FUNDING

It goes without question that government funding of R&D is a political decision. All of the arguments mentioned above are moral/political arguments,
even though they may appeal to historical, economic, or sociological premises.
Although scientists can and should provide the public with advice about the
funding of research, the public still has the power to approve, disapprove, or
modify science budgets (Guston 2000). As a useful analogy for thinking about
these issues, suppose that R&D investments are like financial investments and
the government holds an R&D portfolio analogous to a stock portfolio. One
question relating to the politics of funding that repeatedly arises is the issue
of balancing the research portfolio among different areas of research (such as
biochemistry vs. economics) or different agencies (such as the NSF vs. the
NIH), and between basic and applied research (Merrill and McGeary 1999).
This debate has also existed at least since World War II, and Vannevar Bush
staked out a position in this debate as well. According to Bush, the government should fund basic research in the hard sciences because private industry
would probably fund other types of R&D, such as pharmaceuticals and engineering, and the social sciences did not merit a great deal of funding. It was
with this philosophy in mind that the government established the NSF to
sponsor basic R&D in the hard sciences. The NSF has evolved over the years,
however, and it now sponsors social science research, mathematics research,
biological research, and even research in the history and philosophy of science. These debates have gone back and forth over the years. During the
1960s and 1970s, NASA received a great deal of funding. During the 1970s,
Congress expanded the funding of the FDA and the EPA. Recently, both the
Clinton and G. W. Bush administrations have favored biomedical R&D. In
Bush's 2002 request, the NIH funding increased by 15% while other agencies
held their ground or lost funding (Malakoff 2001).

To determine the exact funding level of any agency, discipline, or program,
one requires a great deal more data than we can present here—as they say, the
devil is in the details. However, consider these general points:

(a) Invest in basic R&D: The government should have a significant level of
commitment to basic R&D because private industry may not sponsor basic
R&D (Bush 1945 [1960], Varmus 1997). Corporations sponsor R&D to make
a solid return on their investments. Because applied research is more likely to
lead to profitable products or services, companies tend to sponsor applied research and product development. There have been some notable exceptions,
of course. For example, for years IBM, Texas Instruments, Bell Telephone,
and GE have sponsored some basic research, but most companies do not.
Therefore, the burden of sponsoring basic R&D falls on the government. In
economic terms, basic research is a type of "public good." A public good is
something that benefits many people although few people have the incentives
or resources to provide the good. For instance, roads, bridges, airports, and
law enforcement are public goods. Most companies would rather benefit from
basic research without investing in it.

(b) Diversify: Because research often involves a great deal of collaboration across different disciplines, the government should ensure that these different disciplines have a sufficient level of funding to sustain a "critical mass" of researchers (Merrill and McGeary 1999). For example, if the government sank most of its money into genetics and did not provide enough funding for cytology, this could hamper collaborations between geneticists and cytologists due to a lack of cytologists and a lack of funding for cytology. Again, using the portfolio analogy, one key principle of investing is diversification. Diversity makes sense in investing because it is hard to tell in advance which area will give the best return on investment or which area will have a down year. In science, diversity is important because it is impossible to tell in advance which collaborations are likely to occur. So to ensure that collaborations can occur, funds should be spread across different areas.

(c) Invest for the long term: Many projects require several years or more time to come to fruition (Gingrich 2000, Varmus 1997). Some disciplines reach conceptual or technical roadblocks before making progress. Therefore, the government needs to have some patience when it comes to R&D investments.

(d) Have some flexibility: Another principle of investing is to have some money that can be easily liquidated to take advantage of investment opportunities. In research, opportunities may include emerging diseases, public health emergencies, major breakthroughs, or hot new fields (Gingrich 2000, Varmus 1997).

(e) Beware of gimmicks or scams: This investment principle also applies to R&D. Gimmicks might include quackery or junk science, as well pork barrel projects that bypass normal peer review channels. If a senator wants to build a marine biology lab in Kansas, something is amiss.

(f) Fund unconventional projects: We need to develop a system of support for research that recognizes the uncertainty of scientific knowledge and the potential fallibility of existing paradigms. The R&D portfolio should therefore leave room for dissenting voices to be heard (May 2001). Chapter 4 argued that controversial projects that run counter to the existing paradigms need to be recognized and sometimes funded. Some funds should be reserved for controversial, creative, or antiparadigm projects. Society should have a way to test market new and unconventional ideas.

(g) Avoid political litmus tests: Debates about government funding have haunted many controversial topics, such as research on fetal tissue, human embryos, stem cells, therapeutic or reproductive cloning, contraception, acupuncture, or the use of marijuana in medical therapy. Although the public has a right to ban funding on any project and should, funding mandates can have unintended adverse impacts on the progress of science. For example, as a result of political resistance to funding research that might find a legitimate use for marijuana, we now have very little good scientific data on the medical benefits of marijuana, even though many patients report that they achieve significant benefits, such as relief of nausea and increased appetite. Regarding our current debates over cloning, there is a danger that cloning legislation might be crafted in such a way that it would prohibit or discourage uses of cloning technology that are not as controversial as reproductive cloning. Political pressure also played a key role in preventing the abortion drug RU-486 from being approved in the United States because the U.S. government did not fund studies on this compound. To avoid adverse impacts on research, any legislation that restricts funding must be crafted carefully and should have a clause requiring the government to reauthorize the legislation so that new developments could be more easily translated into policy.

This concludes this chapter as well as this book. We hope that readers will apply the concepts, principles, and information contained in this book to the problems, issues, and questions that they encounter in the laboratory, the library, the classroom, the office, and the public sphere.

QUESTIONS FOR DISCUSSION

1. How is science similar to and different from philosophy, religion, mathematics, and art?
2. What is your current understanding of the distinction between "objective" and "subjective"?
3. Was the "war on cancer" an appropriate method for funding cancer research by the federal government? Why or why not?
4. Should society have an intense dialogue about the ethical and societal values of major projects such as the atomic bomb and the human genome project before funding? Why and for how long?
5. Should researchers be involved in advocacy for social causes? Why or why not? Should they advocate for causes linked to their own area of research?
6. How would you design a system of research funding to allow for funding unconventional and controversial projects?
7. Should democracy surrender completely to those whom the Greek philosophers called the "knowledgeable" to run the country? In all issues? In some issues? Why? What is the proper place of "expert knowledge" or "expert opinion" in a democratic society?
8. Should scientists or other experts be paid for their testimony? Does payment for testimony pose any conflict of interest problems?

CASES FOR DISCUSSION

Case 1

A train travels through a small town (population 35,000) each day. Several times a month, the train carries hazardous materials used to make fertilizer. Although no derailments or wrecks have occurred during any of these shipments, many citizens are concerned about this potential hazard. The train tracks pass close to a high school and a hospital. Dr. Wilson is an environmental toxicologist at a university located in this small town. He alerted a local citizens group about the dangers of the train and has written letters to the editor of the local newspaper. He has been asked to testify on a panel convened by the city council to address the issue.

- How should Dr. Wilson participate in this policy debate?
- Has he done anything wrong or morally questionable to this point, or has he been acting as a socially responsible researcher?
- Would it be wrong for him to bias his testimony at the meeting?

Case 2

Ms. Carter teaches biology at a large high school (3,000 students). In senior year biology classes, students are introduced to topics in population genetics, evolution, and ecology. She teaches Darwin's theory of evolution by natural selection as well as its social and historical context. Although she does not teach the details of creation science, Ms. Carter explains why so many people opposed Darwinism despite strong scientific evidence for the theory, and she discusses creationism as a philosophical or religious theory. She explains that most scientists prior to Darwin believed that species were created by God and did not evolve but that most scientists now accept his theory.

- Should Ms. Carter teach evolution in the classroom?
- Should she teach creationism?
- If she discusses creationism, should she describe it as a scientific theory that competes with evolutionary theory, or should she describe it as a mere philosophical or religious idea?

Case 3

Dr. Vorcas works for a pharmaceutical company that specializes in drugs to treat asthma. While reviewing some of the company's research records as part of routine quality assurance procedures, he discovers that the company has data on a dozen unreported adverse events from a new medication that it did not report to the FDA. Although no one died from these adverse events, the adverse events resulted in hospitalizations for tachycardia. The FDA recently approved the medication. Dr. Vorcas signed a contract with the company when he was hired in which he agreed not to disclose confidential information.

- How should Dr. Vorcas proceed?
- Should he ignore these adverse events or report them to the FDA?

Case 4

Dr. Wilcox and her associates at a university medical school have been testing a new contraceptive in mice that functions like a morning-after pill. The drug has been 95% effective at preventing implantation when taken within 24 hours of insemination. She has developed a research proposal for testing the drug in human subjects and has a contract with a pharmaceutical company to begin clinical trials. She submitted an application to the NIH, which was rejected. She submitted her proposal to her university's institutional review board, which tabled her proposal. The chair of the IRB said that the members decided that the benefits of the research did not outweigh the risks and that the protocol is immoral. The university is a public university located in a conservative, southern town. It receives many large donations from religious conservatives and fundamentalist Christians who are opposed to abortion and birth control.

- Is Dr. Wilcox's research worth pursuing?
- Should the IRB have tabled her proposal?
- Should the NIH have funded her research?
- Does the IRB have a conflict of interest?

Case 5

There have been no cases of smallpox in the world for over a decade, but several laboratories have kept strains of the virus. It is not known whether any strains of the virus exist in countries with biological weapons programs.

- Should the strains be preserved or destroyed?

Case 6

Many transplantation researchers believe that pigs will be an important resource for human organs once it is possible to overcome organ rejection problems. To develop pigs that are immunologically compatible with human beings, researchers have created populations of genetically engineered pigs. The pigs have human antigens to enable them to be immunologically similar human beings. There is a small but real risk of transferring viruses from pigs to human beings, which would pose a risk to transplant recipients and the public's health. In preliminary studies of pig to human skin transplants, none of the recipients developed pig viruses.

- Should this research be continued?
- When, if ever, should clinical trials in human beings begin?

Case 7

Researchers working for a Dutch pharmaceutical company are developing a lotion that couples could use to control the sex of the child. The lotion contains a drug that kills or immobilizes sperm carrying the X-chromosome. In animal studies, it has been 95% effective in producing male offspring. The lotion would be administered in the same manner as spermicidal gels used today.

- Should the drug be developed for human use?
- Should governments sponsor research on this drug?

Case 8

An anthropologist has been studying for several years a Native-American community that lives on an island off the coast of Canada. The community is currently involved in a dispute with the Canadian government concerning the ownership of the island. The community claims that they have been living on the island for hundreds of years, long before any white settlers arrived in Canada. In her discussions with some of the elders of the community, the anthropologist is able to get a better estimate of how long they have been living on the island. She discovers that they actually arrived on the island a little more than 100 years ago. This fact, if disclosed to the public, would undermine their ownership claims.

- Should the anthropologist publish or otherwise disseminate what she has learned about the community's ownership claims?
- If she is asked to appear in court, how should she testify? Should she disclose information in court that could harm the community?

Appendix 1

Office of Research Integrity (ORI) Model Policy for Responding to Allegations of Scientific Misconduct

I. INTRODUCTION

A. General Policy

[*NOTE*: Institution should insert general statements about its philosophy and that of the scientific community related to ethics in research in this section. These might include institutional values related to scientific integrity, a statement of principles, and the institution's position on preventing misconduct in research and supporting good faith whistleblowers.]

B. Scope

This policy and the associated procedures apply to all individuals at [*Institution*] engaged in research that is supported by or for which support is requested from PHS. The PHS regulation at 42 CFR Part 50, Subpart A, applies to any research, research-training or research-related grant or cooperative agreement with PHS. This policy applies to any person paid by, under the control of, or affiliated with the institution, such as scientists, trainees, technicians and other staff members, students, fellows, guest researchers, or collaborators at [*Institution*].

The policy and associated procedures will normally be followed when an allegation of possible misconduct in science is received by an institutional official. Particular circumstances in an individual case may dictate variation from the normal procedure deemed in the best interests of [*Institution*] and PHS. Any change from normal procedures also must ensure fair treatment to the subject of the inquiry or investigation. Any significant variation should be approved in advance by the [*designated official*] of [*Institution*].

II. DEFINITIONS

A. *Allegation* means any written or oral statement or other indication of possible scientific misconduct made to an institutional official.

B. *Conflict of interest* means the real or apparent interference of one person's interests with the interests of another person, where potential bias may occur due to prior or existing personal or professional relationships.

C. *Deciding Official* means the institutional official who makes final determinations on allegations of scientific misconduct and any responsive institutional actions. [*Optional addition*: The Deciding Official will not be the same individual as the Research Integrity Officer and should have no direct prior involvement in the institution's inquiry, investigation, or allegation assessment.]

Sections that are based on requirements of the U.S. Public Health Service regulations codified at 42 CFR Part 50, Subpart A have endnotes that indicate the applicable section number, e.g., 42 CFR 50.103(d)(1).

D. *Good faith allegation* means an allegation made with the honest belief that scientific misconduct may have occurred. An allegation is not in good faith if it is made with reckless disregard for or willful ignorance of facts that would disprove the allegation.

E. *Inquiry* means gathering information and initial fact-finding to determine whether an allegation or apparent instance of scientific misconduct warrants an investigation.[1]

F. *Investigation* means the formal examination and evaluation of all relevant facts to determine if misconduct has occurred, and, if so, to determine the responsible person and the seriousness of the misconduct.[2]

G. *ORI* means the Office of Research Integrity, the office within the U.S. Department of Health and Human Services (DHHS) that is responsible for the scientific misconduct and research integrity activities of the U.S. Public Health Service.

H. *PHS* means the U.S. Public Health Service, an operating component of the DHHS.

I. *PHS regulation* means the Public Health Service regulation establishing standards for institutional inquiries and investigations into allegations of scientific misconduct, which is set forth at 42 CFR Part 50, Subpart A, entitled "Responsibility of PHS Awardee and Applicant Institutions for Dealing With and Reporting Possible Misconduct in Science."

J. *PHS support* means PHS grants, contracts, or cooperative agreements or applications therefore.

K. *Research Integrity Officer* means the institutional official responsible for assessing allegations of scientific misconduct and determining when such allegations warrant inquiries and for overseeing inquiries and investigations. [*Option*: A multi-campus institution or an institution with several large research components may wish to delegate these functions to more than one individual.]

L. *Research record* means any data, document, computer file, computer diskette, or any other written or non-written account or object that reasonably may be expected to provide evidence or information regarding the proposed, conducted, or reported research that constitutes the subject of an allegation of scientific misconduct. A research record includes, but is not limited to, grant or contract applications, whether funded or unfunded; grant or contract progress and other reports; laboratory notebooks; notes; correspondence; videos; photographs; X-ray film; slides; biological materials; computer files and printouts; manuscripts and publications; equipment use logs; laboratory procurement records; animal facility records; human and animal subject protocols; consent forms; medical charts; and patient research files.

M. *Respondent* means the person against whom an allegation of scientific misconduct is directed or the person whose actions are the subject of the inquiry or investigation. There can be more than one respondent in any inquiry or investigation.

N. *Retaliation* means any action that adversely affects the employment or other institutional status of an individual that is taken by an institution or an employee because the individual has in good faith made an allegation of scientific misconduct or of inadequate institutional response thereto or has cooperated in good faith with an investigation of such allegation. [*Option*: The institution may wish to define more specifically the standard to be applied in its determination of whether an adverse action was taken in response to a good faith allegation or cooperation.]

O. *Scientific misconduct or misconduct in science* means fabrication, falsification, plagiarism, or other practices that seriously deviate from those that are commonly accepted within the scientific community for proposing, conducting, or reporting research. It does not include honest error or honest differences in interpretations or judgments of data.[3]

P. *Whistleblower* means a person who makes an allegation of scientific misconduct.

III. RIGHTS AND RESPONSIBILITIES

A. Research Integrity Officer

The [*designated institutional official*] will appoint [*Option*: will serve as] the Research Integrity Officer, who will have primary responsibility for implementation of the procedures set forth in this document. The Research Integrity Officer will be an institutional official who is well qualified to handle the procedural requirements involved and is sensitive to the varied demands made on those who conduct research, those who are accused of misconduct, and those who report apparent misconduct in good faith.

The Research Integrity Officer will appoint the inquiry and investigation committees and ensure that necessary and appropriate expertise is secured to carry out a thorough and authoritative evaluation of the relevant evidence in an inquiry or investigation. The Research Integrity Officer will attempt to ensure that confidentiality is maintained.

The Research Integrity Officer will assist inquiry and investigation committees and all institutional personnel in complying with these procedures and with applicable standards imposed by government or external funding sources. The Research Integrity Officer is also responsible for maintaining files of all documents and evidence and for the confidentiality and the security of the files.

The Research Integrity Officer [*Option*: Deciding Official] will report to ORI as required by regulation and keep ORI apprised of any developments during the course of the inquiry or investigation that may affect current or potential DHHS funding for the individual(s) under investigation or that PHS needs to know to ensure appropriate use of Federal funds and otherwise protect the public interest.[4]

B. Whistleblower

The whistleblower will have an opportunity to testify before the inquiry and investigation committees, to review portions of the inquiry and investigation reports pertinent to his/her allegations or testimony, to be informed of the results of the inquiry and investigation, and to be protected from retaliation. Also, if the Research Integrity Officer has determined that the whistleblower may be able to provide pertinent information on any portions of the draft report, these portions will be given to the whistleblower for comment.

The whistleblower is responsible for making allegations in good faith, maintaining confidentiality, and cooperating with an inquiry or investigation.

C. Respondent

The respondent will be informed of the allegations when an inquiry is opened and notified in writing of the final determinations and resulting actions. The respondent will also have the opportunity to be interviewed by and present evidence to the inquiry and investigation committees, to review the draft inquiry and investigation reports, and to have the advice of counsel.

The respondent is responsible for maintaining confidentiality and cooperating with the conduct of an inquiry or investigation. If the respondent is not found guilty of scientific misconduct, he or she has the right to receive institutional assistance in restoring his or her reputation.[5]

D. Deciding Official

The Deciding Official will receive the inquiry and/or investigation report and any written comments made by the respondent or the whistleblower on the draft report. The Deciding Official will consult with the Research Integrity Officer or other appropriate officials and will determine whether to conduct an investigation, whether misconduct occurred, whether to impose sanctions, or whether to take other appropriate administrative actions [see section X].

IV. GENERAL POLICIES AND PRINCIPLES

A. Responsibility to Report Misconduct

All employees or individuals associated with [*Institution*] should report observed, suspected, or apparent misconduct in science to the Research Integrity Officer [*Option*: also list other officials]. If an individual is unsure whether a suspected incident falls within the definition of scientific misconduct, he or she may call the Research Integrity Officer at [*telephone number*] to discuss the suspected misconduct informally. If the circumstances described by the individual do not meet the definition of scientific misconduct, the Research Integrity Officer will refer the individual or allegation to other offices or officials with responsibility for resolving the problem.

At any time, an employee may have confidential discussions and consultations about concerns of possible misconduct with the Research Integrity Officer [*Option*: also list other officials] and will be counseled about appropriate procedures for reporting allegations.

B. Protecting the Whistleblower

The Research Integrity Officer will monitor the treatment of individuals who bring allegations of misconduct or of inadequate institutional response thereto, and those who cooperate in inquiries or investigations. The Research Integrity Officer will ensure that these persons will not be retaliated against in the terms and conditions of their employment or other status at the institution and will review instances of alleged retaliation for appropriate action.

Employees should immediately report any alleged or apparent retaliation to the Research Integrity Officer.

Also the institution will protect the privacy of those who report misconduct in good faith[6] to the maximum extent possible. For example, if the whistleblower requests anonymity, the institution will make an effort to honor the request during the allegation assessment or inquiry within applicable policies and regulations and state and local laws, if any. The whistleblower will be advised that if the matter is referred to an investigation committee and the whistleblower's testimony is required, anonymity may no longer be guaranteed. Institutions are required to undertake diligent efforts to protect the positions and reputations of those persons who, in good faith, make allegations.[7]

C. Protecting the Respondent

Inquiries and investigations will be conducted in a manner that will ensure fair treatment to the respondent(s) in the inquiry or investigation and confidentiality to the extent possible without compromising public health and safety or thoroughly carrying out the inquiry or investigation.[8]

Institutional employees accused of scientific misconduct may consult with legal counsel or a nonlawyer personal adviser (who is not a principal or witness in the case) to seek advice and may bring the counsel or personal adviser to interviews or meetings on the case. [*Option*: Some institutions do not permit the presence of lawyers at interviews or meetings with institutional officials.]

D. Cooperation with Inquiries and Investigations

Institutional employees will cooperate with the Research Integrity Officer and other institutional officials in the review of allegations and the conduct of inquiries and investigations. Employees have an obligation to provide relevant evidence to the Research Integrity Officer or other institutional officials on misconduct allegations.

E. Preliminary Assessment of Allegations

Upon receiving an allegation of scientific misconduct, the Research Integrity Officer will immediately assess the allegation to determine whether there is sufficient evidence to warrant an inquiry, whether PHS support or PHS applications for funding are involved, and whether the allegation falls under the PHS definition of scientific misconduct.

V. CONDUCTING THE INQUIRY

A. Initiation and Purpose of the Inquiry

Following the preliminary assessment, if the Research Integrity Officer determines that the allegation provides sufficient information to allow specific follow-up, involves PHS support, and falls under the PHS definition of scientific misconduct, he or she will immediately initiate the inquiry process. In initiating the inquiry, the Research Integrity Officer should identify clearly the original allegation and any related issues that should be evaluated. The purpose of the inquiry is to make a preliminary evaluation of the available evidence and testimony of the respondent, whistleblower, and key witnesses to determine whether there is sufficient evidence of possible scientific misconduct to warrant an investigation. The purpose of the inquiry is not to reach a final conclusion about whether misconduct definitely occurred or who was responsible. The findings of the inquiry must be set forth in an inquiry report.

B. Sequestration of the Research Records

After determining that an allegation falls within the definition of misconduct in science and involves PHS funding, the Research Integrity Officer must ensure that all original research records and materials relevant to the allegation are immediately secured. The Research Integrity Officer may consult with ORI for advice and assistance in this regard.

C. Appointment of the Inquiry Committee

The Research Integrity Officer, in consultation with other institutional officials as appropriate, will appoint an inquiry committee and committee chair within [*suggested*: 10 days] of the initiation of the inquiry. The inquiry committee should consist of individuals who do not have real or apparent conflicts of interest in the case, are unbiased, and have the necessary expertise to evaluate the evidence and issues related to the allegation, interview the principals and key witnesses, and conduct the inquiry. These individuals may be scientists, subject matter experts, administrators, lawyers, or other qualified persons, and they may be from inside or outside the institution. [*Option*: As an alternative, the institution may appoint a standing committee authorized to add or reuse members or use experts when necessary to evaluate specific allegations.]

The Research Integrity Officer will notify the respondent of the proposed committee membership in [*suggested*: 10 days]. If the respondent submits a written objection to any appointed member of the inquiry committee or expert based on bias or conflict of interest within [*suggested*: 5 days], the Research Integrity Officer will determine whether to replace the challenged member or expert with a qualified substitute.

D. Charge to the Committee and the First Meeting

The Research Integrity Officer will prepare a charge for the inquiry committee that describes the allegations and any related issues identified during the allegation assessment and states that the purpose of the inquiry is to make a preliminary evaluation of the evidence and testimony of the respondent, whistleblower, and key witnesses to determine whether there is sufficient evidence of possible scientific misconduct to warrant an investigation as required by the PHS regulation. The purpose is not to determine whether scientific misconduct definitely occurred or who was responsible.

At the committee's first meeting, the Research Integrity Officer will review the charge with the committee; discuss the allegations, any related issues, and the appropriate procedures for conducting the inquiry; assist the committee with organizing plans for the inquiry; and answer any questions raised by the committee. The Research Integrity Officer and institutional counsel will be present or available throughout the inquiry to advise the committee as needed.

E. Inquiry Process

The inquiry committee will normally interview the whistleblower, the respondent, and key witnesses as well as examining relevant research records and materials. Then the inquiry committee will evaluate the evidence and testimony obtained during the inquiry. After consultation with the Research Integrity Officer and institutional counsel, the committee members will decide whether there is sufficient evidence of possible scientific misconduct to recommend further investigation. The scope of the inquiry does not include deciding whether misconduct occurred or conducting exhaustive interviews and analyses.

VI. THE INQUIRY REPORT

A. Elements of the Inquiry Report

A written inquiry report must be prepared that states the name and title of the committee members and experts, if any; the allegations; the PHS support; a summary of the inquiry process used; a list of the research records reviewed; summaries of any interviews; a description of the evidence in sufficient detail to demonstrate whether an investigation is warranted or not; and the committee's determination as to whether an investigation is recommended and whether any other actions should be taken if an investigation is not recommended. Institutional counsel will review the report for legal sufficiency.

B. Comments on the Draft Report by the Respondent and the Whistleblower

The Research Integrity Officer will provide the respondent with a copy of the draft inquiry report for comment and rebuttal and will provide the whistleblower, if he or she is identifiable, with portions of the draft inquiry report that address the whistleblower's role and opinions in the investigation. [*Option*: The institution may provide the whistleblower with a summary of the inquiry findings for comment instead of portions of the draft report.]

1. Confidentiality   The Research Integrity Officer may establish reasonable conditions for review to protect the confidentiality of the draft report.

2. Receipt of Comments   Within [*suggested*: 14] calendar days of their receipt of the draft report, the whistleblower and respondent will provide their comments, if any, to the inquiry committee. Any comments that the whistleblower or respondent submits on the draft report will become part of the final inquiry report and record.[9] Based on the comments, the inquiry committee may revise the report as appropriate.

C. Inquiry Decision and Notification

1. Decision by Deciding Official   The Research Integrity Officer will transmit the final report and any comments to the Deciding Official, who will make the determination of whether findings from the inquiry provide sufficient evidence of possible scientific misconduct to justify conducting an investigation. The inquiry is completed when the Deciding Official makes this determination, which will be made within 60 days of the first meeting of the inquiry committee. Any extension of this period will be based on good cause and recorded in the inquiry file.

2. Notification   The Research Integrity Officer will notify both the respondent and the whistleblower in writing of the Deciding Official's decision of whether to proceed to an investigation and will remind them of their obligation to cooperate in the event an investigation is opened. The Research Integrity Officer will also notify all appropriate institutional officials of the Deciding Official's decision.

D. Time Limit for Completing the Inquiry Report

The inquiry committee will normally complete the inquiry and submit its report in writing to the Research Integrity Officer no more than 60 calendar days following its first meeting,[10] unless the Research Integrity Officer approves an extension for good cause. If the Research Integrity Officer approves an extension, the reason for the extension will be entered into the records of the case and the report.[11] The respondent also will be notified of the extension.

VII. CONDUCTING THE INVESTIGATION

A. Purpose of the Investigation

The purpose of the investigation is to explore in detail the allegations, to examine the evidence in depth, and to determine specifically whether misconduct has been committed, by whom, and to what extent. The investigation will also determine whether there are additional instances of possible misconduct that would justify broadening the scope beyond the initial allegations. This is particularly important where the alleged misconduct involves clinical trials or potential harm to human subjects or the general public or if it affects research that forms the basis for public policy, clinical practice, or public health practice. The findings of the investigation will be set forth in an investigation report.

B. Sequestration of the Research Records

The Research Integrity Officer will immediately sequester any additional pertinent research records that were not previously sequestered during the inquiry. This sequestration should occur before or at the time the respondent is notified that an investigation has begun. The need for additional sequestration of records may occur for any number of reasons, including the institution's decision to investigate additional allegations not considered during the inquiry stage or the identification of records during the inquiry process that had not been previously secured. The procedures to be followed for sequestration during the investigation are the same procedures that apply during the inquiry.

C. Appointment of the Investigation Committee

The Research Integrity Officer, in consultation with other institutional officials as appropriate, will appoint an investigation committee and the committee chair within [*suggested*: 10 days] of the notification to the respondent that an investigation is planned or as soon thereafter as practicable. The investigation committee should consist of at least three individuals who do not have real or apparent conflicts of interest in the case, are unbiased, and have the necessary expertise to evaluate the evidence and issues related to the allegations, interview the principals and key witnesses, and conduct the investigation.[12] These individuals may be scientists, administrators, subject matter experts, lawyers, or other qualified persons, and they may be from inside or outside the institution. Individuals appointed to the investigation committee may also have served on the inquiry committee. [*Option*: As an alternative, the institution may appoint a standing committee authorized to add or reuse members or use consultants when necessary to evaluate specific allegations].

The Research Integrity Officer will notify the respondent of the proposed committee membership within [*suggest*: 5 days]. If the respondent submits a written objection to any appointed member of the investigation committee or expert, the Research Integrity Officer will determine whether to replace the challenged member or expert with a qualified substitute.

D. Charge to the Committee and the First Meeting

1. Charge to the Committee   The Research Integrity Officer will define the subject matter of the investigation in a written charge to the committee that describes the allegations and related issues identified during the inquiry, defines scientific misconduct, and identifies the name of the respondent. The charge will state that the committee is to evaluate the evidence and testimony of the respondent, whistleblower, and key witnesses to determine whether, based on a preponderance of the evidence, scientific misconduct occurred and, if so, to what extent, who was responsible, and its seriousness.

During the investigation, if additional information becomes available that substantially changes the subject matter of the investigation or would suggest additional respondents, the committee will notify the Research Integrity Officer, who will determine whether it is necessary to notify the respondent of the new subject matter or to provide notice to additional respondents.

2. The First Meeting   The Research Integrity Officer, with the assistance of institutional counsel, will convene the first meeting of the investigation committee to review the charge, the inquiry report, and the prescribed procedures and standards for the conduct of the investigation, including the necessity for confidentiality and for developing a specific investigation plan. The investigation committee will be provided with a copy of these instructions and, where PHS funding is involved, the PHS regulation.

E. Investigation Process

The investigation committee will be appointed and the process initiated within 30 days of the completion of the inquiry, if findings from that inquiry provide a sufficient basis for conducting an investigation.[13]

The investigation will normally involve examination of all documentation including, but not necessarily limited to, relevant research records, computer files, proposals, manuscripts, publications, correspondence, memoranda, and notes of telephone calls.[14] Whenever possible, the committee should interview the whistleblower(s), the respondents(s), and other individuals who might have information regarding aspects of the allegations.[15] Interviews of the respondent should be tape recorded or transcribed. All other interviews should be transcribed, tape recorded, or summarized. Summaries or transcripts of the interviews should be prepared, provided to the interviewed party for comment or revision, and included as part of the investigatory file.[16]

VIII. THE INVESTIGATION REPORT

A. Elements of the Investigation Report

The final report submitted to ORI must describe the policies and procedures under which the investigation was conducted, describe how and from whom information relevant to the investigation was obtained, state the findings, and explain the basis for the findings. The report will include the actual text or an accurate summary of the views of any individual(s) found to have engaged in misconduct as well as a description of any sanctions imposed and administrative actions taken by the institution.[17]

B. Comments on the Draft Report

1. Respondent The Research Integrity Officer will provide the respondent with a copy of the draft investigation report for comment and rebuttal. The respondent will be allowed [ ] days to review and comment on the draft report. The respondent's comments will be attached to the final report. The findings of the final report should take into account the respondent's comments in addition to all the other evidence.

2. Whistleblower The Research Integrity Officer will provide the whistleblower, if he or she is identifiable, with those portions of the draft investigation report that address the whistleblower's role and opinions in the investigation. The report should be modified, as appropriate, based on the whistleblower's comments.

3. Institutional Counsel The draft investigation report will be transmitted to the institutional counsel for a review of its legal sufficiency. Comments should be incorporated into the report as appropriate.

4. Confidentiality In distributing the draft report, or portions thereof, to the respondent and whistleblower, the Research Integrity Officer will inform the recipient of the confidentiality under which the draft report is made available and may establish reasonable conditions to ensure such confidentiality. For example, the Research Integrity Officer may request the recipient to sign a confidentiality statement or to come to his or her office to review the report.

C. Institutional Review and Decision

Based on a preponderance of the evidence, the Deciding Official will make the final determination whether to accept the investigation report, its findings, and the recommended institutional actions. If this determination varies from that of the investigation committee, the Deciding Official will explain in detail the basis for rendering a decision different from that of the investigation committee in the institution's letter transmitting the report to ORI. The Deciding Official's explanation should be consistent with the PHS definition of scientific misconduct, the institution's policies and procedures, and the evidence reviewed and analyzed by the investigation committee. The Deciding Official may also return the report to the investigation committee with a request for further fact-finding or analysis. The Deciding Official's determination, together with the investigation committee's report, constitutes the final investigation report for purposes of ORI review.

When a final decision on the case has been reached, the Research Integrity Officer will notify both the respondent and the whistleblower in writing. In addition, the Deciding Official will determine whether law enforcement agencies, professional societies, professional licensing boards, editors of journals in which falsified reports may have been published, collaborators of the respondent in the work, or other relevant parties should be notified of the outcome of the case. The Research Integrity Officer is responsible for ensuring compliance with all notification requirements of funding or sponsoring agencies.

D. Transmittal of the Final Investigation Report to ORI

After comments have been received and the necessary changes have been made to the draft report, the investigation committee should transmit the final report with attachments, including the respondent's and whistleblower's comments, to the Deciding Official, through the Research Integrity Officer.

E. Time Limit for Completing the Investigation Report

An investigation should ordinarily be completed within 120 days of its initiation,[18] with the initiation being defined as the first meeting of the investigation committee. This includes conducting the investigation, preparing the report of findings, making the draft report available to the subject of the investigation for comment, submitting the report to the Deciding Official for approval, and submitting the report to the ORI.[19]

IX. REQUIREMENTS FOR REPORTING TO ORI

A. An institution's decision to initiate an investigation must be reported in writing to the Director, ORI, on or before the date the investigation begins.[20] At a minimum, the notification should include the name of the person(s) against whom the allegation has been made, the general nature of the allegation as it relates to the PHS definition of scientific misconduct, and the PHS applications or grant number(s) involved.[21] ORI must also be notified of the final outcome of the investigation and must be provided with a copy of the investigation report.[22] Any significant variations from the provisions of the institutional policies and procedures should be explained in any reports submitted to ORI.

B. If an institution plans to terminate an inquiry or investigation for any reason without completing all relevant requirements of the PHS regulation, the Research Integrity Officer will submit a report of the planned termination to ORI, including a description of the reasons for the proposed termination.[23]

C. If the institution determines that it will not be able to complete the investigation in 120 days, the Research Integrity Officer will submit to ORI a written request for an extension that explains the delay, reports on the progress to date, estimates the date of completion of the report, and describes other necessary steps to be taken. If the request is granted, the Research Integrity Officer will file periodic progress reports as requested by the ORI.[24]

D. When PHS funding or applications for funding are involved and an admission of scientific misconduct is made, the Research Integrity Officer will contact ORI for consultation and advice. Normally, the individual making the admission will be asked to sign a statement attesting to the occurrence and extent of misconduct. When the case involves PHS funds, the institution cannot accept an admission of scientific misconduct as a basis for closing a case or not undertaking an investigation without prior approval from ORI.[25]

E. The Research Integrity Officer will notify ORI at any stage of the inquiry or investigation if:

1. there is an immediate health hazard involved;[26]
2. there is an immediate need to protect Federal funds or equipment;[27]
3. there is an immediate need to protect the interests of the person(s) making the allegations or of the individual(s) who is the subject of the allegations as well as his/her co-investigators and associates, if any;[28]
4. it is probable that the alleged incident is going to be reported publicly;[29]
5. the allegation involves a public health sensitive issue, e.g., a clinical trial; or
6. there is a reasonable indication of possible criminal violation. In this instance, the institution must inform ORI within 24 hours of obtaining that information.[30]

X. INSTITUTIONAL ADMINISTRATIVE ACTIONS

[*Institution*] will take appropriate administrative actions against individuals when an allegation of misconduct has been substantiated.[31]

If the Deciding Official determines that the alleged misconduct is substantiated by the findings, he or she will decide on the appropriate actions to be taken, after consultation with the Research Integrity Officer. The actions may include:

A. withdrawal or correction of all pending or published abstracts and papers emanating from the research where scientific misconduct was found;
B. removal of the responsible person from the particular project, letter of reprimand, special monitoring of future work, probation, suspension, salary reduction, or initiation of steps leading to possible rank reduction or termination of employment;
C. restitution of funds as appropriate.

XI. OTHER CONSIDERATIONS

A. Termination of Institutional Employment or Resignation Prior to Completing Inquiry or Investigation

The termination of the respondent's institutional employment, by resignation or otherwise, before or after an allegation of possible scientific misconduct has been reported, will not preclude or terminate the misconduct procedures.

If the respondent, without admitting to the misconduct, elects to resign his or her position prior to the initiation of an inquiry, but after an allegation has been reported, or during an inquiry or investigation, the inquiry or investigation will proceed. If the respondent refuses to participate in the process after resignation, the committee will use its best efforts to reach a conclusion concerning the allegations, noting in its report the respondent's failure to cooperate and its effect on the committee's review of all the evidence.

B. Restoration of the Respondent's Reputation

If the institution finds no misconduct and ORI concurs, after consulting with the respondent, the Research Integrity Officer will undertake reasonable efforts to restore the respondent's reputation. Depending on the particular circumstances, the Research Integrity Officer should consider notifying those individuals aware of or involved in the investigation of the final outcome, publicizing the final outcome in forums in which the allegation of scientific misconduct was previously publicized, or expunging all reference to the scientific misconduct allegation from the respondent's personnel file. Any institutional actions to restore the respondent's reputation must first be approved by the Deciding Official.

C. Protection of the Whistleblower and Others[32]

Regardless of whether the institution or ORI determines that scientific misconduct occurred, the Research Integrity Officer will undertake reasonable efforts to protect whistleblowers who made allegations of scientific misconduct in good faith and others who cooperate in good faith with inquiries and investigations of such allegations. Upon completion of an investigation, the Deciding Official will determine, after consulting with the whistleblower, what steps, if any, are needed to restore the position or reputation of the whistleblower. The Research Integrity Officer is responsible for implementing any steps the Deciding Official approves. The Research Integrity Officer will also take appropriate steps during the inquiry and investigation to prevent any retaliation against the whistleblower.

D. Allegations Not Made in Good Faith

If relevant, the Deciding Official will determine whether the whistleblower's allegations of scientific misconduct were made in good faith. If an allegation was not made in good faith, the Deciding Official will determine whether any administrative action should be taken against the whistleblower.

E. Interim Administrative Actions

Institutional officials will take interim administrative actions, as appropriate, to protect Federal funds and ensure that the purposes of the Federal financial assistance are carried out.[33]

XII. RECORD RETENTION

After completion of a case and all ensuing related actions, the Research Integrity Officer will prepare a complete file, including the records of any inquiry or investigation and copies of all documents and other materials furnished to the Research Integrity Officer or committees. The Research Integrity Officer will keep the file for three years after completion of the case to permit later assessment of the case. ORI or other authorized DHHS personnel will be given access to the records upon request.[34]

Issued April 1995
Revised February 1997

ENDNOTES

1. 42 CFR 50.102.
2. 42 CFR 50.102.
3. 42 CFR 50.102.
4. 42 CFR 50.103(d)(12).
5. 42 CFR 50.103(d)(13).
6. 42 CFR 50.103(d)(2).
7. 42 CFR 50.103(d)(13).
8. 42 CFR 50.103(d)(3).
9. 42 CFR 50.103(d)(1).
10. 42 CFR 50.103(d)(1).
11. 42 CFR 50.103(d)(1).
12. 42 CFR 50.103(d)(8).
13. 42 CFR 50.103(d)(7).
14. 42 CFR 50.103(d)(7).
15. 42 CFR 50.103(d)(7).
16. 42 CFR 50.103(d)(7).
17. 42 CFR 50.104(a)(4); 42 CFR 50.103(d)(15).
18. 42 CFR 50.104(a)(2).
19. 42 CFR 50.104(a)(2).
20. 42 CFR 50.104(a)(1).
21. 42 CFR 50.104(a)(1).
22. 42 CFR 50.103(d)(15).
23. 42 CFR 50.104(a)(3).
24. 42 CFR 50.104(a)(5).
25. 42 CFR 50.104(a)(3).
26. 42 CFR 50.104(b)(1).
27. 42 CFR 50.104(b)(2).
28. 42 CFR 50.104(b)(3).
29. 42 CFR 50.104(b)(4).
30. 42 CFR 50.104(b)(5).
31. 42 CFR 50.103(d)(14).
32. 42 CFR 50.103(d)(14).
33. 42 CFR 50.103(d)(11).
34. 42 CFR 50.103(d)(10).

Appendix 2

Resources

CODES AND REGULATIONS

Code of Federal Regulations

21 CFR 50. 1997. Food and Drug Administration: Protection of Human Subjects.

21 CFR 54. Food and Drug Administration: Financial Disclosure by Clinical Investigators.

21 CFR 56. 1996. Food and Drug Administration: Institutional Review Boards.

45 CFR 46, part A. 1991. Department of Health and Human Services: Basic Policy for Protection of Human Research Subjects.

45 CFR 46, part B. 1991. Department of Health and Human Services: Additional Protections Relating to Research, Development, and Related Activities Involving Fetuses, Pregnant Women, and Human In Vitro Fertilization.

45 CFR 46, part C. 1991. Department of Health and Human Services: Additional Protections Pertaining to Biomedical and Behavioral Research Involving Prisoners as Subjects.

45 Code of Federal Regulations 46, part D. 1991. Department of Health and Human Services: Additional Protections for Children Involved as Subjects in Research.

Federal Register

56 *Federal Register* 28012. 1991. The Common Rule.

59 *Federal Register* 14508. 1994. NIH Guidelines on the Inclusion of Women and Minorities in Research.

60 *Federal Register* 35810. 1995. Objectivity in Research.

Medical Associations

Council of the International Organization of Medical Sciences (CIOMS). 1993. International Ethical Guidelines for Biomedical Research Involving Human Subjects. Geneva: CIOMS.

World Medical Association (WMA). 1964, 1975, 1983, 1989, 1996, 2000. Declaration of Helsinki: Recommendations Guiding Physicians in Biomedical Research Involving Human Subjects. Ferney-Voltaire Cedex, France: WMA.

Books and Articles

Association of Academic Health Centers (AAHC). 1994. Conflicts of Interest in Institutional Decision-Making. Washington, DC: AAHC.

Cape, R. 1984. Academic and Corporate Values and Goals: Are They Really in Conflict? In: Runser, D. (ed.), Industrial-Academic Interfacing. Washington, DC: American Chemical Society, pp. 1–21.

Committee on Life Sciences and Health of the Federal Coordinating Council for Science, Engineering and Technology (FCCSET). 1993. Biotechnology for the 21st Century: Realizing the Promise. Washington, DC: FCCSET.

Davis, M. 1999. Ethics and the University. New York: Routledge.

Haber, E. 1996. Industry and the University. Nature Biotechnology 14:1501–1502.

Huth, E. 1996. Conflicts of Interest in Industry-Funded Research. In: Spece, R., Shimm, D., and Buchanan, A (eds.), Conflicts of Interest in Clinical Practice and Research. New York: Oxford University Press, pp. 407–417.

Kreeger, K.Y. 1997. Studies Call Attention To Ethics of Industry Support. The Scientist 11:1–5.

Lomasky, L. 1987. Public Money, Private Gain, Profit for All. Hastings Center Report 17(3): 5–7.

McCain, K. 1996. Communication, Competition and Secrecy: The Production and Dissemination of Research Related Information in Genetics. Science, Technology and Human Values 16:492–510.

Snapper, J. (eds.). 1989. Owning Scientific and Technical Information. Brunswick, NJ: Rutgers University Press, pp. 29–39.

Williams, T. 1987. The History of Invention. New York: Facts on File Publications.

Web Sites

The Belmont Report, Department of Health and Human Services
http://ohrp.osophs.dhhs.gov/humansubjects/guidance/belmont.htm

Bibliographic materials
http://onlineethics.org/bib/index.html

Guidelines, Council of the International Organization of Medical Sciences (CIOMS)
http://www.cdc.gov/od/ads/intlgui3.htm

Declaration of Helsinki, World Medical Association
http://www.wma.net/e/policy/17-c_e.html

Women, Minorities, and Persons with Disabilities in Science and Engineering, National Science Foundation
http://www.nsf.gov/sbe/srs/nsf99338/foreword.htm

Freedom of Information Act (5 U.S.C. '552)
http://www.usdoj.gov/oip/foia_updates/Vol XVII 4/page2.htm

Guide to Mentoring and Training, National Institutes of Health
http://www1.od.nih.gov/oir/sourcebook/ethic-conduct/mentor-guide.htm#supervisors

Guide to Sharing Resources, National Institutes of Health
http://www.nih.gov./od/ott/Rtguide_final.htm

Institutional Review Board Guidebook, Department of Health and Human
    Services
http://ohrp.osophs.dhhs.gov/irb/irb_guidebook.htm

Mentoring Students in Science and Engineering
National Academy of Sciences, On Being a Mentor to Students in
    Science and Engineering (1997). Available at http://www.search.nap.
    edu/readingroom/books/mentor.

Nuremberg Code
http://ohsr.od.nih.gov/nuremberg.php3

Office for Human Research Protections (OHRP)
http://ohrp.osophs.dhhs.gov/index.htm

Office of Research Integrity
http://ori.dhhs.gov/

Protection of Human Subjects (45CFR46)
http://ohrp.osophs.dhhs.gov/humansubjects/guidance/45cfr46.htm

Secrecy in Science, Colloquium of the American Association for the
    Advancement of Science Colloquium
http://www.aaas.org/spp/secrecy/AAASMIT.htm

Uniform Requirements, International Committee of Medical Journal
    Editors
http://www.acponline.org/journals/annals/01jan97/unlfreqr.htm

University of Maryland COI Procedures
http://www.ord.umaryland.edu/resources/COI.html

References

References that we also suggest for further reading are marked with an asterisk (*).

42 CFR 50, subpart A, August 8, 1989.

1995. 42 CFR part 50.

1995. 45 CFR part 64.

Abby, M., et al., 1994. Peer Review Is an Effective Screening Process to Evaluate Medical Manuscripts. JAMA 272: 105–107.

Actuarial Foundation. 1998. Genetic Testing: Implications for Insurance. Actuarial Foundation, Schaumburg, IL.

Adler, R.G., 1993. Choosing the Form of Legal Protection. In Understanding Biotechnology Law, Gale R. Peterson, ed., Marcel Deckker, New York, wpp. 63–86.

Advisory Committee on Human Radiation Experiments (ACHRE), 1995. Final Report. Stock No. 061-000-00-848-9, Superintendent of Documents, U.S. Government Printing Office, Washington, DC.

Agnew, B., 1999a. NIH Eyes Sweeping Reform of Peer Review. Science 286: 1074–76.

Agnew, B., 1999b. NIH Invites Activists into the Inner Sanctum. Science 283: 1999–2001.

Agnew, B., 2000. Financial Conflicts Get more Scrutiny at Clinical Trials. Science 289: 1266–67.

Aller, R., and Aller, C., 1997. An Institutional Response to Patient/Family Complaints. In Ethics in Neurobiological Research with Human Subjects, A. E. Shamoo, (ed.), Gordon and Breach, Amsterdam, The Netherlands, pp. 155–1172.

Altman, L., 1995. Promises of Miracles: News Releases Go Where Journals Fear to Tread. New York Times, January 10, C2–C3.

Altman, L.K., 1997. Experts See Bias In Drug Data. New York Times, April 29, C1–C8.

American Association for the Advancement of Science (AAAS), 1980. Principles of Scientific Freedom and Responsibility. AAAS, Washington, DC.

American Association for the Advancement of Science (AAAS), 1991. Misconduct in Science. AAAS, Washington, DC.

American Association for the Advancement of Science (AAAS), 2000. Inheritable Genetic Modifications. AAAS, Washington, DC.

American Association for the Advancement of Science (AAAS)–American Bar Association (ABA), 1988. Project on Scientific Fraud and Misconduct. National Conference of Lawyers and Scientists, Report on Workshop No. 1, AAAS, Washington, DC.

American Psychological Association. 1992. Ethical Principles of Psychologists and Code of Conduct. American Psychologist 47: 1597–611.

*American Statistical Association (ASA), 1999. Ethical Guidelines for Statistical Practice. ASA, Alexandria, VA.

Anderson, W., 1989. Why Draw a Line? Journal of Medicine and Philosophy 14(4): 681–93.

Andrews, L., 2000. The Clone Age. Henry Holt, New York.

Andrews, L., and Nelkin, D., 2001. Body Bazaar. Crown Publishers, New York.

Angell, M., 1997a. The Ethics of Clinical Research in the Third World. New England Journal of Medicine 337: 847–49.

Angell, M., 1997b. Science on Trial. Norton, New York.

Angell, M., 2000. Is Academic Medicine for Sale? New England Journal of Medicine 342: 1516–18.

Angell, M., 2001. Medicine in the Noise Age: What Can We Believe? Accountability in Research, 8: 189–196.

Annas, G.J., 1994. Regulatory Model for Human Embryo Cloning: The Free Market Professional Guidelines and Government Restrictions. Kennedy Institute of Ethics Journal 4: 235–49.

Animal Welfare Act, 1966, 1996. Title 7 U.S. Code, 2131–56.

Annas, G.J., and Elias, S., 1992. Gene Mapping. Oxford University Press, New York.

Applebaum, P., et al., 1987. False Hopes and Best Data: Consent to Research and the Therapeutic Misconception. Hastings Center Report 17(2): 20–24.

Aristotle, 330 BC [1984]. Nichomachean Ethics. In Complete Works of Aristotle, J. Barnes, (ed.), Princeton University Press, Princeton, NJ.

Armstrong, J., 1997. Peer Review for Journals: Evidence of Quality Control, Fairness, and Innovation. Science and Engineering Ethics 3(1): 63–84.

Associated Press, 1997. Test of AIDS Vaccine Sought. Denver Post, September 22, A3.

Associated Press, 2001. FBI Mistakenly Withheld Boxes of Documents from McVeigh. New York Times, May 10, A1.

Association of Academic Health Centers (AAHC), 1994. Conflict of Interest in Institutional Decision-Making. AAHC, Washington, DC.

Association of Academic Health Centers (AAHC), 1990. Conflict of Interest in Academic Health Centers. AAHC, Washington, DC.

Babbage, C., 1830 [1970]. Reflections on the Decline of Science in England. Augustus Kelley, New York.

Bailar, J., 1986. Science, Statistics, and Deception. Annals of Internal Medicine 105: 259–60.

Baldessarini, R.J., and Viguera, A.C., 1995. Neuroleptic Withdrawal in Schizophrenic Patients. Archives of General Psychology 52: 189–91.

Baltimore, D., 1991. Baltimore Declares O'Toole Mistaken, Nature 351: 341–343.

Banoub-Baddour, S., and Gien, L.T., 1991. Student-Faculty Joint-Authorship: Mentorship in Publication. Canadian Journal of Nursing Research 23: 5–14.

Barbash, F., 1996. Piltdown Meltdown: A Hoaxer Revealed. Washington Post, May 24, A1, A34.

Barber, B., 1961. Resistance by Scientists to Scientific Discovery. Science 134: 596–602.

Barinaga, M., 2000. Soft Money's Hard Realities. Science 289: 2024–28.

*Barnard, N., and Kaufman, S., 1997. Animal Research Is Wasteful and Misleading. Scientific American 276(2): 80–82.

Bayles, M., 1988. Professional Ethics, 2nd ed. Wadsworth, Belmont, CA.

Bean, W.B., 1977. Walter Reed and the Ordeal of Human Experiments. Bulletin of the History of Medicine 51: 75–92.

Beardsley, T., 1994. Big-Time Biology. Scientific American 271(5): 90–97.

Beauchamp, T.L., 1996. Looking Back and Judging Our Predecessors. Kennedy Institute of Ethics Journal 6: 251–70.

Beauchamp, T.L., and Childress, J.F., 1994. Principles of Biomedical Ethics, 4th ed. Oxford University Press, New York.

*Beaudet, A.L., et al., 1995. Genetics, Biochemistry, and Molecular Basis of Variant Human Phenotypes. In The Metabolic and Molecular Basis of Inherited Disease, Scriver et al., eds., McGraw-Hill, New York pp. 53–130.

Beaudette, C.G., 2000. Excess Heat—Why Cold Fusion Research Prevailed. Oak Grove Press, South Bristol, ME.

Beecher, H., 1966. Ethics and Clinical Research. New England Journal of Medicine 274: 1354–60.

Bennett, T., 1994. Regulations and Requirements. In Essentials for Animals Research, T. Bennett, et al., (eds.), National Agricultural Library, Beltsville, MD.

Bentham, J., 1789 [1988]. Introduction to Principles of Morals and Legislation. New York, Penguin.

Berger, E., and Gert, B., 1997. Institutional Responsibility. In Research Ethics: A Reader, D. Elliot, and J. Stern (eds.), University Press of New England, Hanover, NH, pp. 197–212.

Bernard, C., 1865 [1957]. An Introduction to the Study of Experimental Medicine, H. Green (trans). Dover, New York.

Bero, L.A., et al., 1994. Publication Bias and Public Health on Environmental Tobacco Smoke. JAMA 272: 133–36.

Bingham, C., 2000. Peer Review and the Ethics of Internet Publishing. In Ethical Issues in Biomedical Publication, A. Jones, and F. McLellan, (eds.). Johns Hopkins University Press, Baltimore, pp. 85–112.

Bird, S., 1993. Teaching Ethics in Science: Why, How, and What. In Ethics, Values, and the Promise of Science, Sigma Xi, Research Triangle Park, NC, pp. 228–32.

Blank, R., 1991. The Effects of Double Blind Versus Single Blind Reviewing: Experimental Evidence from American Economic Review. American Economic Review 81: 1041–67.

Blinderman, C., 1986. The Piltdown Inquest. Prometheus Books, Buffalo, NY.

Blumenthal, D., 1995. Academic-Industry Relationships in the 1990s: Continuity and Change. Paper presented at the symposium Ethical Issues in Research Relationships between Universities and Industry, Baltimore, MD, November 3–5.

*Blumenthal, D., 1997. Withholding Research Results in Academic Life Science: Evidence from a National Survey of Faculty. JAMA 277: 1224–28.

Blumenthal, D., et al., 1986. University-Industry Research Relationships in Biotechnology: Implications for the University. Science 232: 1361–66.

Blumenthal, D., et al., 1996a. Participation of Life-Science Faculty in Relationships with Industry. New England Journal of Medicine 335: 1734–39.

Blumenthal, D., et al., 1996b. Relationship between Academic Institutions and Industry in the Life Sciences—An Industry Survey. New England Journal of Medicine 334: 368–73.

Bodenheimer, T., 2000. Uneasy Alliance: Clinical Investigators and the Pharmaceutical Industry. New England Journal of Medicine 342: 1539–44.

Bok, D., 1994. The Commercialized University. In N. Bowie, University-Business Partnerships: an Assessment. Rowman and Littlefield, Lanham, MD, pp. 116–122.

Bonner, J., 1980. The Evolution of Culture in Animals. Princeton University Press, Princeton, NJ.

Boozang, K., 1998. Western Medicine Opens the Door to Alternative Medicine. American Journal of Law and Medicine 25(2/3): 185–212.

Botting, J., and Morrison, A., 1997. Animal Research Is Vital to Medicine. Scientific American 276(2): 83–85.

Bower, B., 1991. Peer Review Under Fire. Science News 139: 394–95.

Bowie, N., 1994. University-Business Partnerships: An Assessment. Rowman and Littlefield, Lanham, MD.

Boyd, R., 1988. How to Be a Moral Realist. In Essay on Moral Realism, J. Sayre-McCord (ed.), Cornell University Press, Ithaca, NY, pp. 181–228.

Bradley, G., 2000. Managing Conflicting Interests. In Scientific Integrity, Francis Macrina, (ed.), American Society for Microbiology Press, Washington, DC, pp. 131–56.

Bradley, S.G., 1995. Conflict of Interest. In Scientific Integrity, Francis L. Macrina (ed.), American Society for Microbiology Press, Washington, DC.

Broad, W.J., 1981. "The Publishing Game: Getting More for Less," Science 211:1137–1139.

*Broad, W., and Wade, N., 1982 [1993]. Betrayers of the Truth: Fraud and Deceit in the Halls of Science. Simon and Schuster, New York.

Bronowski, J., 1956. Science and Human Values. Harper and Rowe, New York.

Browing, T., 1995. Reaching for the "Low Hanging Fruit": The Pressure for Results in Scientific Research—a Graduate Student's Perspective. Science and Engineering Ethics 1: 417–26.

Brown, J., 2000. Privatizing the University—the New Tragedy of the Commons. Science 290: 1701–702.

Bulger, R., 1987. Use of Animals in Experimental Research: A Scientist's Perspective. Anatomical Record 219: 215–20.

Burke, J., 1995. The Day the Universe Changed. Little, Brown, Boston.

Burnham, J.C., 1990. The Evolution of Editorial Peer Review. JAMA 263: 1323–29.

Bush, V., 1945 [1960]. Science: The Endless Frontier. National Science Foundation, Washington, DC.

Butler, D., 1999a. The Writing Is on the Web for Science Journals in Print. Nature 397: 195–99.

Butler, D., 1999b. NIH Plan Brings Global Electronic Journal a Step Nearer Reality. Nature 398: 735.

Butterfield, H., 1957. The Origins of Modern Science. Free Press, New York.

Buzzelli, D., 1993. NSF's Approach to Misconduct in Science. Accountability in Research 3: 215–22.

Byrne, R., 1988. 637 Best Things Anybody Said. Fawcett Crest, New York.

Callaham, M., et al., 1998. Reliability of Editors' Subjective Quality Rating of Peer Review of Manuscripts. JAMA 280: 229–31.

Callahan, S., 1998. The Ethical Challenge of the New Reproductive Technology. In Health Care Ethics—Critical Issues for the 21st Century, J. Monagle and D. Thomasma, (eds.), Aspen Publishers, Boulder, CO, pp. 45–55.

Caplan, A., 1983. Beastly Conduct: Ethical Issues in Animal Experimentation. Annals of the NY Academy of Science 406: 159–69.

Caplan, A.L. (ed.), 1992. When Medicine Went Mad—Bioethics and the Holocaust. Humana Press, Totowa, NJ, pp. 1–358.

*Capron, A.M., 1989. Human Experimentation. In Medical Ethics, R.M. Veatch (ed.), Jones and Bartlett, Boston, pp, 125–72.

Carey, J., et al., 1997. The Biotech Century. Business Week, March 10, 79–88.

Carruthers, P., 1992. The Animals Issue. Cambridge University Press, Cambridge.

Carson, R., 1961. Silent Spring. Houghton Mifflin, Boston.

Cassell, E., 1991. The Nature of Suffering. Oxford University Press, New York.

Cech, T., and Leonard, J., 2001. Conflicts of Interest: Moving beyond Disclosure. Science 291: 989.

Celera Genomics, 2001. http://www.celera.com. Accessed April 26, 2001.

Chalmers, T.C., et al., 1990. Minimizing the Three Stages of Publication Bias. JAMA 263: 1392–95.

Chapman, A. (ed.), 1999. Perspectives on Genetic Patenting. AAAS, Washington, DC.

*Cheny, D., (ed.), 1993. Ethical Issues in Research. University Press, Frederick, MD.

Chernow, R., 1998. Titan—the Life of John D. Rockefeller, Jr. Vantage Books, New York.

Chickering, R.B., and Hartman, S., 1980. How to Register a Copyright and Protect Your Creative Work. Charles Scribner's Sons, New York.

Cho, M.K., 1997. Letters to the Editor, Disclosing Conflicts of Interest. Lancet 350: 72–73.

Cho, M.K., 1998. Fundamental Conflict of Interest. HMS Beagle: The BioMedNet Magazine, issue 24, http://biomednet.com/hms beagle/1998/24/people/op-ed.htm.

Cho, M.K., and Bero, L.A., 1996. The Quality of Drug Studies Published in Symposium Proceedings. Annals of Internal Medicine 124: 485–489.

Cho, M.K., and Billings, P., 1997. Conflict of Interest and Institutional Review Boards. Journal of Investigative Medicine 45: 154–59.

Cho, M., et al., 2000. Policies on Faculty Conflicts of Interest at US Universities. JAMA 284: 2203–208.

Chubb, S., 2000. Introduction to the Series of Papers in Accountability in Research Dealing with "Cold Fusion." Accountability in Research 8: 1–18.

Chubin, D., and Hackett, E., 1990. Peerless Science. State University of New York Press, Albany.

Claverie, J., 2001. What if There Are Only 30,000 Human Genes? Science 291: 1255–57.

Clayton E., 2001. Bioethics of Genetic Testing. Encyclopedia of Life Sciences. Nature Publishing Group, Macmillan, London. Available at: http://www.els.net.

Clayton, E., et al., 1995. Informed Consent for Genetic Research on Stored Tissue Samples. JAMA 274: 1786–92.

Cohen, C., 1986. The Case for the Use of Animals in Biomedical Research. New England Journal of Medicine 315: 865–70.

Cohen, J., 1991. What Next in the Gallo Case? Science 254: 944–49.

Cohen, J., 1994. US-French Patent Dispute Heads for Showdown. Science 265: 23–25.

Cohen, L., and Hahn, R., 1999. A Solution to Concerns over Public Access to Scientific Data. Science 285: 535–36.

Cole, S., and Cole, J.R., 1981. Peer Review in the NSF: Phase Two. National Academy of Sciences, Washington, DC.

Cole, S., et al., 1978. Peer Review in the NSF: Phase One. National Academy of Sciences, Washington, DC.

Commission on Research Integrity (CRI), 1995. Integrity and Misconduct in Research. U.S. Department of Health and Human Services, Washington, DC.

Commoner, B., 1963. Science and Survival. Viking Press, New York.

Common Rule, 1991. 56 Federal Register 28012.

Copernicus, N., 1542 [1995]. On the Revolutions of the Heavenly Spheres, C. Wallis (trans.). Prometheus Books, Amherst, NY.

Council for International Organizations of Medical Sciences (CIOMS), 1993. International Ethical Guidelines for Biomedical Research Involving Human Subjects. Geneva, CIOMS.

Cranston, M., 1967. Bacon, Francis. In The Encyclopedia of Philosophy, vols. 1 and 2, P. Edwards, (ed.), Macmillan, New York, pp. 235–40.

Cromer, A., 1993. Uncommon Sense: The Heretical Nature of Science. Oxford University Press, New York.

Crossen, C., 1994. Tainted Truth. Simon and Schuster, New York.

Crow, T.J., J.F. MacMillian, A.L. Johnson, and B.C. Johnstone, 1986. "A Randomised Controlled Trial of Prophylatic Neuroleptic Treatment," British Journal of Psychiatry 148: 120–27.Culliton, B.J., 1990. Gallo Inquiry Takes Puzzling Turn. Science 250: 202–203.

Culliton, J., 1977. Harvard and Monsanto: The $23 Million Alliance. Science 195: 759–63.

D'Agostino, L.J., et al. (eds.), 1988. Personal Conflicts of Interest in Government Contracting. American Bar Association, Washington, DC.

Dalton, R., 1999. Kansas Kicks Evolution out the Classroom. Nature 400: 701.

Daubert v. Merrell Dow Pharmaceutical, 1993. 113 S CT 2768: 92–102.

Debus A. 1978. Man and Nature in the Renaissance. Cambridge University Press, Cambridge.

Davidson, R., 1986. Source of Funding and Outcome of Clinical Trials. Journal of General Internal Medicine 1: 155–58.

Davis, M., 1982. Conflict of Interest. Business and Professional Ethics Journal 1(4): 17–27.

*Davis, M., 1990. The Discipline of Science: Law or Profession. Accountability in Research 1: 137–45.

Davis, M., 1991. University Research and the Wages of Commerce. Journal of College and University Law 18: 29–39.

Davis, M., 1995a. A Preface to Accountability in the Professions. Accountability in Research 4: 81–90.

Davis, M., 1995b. Panel discussion at the symposium Ethical Issues in Research Relationships between Universities and Industry, Baltimore, MD.

DeAngelis, C., 2000. Conflict of Interest and the Public Trust. JAMA 284: 2237–38.

DeBakey, L., 1990. Journal Peer Reviewing. Archives of Ophthalmology 108: 345–49.

Debus, A., 1978. Man and Nature in Renaissance. Cambridge University Press, Cambridge.

De George, R., 1995. Business Ethics, 4th ed. Prentice-Hall, Englewood Cliffs, NJ.

DeGrazia, D., 1991. The Moral Status of Animals and Their Use in Research. Kennedy Institute of Ethics Journal 1: 48–70.

DeMets, D., 1999. Statistics and Ethics in Medical Research. Science and Engineering Ethics 5: 97–117.

Dennett, D., 1995. Darwin's Dangerous Idea. Simon and Schuster, New York.

Descartes, R., [1970]. Descartes: Philosophical Letters, A. Kenny (trans. and ed.). Oxford University Press, Oxford.

de Waal, F., 1996. Good Natured: The Origins of Right and Wrong in Humans and Other Animals. Harvard University Press, Cambridge, MA.

Deyo, R.A., et al., 1997. The Messenger under Attack—Intimidation of Research by Special-Interest Groups. New England Journal of Medicine 336: 1176–80.

Diamond v. Chakrabarty, 1980. 447 US 303–310.

Dickson, D., 1988. The New Politics of Science. University of Chicago Press, Chicago.

Dickson, D., 1995. Between Politics and Science. Cambridge University Press, Cambridge.

Diguisto, E., 1994. Equity in Authorship: A Strategy for Assigning Credit when Publishing. Social Science and Medicine 38: 55–58.

Djerassi, C., 1999. Who Will Mentor the Mentors? Nature 397: 291.

Doucet, M.S., et al., 1994. An Application of Stratified Sampling Techniques for Research Data. Accountability in Research 3: 237–47.

Drenth, J., 1996. Proliferation of Authors on Research Reports in Medicine. Science and Engineering Ethics 2: 469–80.

Dresser, R., 1992. Wanted: Single, White Male for Medical Research. Hastings Center Report 22(1): 24–29.

Dreyfuss, R., 2000. Collaborative Research: Conflicts on Authorship, Ownership, and Accountability. Vanderbilt Law Review 53: 1161–232.

Ducor, P., 2000. Coauthorship and Coinventorship. Science 289: 873–75.

Duft, B.J., 1993. Preparing Patent Application. In Understanding Biotechnology Law, Gale R. Peterson, (ed.), Marcel Dekker, New York, pp. 87–186.

Dustira, A.K., 1992. The Funding of Basic and Clinical Biomedical Research. In Biomedical Research: Collaboration and Conflict of Interest, R.J. Porter, and T. E. Malone, (eds.), Johns Hopkins University Press, Baltimore, MD.

Egilman, D., et al., 1998a. Ethical Aerobics: ACHREs Fleight from Responsibility. Accountability in Research 6: 15–62.

Egilman, D., et al., 1998b. A Little Too Much of the Buchenwald Touch? Military Radiation Research at the University of Cincinnati, 1960–1972. Accountability in Research 6: 63–102.

Eisen, H.N., 1991. Origins of MIT Inquiry. Nature 351: 343–44.

Eisenberg, R., 1995. Patenting Organisms. In Encyclopedia of Bioethics, rev. ed., Simon and Schuster, New York, pp. 1911–14.

Emanuel, E., et al., 2000. What Makes Clinical Research Ethical? JAMA 283: 2701–11.

Engler, R.L., et al., 1987. Misrepresentation and Responsibility in Medical Research. New England Journal of Medicine 317: 1383–89.

Enriquez, J., 1998. Genomics and the World's Economy. Science 281: 925–26.

Enserink, M., 2000. Patent Office May Raise the Bar on Gene Claims. Science 287: 1196–97.

Etkowitz, H., et al., 1994. The Paradox of Critical Mass for Women in Science. Science 266: 51–54.

Faden, R.R., and Beauchamp, T. L., 1986. A History of Informed Consent. Oxford University Press, New York.

Federal Register 56: 22286–90, May 14, 1991.

Feinberg, J., 1973. Social Philosophy. Prentice-Hall, Englewood Cliffs, NJ.

Fields, K.L., and Price, A.R., 1993. Problems in Research Integrity Arising from Misconceptions about the Ownership of Research. Academe Medicine Suppl. 3: S60–S64.

Flanagin, A., et al., 1998. Prevalence of Articles with Honorary and Ghost Authors in Peer-Reviewed Medical Journals. JAMA 280: 222–24.

Fleischmann, M., 2000. Reflections on the Sociology of Science and Social Responsibility in Science, in Relationship to Cold Fusion. Accountability in Research 8: 19–54.

Fleischmann, M., and Pons, S., 1989. Electrochemically Induced Nuclear Fusion of Deuterium. Journal of Electroanalytical Chemistry 261: 301.

Fleishman, J.L., 1982. The Delicate Dichotomy of Judical Ethics. In Ethics and Government, Final Report, Annual Chief Justice Earl Warren Conference on Advocacy in United States, Roscoe Pound–American Trial Lawyers Foundations, Washington, DC, pp. 37–52.

Fletcher, J.C., 1989. Where in the World Are We Going with the New Genetics? Journal of Contemporary Health Law and Policy 5: 33–51.

Fletcher, R. and Fletcher, S., 1997. Evidence for the Effectiveness of Peer Review. Science and Engineering Ethics 3(1): 35–50.

Forkenflick, D., 1996. Academic Career Unravels. Baltimore Sun, July 24, 1A, 7A.

Foster, F., and Shook, R., 1993. Patents, Copyrights, and Trademarks, 2nd ed. John Wiley, New York.

Fox, J.L., 1981. Theory Explaining Cancer Partly Retracted. Chemical and Engineering News 59: 35–36.

Fox, R., and DeMarco, J., 1990. Moral Reasoning. Holt, Rinehart, and Winston, Chicago.

Fox, S., 1999. Pharmacogeomics Thrives in Europe. Genetic Engineering News, June 15, 19, 21, 49.

Fraedrich, F., 1991. Business Ethics. Houghton Mifflin, Boston.

Francis, L., 1996. IRBs and Conflict of Interest. In Conflict of Interest in Clinical Practice and Research, Spece, R., et al. (eds.), Oxford University Press, New York, pp. 418–36.

Frankel, M., 1999. Public Access to Data. Science 283: 1114.

Frankena, W., 1973. Ethics, 2nd ed. Prentice-Hall, Englewood Cliffs, NJ.

Freedman, B. 1987. Equipoise and the Ethics of Clinical Research. New England Journal of Medicine 317: 141–45.

Frey, R., 1980. Interests and Rights: The Case against Animals. Oxford University Press, New York.

Frey, R., 1994. The Ethics of the Search for Benefits: Experimentation in Medicine. In Principles of Health Care Ethics, R. Gillon, (ed.), John Wiley, Chichester, pp. 1067–75.

Friedberg, M., 1999. Evaluation of Conflict of Interest in Economic Analyses of New Drugs Used in Oncology. JAMA 282: 1453–57.

Friedly, J., 1996a. How Congressional Pressure Shaped the Baltimore Case. Science 273: 873–75.

Friedly, J., 1996b. After 9 Years, a Tangled Case Lurches toward a Close. Science 272: 947–48.

Friedman, P.J., 1990. Correcting the Literature following Fraudulent Publication, JAMA 263: 1416–19.

Friedman, S., et al. (eds.), 1999. Communicating Uncertainty: Media Coverage of New and Controversial Science. Mahwah, NJ: Lawrence Erlbaum.

Funk Brothers Seed Co. v. Kalo Inculcant Co., 1948. 333 US 127–32.

Galileo, G., 1632 [2001]. Dialogue Concerning the Two Chief World Systems. S. Drak (trans.), Modern Library of Science, New York.

Galileo, G., 1638 [1991]. Dialogues Concerning the Two New Sciences. H. Crew and A. de Salvio (trans.), Prometheus Books, Amherst, NY.

Gardner, H., 1995. Leading Minds—An Anatomy of Leadership. Basic Books, New York.

Gardner, W., and Rosenbaum, J., 1998. Database Protection and Access to Information. Science 281: 786–88.

Garfield, E., 1987. The Anomie-Deviant Behavior Connection: The Theories of Durkheim, Merton, and Srole. Current Contents, September 28, 39: 3–12.

*Garfield, E., 1990. The Impact of Fraudulent Research on the Scientific Literature— the Stephen Breuning Case. JAMA, 263: 1424–26.

Garfunkel, J.M., et al., 1994. Effect of Institutional Prestige on Reviewer's Recommendations and Editorial Decisions. JAMA 272: 137–38.

Garner, B.A., (ed.), 1999. Black's Law Dictionary, 7th ed. West Group, St. Paul, MN.

Geison, G.L., 1978. Pasteur's Work on Rabies: Reexamining the Ethical Issues. Hastings Center Report 8: 26–33.

Geison, G.L., 1995. The Private Science of Louis Pasteur. Princeton University Press, Princeton, NJ.

Gert, B., 1993. Morality and Scientific Research. In Ethics, Values, and the Promise of Science. Sigma Xi, Research Triangle Park, NC.

Gibbs, W., 1996. The Price of Silence: Does Profit-Minded Secrecy Retard Scientific Progress? Scientific American 275(5): 15–16.

Giere, R., 1991. Understanding Scientific Reasoning, 3rd ed. Holt, Rinehart and Winston, Chicago.

Gilbert, P.L., et al., 1995. Neuroleptic Withdrawal in Schizophrenic Patients: A Review of the Literature. Archives of General Psychiatry 52: 173–88.

Gingrich, N., 2000. An Opportunities-Based Science Budget. Science 290: 1303.

Glantz, L., 1998. Research with Children. American Journal of Law and Medicine 24(2/3): 213–44.

Glantz, S.A., and Bero, L.A., 1994. Inappropriate and Appropriate Selection of "Peers" in Grant Review. JAMA 272: 114–16.

Glass, R., et al., 1999. JAMA and Editorial Independence. JAMA 281: 460.

Glick, J.L., 1992. Scientific Data Audit—a Key Management Tool. Accountability in Research, 2: 153–68.

Glick, J.L., 1993. Perceptions Concerning Research Integrity and the Practice of Data Audit in the Biotechnology Industry. Accountability in Research 3: 187–95.

Glick, J.L., 1997. Rationale and Methodology for Investing in the Biotechnology Industry. Technology Management 3: 343–58.

Glick, J.L., and Shamoo, A.E., 1991. Auditing Biochemical Research Data: A Case Study. Accountability in Research 1: 223–43.

Glick, J.L., and Shamoo, A.E., 1993. A Call For the Development of "Good Research Practices" (GRP) Guidelines. Accountability in Research 2: 231–35.

Glick, J.C.L., and Shamoo, A.E., 1994. Results of a Survey on Research Practices, Completed by Attendees at the Third Conference on Research Policies and Quality Assurance. Accountability in Research 3: 275–80.

Godlee, F., 2000. The Ethics of Peer Review. In Ethical Issues in Biomedical Publication, A. Jones, and F. McLellan (eds.), Johns Hopkins University Press, Baltimore, MD, pp. 59–84.

Gold, R., 1996. Body Parts: Property Rights and the Ownership of Human Biological Materials. Georgetown University Press, Washington, DC.

*Goode, S., 1993. Trying to Declaw the Campus Copycats. Insight Magazine, April 18, 10–29.

Goodman, B., 2000. New Definition for Misconduct a Step Closer. The Scientist, January 24, 14: 1, 2.

Goodman, S., 1994. Manuscript Quality before and after Peer Review and Editing at the Annals of Internal Medicine. Annals of Internal Medicine 121: 11–21.

Goodstein, D., 1992. What Do We Mean When We Use the Term Scientific Fraud? Scientist, March 2, 11–13.

Goodstein, D.L., 1994. Whatever Happened to Cold Fusion? American Scholar 63: 527.

Goldstein, T., 1980. Dawn of Modern Science. Houghton Mifflin, Boston.

Gould S., 1981. The Mismeasure of Man. Norton, New York.

Graham, G., 1999. The Internet: A Philosophical Inquiry. Routledge, London.

*Green, E.D., et al., 1995. The Human Genome Project and Its Impact on the Study of Human Beings. In The Metabolic and Molecular Basis of Inherited Disease, Scriver et al. (eds.), pp. 401–55.

Griffin, P., 1992. Animal Minds. University of Chicago Press, Chicago.

Grimlund, R.A., and Doucet, M.S., 1992. Statistical Auditing Techniques for Research Data: Financial Auditing Parallels and New Requirements. Accountability in Research 2: 25–53.

Grinnell, F., 1992. The Scientific Attitude, 2nd ed. Guilford Press, New York.

Grinnell, F., 1999. Ambiguity, Trust, and Responsible Conduct of Research. Science and Engineering Ethics 5(2): 205–14.

Gross, C., et al., 1999. The Relation between Funding at the National Institutes of Health and the Burden of Disease. New England Journal of Medicine 340: 1881–87.

Guston, D., 2000. Between Politics and Science. Cambridge University Press, Cambridge.

Guttman, D., 1998. Disclosure and Consent: Through the Cold War Prism. Accountability in Research, 6: 1–14.

Hamilton, D.P., 1991. NIH Finds Fraud in Cell Paper. Science 25: 1552–54.

Harris, N., 1999. It's Time to "Out" the Selfish Researchers. Nature 398: 102.

Harvey W., 1628 [1993]. On the Motion of the Heart and Blood in Animals. Prometheus Books, Buffalo, NY.

Heisenberg, W., 1971. Physics and Beyond. Harper, New York.

Hempel, C., 1965. Philosophy of Natural Science. Prentice-Hall, Englewood Cliffs, NJ.

Herrnstein, R and Murray, C., 1994. The Bell Curve: Intelligence and Class Structure in American Life. Free Press, New York.

Hilts, P., 1994. Philip Morris Blocked '83 Paper Showing Tobacco is Addictive, Panel Finds. New York Times, April 1, A1.

Hilts, P., 2000. Medical-Research Official Cites Ethics Woes. New York Times, August 17, A1.

Hirst, R., 1967. Primary and Secondary Qualities. In The Encyclopedia of Philosophy, vols. 5 and 6, P. Edwards (ed.), MacMillan, New York, pp. 455–57.

Hobbes, T., 1651 [1962]. Leviathan. MacMillan, New York.

Holden, C., 2000. NSF Searches for Right Way to Help Women. Science 289: 379–81.

Hollander, R., et al., 1996. Why Teach Ethics in Science and Engineering? Science and Engineering Ethics 1: 83–87.

Holton, G., 1978. Subelectrons, Presuppositions, and the Millikan-Ehrenhaft Dispute. Historical Studies in the Physical Sciences 9: 166–224.

Holtug, N., 1997. Altering Humans—The Case for and against Human Gene Therapy. Cambridge Quarterly of Healthcare Ethics 6: 157–74.

Holtzman, N.A., 1989. Proceed with Caution. Johns Hopkins University Press, Baltimore, MD.

Hoppe, S.K., 1996. Institutional Review Boards and Research on Individuals with Mental Disorders. Accountability in Research 4: 187–196.

*Hornblum, A.M., 1998. Acres of Skin. Routledge, New York.

Huber P., 1991. Galileo's Revenge: Science in the Courtroom. Basic Books, New York.

Hull, D., 1988. Science as a Process. University of Chicago Press, Chicago.

Humbr, J., and Almeder, R. (eds.), 1997. What Is Disease? Humana Press, Totowa, NJ.

Hurt, R., and Robertson, C., 1998. Prying Open the Door to the Tobacco Industry's Secrets about Nicotine. JAMA 280: 1173–81.

Huth, E., 1986a. Irresponsible Authorship and Wasteful Publication. Annals of Internal Medicine 104: 257–59.

Huth, E., 1986b. Guidelines on Authorship of Medical Papers. Annals of Internal Medicine 104: 269–74.

Huth, E., 2000. Repetitive and Divided Publication. In Ethical Issues in Biomedical Publication, A. Jones, and F. McLellan (eds.), Johns Hopkins University Press, Baltimore, MD, pp. 112–36.

Imanishi-Kari, T., 1991. OSI's Conclusions Wrong. Nature 351: 344–45.

*Inglefinger, F., 1972. Informed (but Uneducated) Consent. New England Journal of Medicine 287: 465–66.

Inspector General, U.S. Department of Health and Human Services (DHHS), 1998. Institutional Review Boards: A System in Jeopardy? DHHS, Washington, DC.

International Committee of Medical Journal Editors (ICMJE), 1997. Uniform Requirements for Manuscripts Submitted to Biomedical Journals. JAMA 277: 927–34.

Irving, D.N., and Shamoo, A.E., 1993. Which Ethics for Science and Public Policy. Accountability in Research 3: 77–100.

ISLAT Working Group, 1998. ART into Science: Regulation of Fertility Techniques. Science 281: 651–52.

Jacob, M., 1997. Scientific Culture and the Making of the Industrial West. Oxford University Press, New York.

Jaffe, A., 1996. Trends and Patterns in Research and Development Expenditures the United States. Proceedings of the National Academy of Sciences of the USA 93: 12658–63.

Jasanoff, S., 1990. The Fifth Branch: Science Advisors as Policy Makers. Harvard University Press, Cambridge, MA.

Jasanoff, S., 1995. Science at the Bar: Law, Science, and Technology in America. Harvard University Press, Cambridge, MA.

Johnson, H., 1993. The Life of a Black Scientist. Scientific American 268 1: 160.

Jonas, H., 1980. Philosophical Essays. Chicago: University of Chicago Press.

*Jonas, H., 1992. Philosophical Reflections on Experimenting with Human Subjects. Reprinted in R. Munson, Intervention and Reflection, 4th ed., Wadsworth, Belmont, CA, pp. 362–71.

Jones, A., 2000. Changing Traditions of Authorship. In Ethical Issues in Biomedical Publication, A. Jones, and F. McLellan (eds), Johns Hopkins University Press, Baltimore, MD, pp. 3–29.

Jones, J.H., 1981. Bad Blood. Free Press, London.

Journal of the American Medical Association (JAMA), 1999. JAMA and Editorial Independence. JAMA 281: 460.

Juengst, E.T., 1998. The Ethics of Prediction: Genetic Risk and the Physician-Patient Relationship. In Health Care Ethics—Critical Issues in the 21st Century, J.F. Monagle, and D.C. Thomasma (eds.), Aspen Publishers, Gaithersburg, MD, pp. 212–27.

Justice, A., et al., 1998. Does Masking the Author Identity Improve Peer Review Quality? Journal of the American Medical Association 280: 240–42.

Kahn, J., Mastroianni, A., Sugarman, J., 1998. Beyond Consent: Seeking Justice in Research. Oxford University Press, New York.

Kaiser, J., 1999. Plan for Divulging Raw Data Eases Fears. Science 283: 914–15.

Kant, I., 1753 [1981]. Grounding for the Metaphysics of Morals, J. Ellington, (transl.). Hackett, Indianapolis.

*Kass, L., 1985. Toward a More Natural Science. Free Press, New York.

Katz, J., 1972. Experimentation with Human Beings. Russell Sage Foundation, New York.

*Katz, J., 1993. Human Experimentation and Human Rights. Saint Louis University Law Journal 38: 7–54.

Katz, J., 1996. Ethics in Neurobiological Research with Human Subjects—Final Reflections. Accountability in Research 4: 277–83.

Kayton, I., 1995. Patent Practice, vol. 1. Patent Resources Institute, Charlottesville, VA.

Kendler, K.S., and Diehl, S.R., 1993. The Genetics of Schizophrenia: A Current Genetic—Epidemiologic Perspective. Schizophrenia Bulletin 19, Special Report 87–112. NIH/NIMH, Rockville, MD.

Kennedy, D., 2001. Accepted Community Standards. Science 291: 789.

*Kevles, D., 1995. In the Name of Eugenics. Harvard University Press, Cambridge, MA.

Kevles, D.J., 1996. The Assault on David Baltimore. New Yorker, May 27, pp. 94–109.

Kevles, D., 1998. The Baltimore Case: A Trial of Politics, Science, and Character. Norton, New York.

King, N., 1995. Experimental Treatment: Oxymoron or Aspiration? Hastings Center Report 25 4: 6–15.

Kirk, R., 1995. Experimental Design, 3rd ed. Brooks/Cole, New York.

Kitcher, P., 1993. The Advancement of Science. Oxford University Press, New York.

Kitcher, P., 1997. The Lives to Come: The Genetic Revolution and Human Possibilities. Simon and Schuster, New York.

Knoll, E., 1990. The Communities of Scientists and Journal Peer Review. JAMA 263: 1330–32.

Koenig, R., 1997. Panel Calls Falsification in German Case "Unprecendented." Science 277: 894–94.

Koenig, R., 1999. European Researchers Grapple with Animal Rights. Science 284: 1604–606.

Koestenbaum, P., 1991. Leadership—the Inner Side of Greatness. Jossey-Bass, Oxford.

*Kong, D., and Whitaker, R., 1998. Doing Harm: Research on the Mentally Ill. The Boston Globe, November 15, A1.

Kopelman, L., 1986. Consent and Randomized Clinical Trials: Are There Moral or Design Problems? Journal of Medicine and Philosophy 11(4): 317–45.

Kopelman, L., 1999. Values and Virtues: How Should They be Taught? Academic Medicine 74(12): 1307–10.

Kopelman, L., 2000. Moral Problems in Assessing Research Risk. IRB: A Review of Human Subjects Research 22(5): 7–10.

Korn, D., 1993. Conflict of Interest: A University Perspective. In Ethical Issues in Research, D. Cheny (ed.), University Press, Frederick, MD, pp. 114–25.

Korsgaard, C., 1996. The Sources of Normativity. Cambridge University Press, Cambridge.

Krimsky, S., et al., 1996a. Financial Interests of Authors in Scientific Publications. Science and Engineering Ethics 2(4): 396–410.

Krimsky, S., 1996b. Financial Interest of Authors in Scientific Journals: A Pilot Study of 14 Publications. Science and Engineering Ethics 2: 1–13.

Kronic, D.A., 1990. Peer Review in 18th-Century Scientific Journalism. JAMA 263: 1321–22.

Kuflik, A., 1989. Moral Foundations of Intellectual Property Rights. In Owning Scientific and Technical Information. V. Weil, and Snapper, J. (eds.), Rutgers University Press, Brunswick, NJ, pp. 29–39.

Kuhn, T., 1970. The Structure of Scientific Revolutions, 2nd ed. University of Chicago Press, Chicago.

Kuhn, T., 1977. The Essential Tension. University of Chicago Press, Chicago.

Kurtz, H., 1995. A Conflict of Wills? Pundit Kept Quiet About Wife's Role as Lobbyist. Washington Post May 23, D1.

Kurtz, H., 1996. Money Talks. Washington Post, January 21, B1.

Kuznik, F., 1991. Fraud Buster. Washington Post Magazine, April 14, 22–26, 31–33.

Laband, D.N., and Piette, M.J., 1994. A Citation Analysis of the Impact of Blinded Peer Review. JAMA 272: 147–49.

*LaFollette, M.C., 1992. Stealing into Print—Fraud, Plagiarism, and Misconduct in Scientific Publishing. University of California Press, Berkley.

LaFollette, M.C., 1994a. The Pathology of Research Fraud: The History and Politics of the US Experience. Journal of Internal Medicine 235: 129–35.

LaFollette, M.C., 1994b. Research Misconduct. Society, March/April, 31: 6–10.

LaFollette, M., 1994c. Measuring Equity—the U.S. General Accounting Office Study of Peer Review. Science Communication 6: 211–20.

LaFollette, M.C., 2000. The Evaluation of the "Scientific Misconduct" Issues: An Historical Overview. Proceedings for the Society for Experimental Biology and Medicine 224: 211–15.

*LaFollette, H., and Shanks, S., 1996. Brute Science. Routledge, New York.

LaFuze, W.L., and Mims, P.E., 1993. Ownership of Laboratory Discoveries and Work Product. In Understanding Biotechnology Law, G.R. Peterson (ed.), Dekker, New York, pp. 203–38.

Lakoff, S. (ed.), 1979. Science and Ethical Responsibility. Addison-Wesley, London.

Lasagna, L., 1992. Some Ethical Problems in Clinical Investigation. In Intervention and Reflection, 4th ed., R. Munson (ed.), Wadsworth, Belmont, CA, pp. 356–62.

Lawler, A., 2000. Silent No Longer: A "Model Minority" Mobilizes. Science 290: 1072–77.

Lebacqz, K., et al., 1999. Geron Ethics Advisory Board. Hastings Center Report 29: 31–36.

Lederer, S., 1995. Subjected to Science: Human Experimentation in America before the Second World War. Johns Hopkins University Press, Baltimore, MD.

Lentz, E.T., 1993. Inventorship in the Research Laboratory. In Understanding Biotechnology Law, G.R. Peterson (ed.), Dekker, New York, pp. 187–202.

Levine, R.J., 1988. Ethics and Regulation of Clinical Research, 2nd ed. Yale University Press, New Haven, CT.

Lloyd, G., 1970. Early Greek Science: Thales to Aristotle. Norton, New York.

Lock, S., 1991. A Difficult Balance: Editorial Peer Review in Medicine. BMJ Publishing, London.

Lock, S., 1993. Research Misconduct: A Resume of Recent Events. In Fraud and Misconduct in Medical Research, S. Lock and F. Wells (eds.), BMJ Publishing, London, pp. 5–24.

Locke, J., 1764 [1980]. Second Treatise of Government, C. Macpherson (ed.). Hackett, Indianapolis, IN.

Loeb, S.E., and Shamoo, A. E., 1989. Data Audit: Its Place in Auditing. Accountability in Research 1: 23–32.

Longino, H., 1990. Science as Social Knowledge. Princeton University Press, Princeton, NJ.

Lucky, R., 2000. The Quickening Pace of Science Communication. Science 289: 259–64.

Lurie, P., and Wolfe, S., 1997. Unethical Trials of Interventions to Reduce Perinatal Transmission of the Human Immunodeficiency Virus in Developing Countries. New England Journal of Medicine 337: 853–56.

Macilwain, C., 1999. Scientists Fight for the Right to Withhold Data. Nature 397: 459.

Macklin, R., 1994. Splitting Embryos on the Slippery Slope. Ethics and Public Policy. Kennedy Institute of Ethics Journal 4: 209–25.

Macklin, R., 1999. International Research: Ethical Imperialism or Ethical Pluralism? Accountability in Research 7: 59–83.

Macrina, F. (ed.), 2000. Scientific Integrity, 2nd ed. American Society for Microbiology Press, Washington, DC.

Malakoff, D., 2000a. Researchers Fight Plan to Regulate Mice, Birds. Science 290: 23.

Malakoff, D., 2000b. Does Science Drive the Productivity Train? Science 289: 1274–76.

Malakoff, D., 2001. For All but the NIH, the Devil Is in the Details. Science 292: 182–83.

Malakoff, D., and Marshall, E., 1999. NIH Wins Big as Congress Lumps Together Eight Bills. Science 282: 598.

Mangan, K.S., 2000. Harvard Weighs a Change in Conflict-of-Interest Rules. Chronicle of Higher Education, May 9, A47–A48.

Manning, K., 1998. Science and Opportunity. Science 282: 1037–38.

Marshall, E., 1983. The Murky World of Toxicity Testing. Science 220: 1130–32.

Marshall, E., 1996. Fraud Strikes Top Genome Lab. Science 274: 908–10.

Marshall, E., 1997a. Even Disclosing Data Can Get You in Trouble. Science 276: 671–72.

Marshall, E., 1997b. The Mouse That Prompted a Roar. Science 277: 24–25.

Marshall, E., 1997c. Need a Reagent? Just Sign Here. Science 278: 212–13.

Marshall, E., 1997d. NIH Plans Peer Review Overhaul. Science 276: 888–89.

Marshall, E., 1998. Embargoes: Good, Bad, or "Necessary Evil"? Science 282: 860–65.

Marshall, E., 1999a. NIH Weighs Bold Plan for Online Preprint Publishing. Science 283: 1610–11.

Marshall, E., 1999b. E-Biomed Morphs to E-Biosci, Focus Shift to Reviewed Papers. Science 285: 810–11.

Marshall, E., 1999c. Two Former Grad Students Sue over Alleged Misuse of Ideas. Science 284: 562–63.

Marshall, E., 1999d. A High-Stakes Gamble on Genome Sequencing. Science 284: 1906–909.

Marshall, E., 2000a. Patent Suit Pits Postdoc Against Former Mentor. Science 287: 2399–2400.

Marshall, E., 2000b. Storm Erupts over Terms for Publishing Celera's Sequence. Science 290: 2042–43.

Marshall, E., 2000c. The Rise of the Mouse, Biomedicine's Model Animal. Science 288: 248–57.

Marshall E., 2000d. Gene Therapy on Trial. Science 288: 951–57.

Marshall E., 2001. Universities Puncture Modest Regulatory Trial Balloon. Science 291: 2060.

Mastroianni, A.C., and Khan, J.P., 1999. Encouraging Accountability in Research: A Pilot Assessment of Training Efforts. Acountability in Research 7: 85–100.

May, R., 2001. Editorial, Science, and Society. Science 292: 1021.

May, R., 1998. The Scientific Investments of Nations. Science 281: 49–51.

Mayr, E., 1982. The Growth of Biological Thought. Harvard University Press, Cambridge, MA.

McCary, V., et al., 2000. A National Survey of Policies on Disclosure of Conflicts of Interest in Biomedical Research. New England Journal of Medicine 343: 1621–26.

McGee, G., 1997. The Perfect Baby. Rownan and Littlefield, Lanham, MD.

McKeon, R. (ed.), 1947. Modern Library. Introduction to Aristotle. New York.

McLellin, F., 1995. Authorship in Biomedical Publications: How Many People Can Wield One Pen? American Medical Writers Association 10: 11.

McNutt, R., et al., 1990. The Effects of Blinding on the Quality of Peer Review: A Randomized Trial. JAMA 263: 1371–76.

McVea, H., 1993. Financial Conglomerates and the Chinese Wall — Regulating Conflicts of Interest. Clarendon Press, Oxford.

Meadows, J., 1992. The Great Scientists. Oxford University Press, New York.

Merrill, S., and McGeary, M., 1999. Who's Balancing the Federal Research Portfolio and How? Science 285: 1679–80.

Merton, R., 1973. The Sociology of Science. University of Chicago Press, Chicago.

Mervis, J., 1999. Efforts to Boost Diversity Face Persistent Problems. Science 284: 1757–58.

Milgram, S., 1974. Obedience to Authority. Harper and Rowe, New York.

Mill, J., 1861, [1979]. Utilitarianism, G. Sher (ed.), Hackett, Indianapolis, IN.

Miller, L., and Bloom, F., 1998. Publishing Controversial Research. Science 282: 1045.

Miller, M., 2000. Phase I Cancer Trials: A Collusion of Misunderstanding. Hastings Center Report 30(4): 34–43.

Monson, N., 1991. How the Scientific Community Protects Its Black Sheep at the Expense of the Whistleblowers and the Public. Health Watch, July/August, 25–33.

Moore v. Regents of the University of California, 1990. 51 Cal 3d 120 134–47.

Moreno, J., 1999. Undue Risk — Secret Experiments on Humans. Freeman, New York.

Moreno, J., et al., 1998. Updating Protections for Human Subjects Involved in Research. JAMA 280: 1951–58.

Morton, J., 1994. Dealing with Conflict of Interest. American Journalism Review 16(10): 52C1.

Moses, H., and Martin, B., 2001. Academic Relationships with Industry: A New Model for Biomedical Research. JAMA 285: 933–35.

Mosimann, J.E., et al., 1995. Data Fabrication: Can People Generate Random Digits? Accountability in Research 4: 31–56.

Müller-Hill, B., 1992. Eugenics: The Science and Religion of the Nazis. In When Medicine Went Mad, A. Caplan (ed.), Humana Press, Totowa, NJ, pp. 43–53.

Munson, R., 1992. Intervention and Reflection, 4th ed. Wadsworth, Belmont, CA.

Munthe, C., and Welin, S., 1996. The Morality of Scientific Openness. Science and Engineering Ethics 2(4): 411–28.

Murphy, P., 1998. 80 Exemplary Ethics Statements. University of Notre Dame Press, Notre Dame, IN.

Myant, N.B., 1990. Cholesterol Metabolism, LDL, and the LDL Receptors. Academic Press, New York.

National Academy of Science (NAS), 1992. Responsible Science—Ensuring the Integrity of the Research Process, vol. 1, Panel on Scientific Responsibility and the Conduct of Research, NAS, Washington, DC.

National Academy of Sciences (NAS), 1994. On Being a Scientist. NAS, Washington, DC.

*National Academy of Science (NAS), 1997. Advisor, Teacher, Role Model, Friend: On Being a Mentor to Students in Science and Engineering. NAS, Washington, DC.

*National Bioethics Advisory Commission (NBAC), 1997. Report on Cloning Human Beings. NBAC, Rockville, MD.

*National Bioethics Advisory Commission (NBAC), 1998. Research Involving Persons with Mental Disorders That May Affect Decisionmaking Capacity, Vol. 1, Report and Recommendations. NBAC, Rockville, MD.

*National Bioethics Advisory Commission (NBAC), 1999. Report on Ethical Issues in Human Stem Cell Research, vol. 1. NBAC, Rockville, MD.

National Commission for the Protection of Human Subjects of Biomedical and Behavioral Research, 1979. The Belmont Report. U.S. Department of Health, Education, and Welfare, Washington, DC.

National Contract Management Association (NCMA), 1989. Ethics/Conflict of Interest—Case Studies. NCMA, Vienna, VA.

National Institutes of Health (NIH), 2000. Guide to Mentoring and Training. NIH, Bethesda, MD.

National Institutes of Health (NIH), 1998. Report of the National Institute of Health Working Group on Research Tools. Available at: http://www.nih.gov/news/researchtools/index.htm.

National Research Council (NRC), 1996. Guide for the Care and Use of Laboratory Animals. National Academy Press, Washington, DC.

National Science Foundation (NSF), 1991. Misconduct in Science and Engineering. Federal Register 56: 22286–90.

National Science Foundation (NSF), 1997. Scientists and Engineers Statistical Data System. Science Resources Studies Division, SESTAT, NSF, Washington, DC.

Nature, 1999. Policy on Papers' Contributors. Nature 399: 393.

Nelkin, D., 1972. The University and Military Research. Cornell University Press, Ithica, NY.

Nelkin, D., 1995. Selling Science. Freeman, New York.

Nelkin, D., and Lindee, S., 1995. The DNA Mystique: The Gene as a Cultural Icon. Freeman, New York.

Newton, I., 1687 [1995]. The Principia, A. Motte (trans.). Prometheus Books, Amhearst, NY.

New York Times News Service, 1997. University Settles Case over Theft of Data. Baltimore Sun, August 10, 9A.

Nurnberger, J.I., Jr., et al., 1994. Genetics of Psychiatric Disorders. In The Medical Basis of Psychiatry, 2nd ed., G. Winokur, and P.J. Clayton (eds.), Saunders, Philadelphia, pp. 459–92.

Office of Research Integrity (ORI), 1995. Guidelines for Institutions and Whistleblowers: Responding to Possible Retaliation against Whistleblowers in Extramural Research. ORI, Rockville, MD.

Office of Research Integrity (ORI), 1998. Responsible Whistleblowing: A Whistle-blower's Bill of Rights. ORI, Rockville, MD.

Office of Research Integrity (ORI), 1996. Annual Report, 1995. Department of Health and Human Services, Rockville, MD.

Office of Research Integrity (ORI), 1999. Scientific Misconduct Investigations, 1993–1997. ORI, Rockville, MD.

Office of Research Integrity (ORI), 2001. Draft Guidelines 9/1/01: Assessing Clinical Research Misconduct. ORI, Rockville, MD.

Office of Science and Technology Policy (OSTP), 1999. Proposed Federal Policy on Research Misconduct to Protect the Integrity of the Research Record. Federal Register 64 (198): 55722–25.

Office of Technology Assessment (OTA), 1986. Alternatives to Animal Use in Research, Testing, and Education. OTA, Washington, DC.

Office of Technology Assessment (OTA), 1990. New Developments in Biotechnology—Patenting Life. Dekker, New York.

O'Harrow, R., Jr., 2000. Harvard Won't Ease Funding Restrictions. The Washington Post, May 26, A16.

Oliver, D.T., 1999. Animal Rights—the Inhumane Crusade. Capital Research Center, Merril Press, Washington, DC.

Ollove, M., 2001. The Lessons of Lynchburg. Baltimore Sun, May 6, 7F.

Oppenheimer, R., 1989. Atom and Void: Essays on Science and Community. Princeton University Press, Princeton, NJ.

Osler, W., 1898. The Principles and Practice of Medicine, 3rd ed. Appleton, New York.

Oxman, A., et al., 1991. Agreement Among Reviewers of Review Articles. Journal of Clinical Epidemiology 44: 91–98.

Panel on Scientific Responsibility and the Conduct of Research, 1992. Responsible Science: Ensuring the Integrity of the Research Process. National Academy Press, Washington, DC.

Parens, E. (ed.), 1999. Enhancing Human Traits: Ethical and Social Implications. Georgetown University Press, Washington, DC.

Parens, E., and Asch, A. (eds.), 2000. Prenatal Testing and Disability Rights. Georgetown University Press, Washington, DC.

Parish, D., 1996. Falsification of Credentials in the Research Setting: Scientific Misconduct? Journal of Law, Medicine and Ethics 24: 260–66.

Pascal, C., 1999. The History and Future of the Office of Research Integrity: Scientific Misconduct and Beyond. Science and Engineering Ethics 5: 183–98.

*Pascal, C., 2000. Scientific Misconduct and Research Integrity for the Bench Scientist. Proceedings of the Society for Experimental Biology and Medicine 224: 220–30.

Pellegrino, E., 1992. Character and Ethical Conduct of Research. Accountability in Research 2: 1–2.

Pence, G., 1995. Animal Subjects. In Classic Cases in Medical Ethics. McGraw-Hill, New York, pp. 203–24.

Pence, G., 1996. Classic Cases in Medical Ethics, 2nd ed. McGraw-Hill, New York.

Pence, G., 1998. Who's Afraid of Human Cloning? Rowman and Littlefield, Lanham, MD.

Pennisi, E., 2001. The Human Genome. Science 291: 1177–80.

Perkins, R.B., 1961. Conflict of Interest in the Executive Branch. In Conference on Conflict of Interest, Feb. 20, 1961, p. 67–79, The Law School, The University of Chicago.

Peters, D., and Ceci, S., 1982. Peer-Review Practices of Psychological Journals: The Fate of Published Articles, Submitted Again. Behavioral and Brain Sciences 5: 187–95.

Pharmaceutical Manufacturers and Research Association (PMRA), 2000. The Pharmaceutical Industry's R&D Investment. PMRA, Washington, DC.

Ph.D. Misconduct Regulation, 1989. 42 CFR 50.101.

*Pimple, K., 1995. General Issues in Teaching Research Ethics. In Research Ethics: Case and Materials, R. Penslar (ed.), Indiana University Press, Indianapolis, IN, pp. 3–16.

Plous, S., and Herzog, H., 2000. Poll Shows Researchers Favor Animal Lab Protection. Science 290: 711.

Pojman, J., 1995. Ethics. Wadsworth, Belmont, CA.

Popper, K., 1959. The Logic of Scientific Discovery. Routledge, London.

*Porter, D., 1993. Science, Scientific Motivation, and Conflict of Interest in Research. In Ethical Issues in Research, D. Cheny (ed.), University Press, Frederick, MD, pp. 114–25.

Porter, R.J., 1992. Conflicts of Interest in Research: The Fundamentals. In Biomedical Research: Collaboration and Conflict of Interest, R.J. Porter and T.E. Malone, (eds.), Johns Hopkins University Press, Baltimore, MD, pp. 122–61.

Porter, R., 1997. The Greatest Benefit to Mankind. Norton, New York.

Pramik, M.J., 1990. NIH Redrafts Its Guidelines to Cover Conflicts of Interest. Genetic and Engineering News 10: 1, 24.

President's Commission for the Study of Ethical Problems in Medicine and Biomedical and Behavioral Research, 1983. Summing Up. U.S. Government Printing Office, Washington, DC.

Press, E., and Washburn, J., 2000. The Kept University. The Atlantic Monthly 285(3): 39–54.

Price, A.R., and Hallum, J.V., 1992. The Office of Scientific Integrity Investigations: The Importance of Data Analysis. Accountability in Research 2: 133–37.

Proctor, R., 1988. Radical Hygiene—Medicine under the Nazis. Harvard University Press, Cambridge, MA.

Proctor, R., 1999. The Nazi War on Cancer. Princeton University Press, Princeton, NJ.

Psaty, B.M., et al., 1995. The Risk of Myocardial Infarction Associated with Antihypertensive Drug Therapies. JAMA 274: 620–25.

Putnam, H., 1981. Reason, Truth, and History. Cambridge University Press, Cambridge.

Quine, W., 1969. Ontological Relativity. Columbia University Press, New York.

Rauh, J.L., 1961. Conflict of Interest in Congress. In Conference on Conflict of Interest—Feb. 20, 1961, University of Chicago Law School, Chicago, pp. 1–12.

Rawls, J., 1971. A Theory of Justice. Harvard University Press, Cambridge, MA.

Ready, T., 1999. Science for Sale. Boston Phoenix, April 29, 60–62.

Regaldo, A., 1995. Multiauthor Papers on the Rise. Science 268: 25–27.

Regan, T., 1983. The Case for Animal Rights. University of California Press, Berkeley.

Regan, T., and Singer, P. (eds.), 1989. Animal Rights and Human Obligations, 2nd ed. Prentice-Hall, Englewood Cliffs, NJ.

Reiss, M., and Straughan, R., 1996. Improving Nature? The Science and Ethics of Genetic Engineering. Cambridge University Press, Cambridge.

Relman, A., 1999. The NIH "E-Biomed" Proposal—a Potential Threat to the Evaluation and Orderly Dissemination of New Clinical Studies. New England Journal of Medicine 340: 1828–29.

Rennie, D., 1989a. How Much Fraud? Let's Do an Experimental Audit. AAAS Observer, no. 3 January (3), 4.

Rennie, D., 1989b. Editors and Auditors [see comments]. JAMA, 261: 2543–45.

Rennie, D., et al., 1997. When Authorship Fails: A Proposal to Make Contributors Accountable. JAMA 278: 579–85.

Rescher, N., 1965. The Ethical Dimension of Scientific Research. In Beyond the Edge of Certainty: Essays on Contemporary Science and Philosophy, N. Rescher (ed.), Prentice-Hall, Englewood Cliffs, NJ, pp. 261–76.

Resnik, M., 1987. Choices: An Introduction to Decision Theory. University of Minnesota Press, Minneapolis.

Resnik, D., 1994. Methodological Conservatism and Social Epistemology. International Studies in the Philosophy of Science 8: 247–64.

Resnik, D., 1996a. Social Epistemology and the Ethics of Research. Studies in the History and Philosophy of Science 27: 565–86.

Resnik, D., 1996b. Data Falsification in Clinical Trials. Science Communication 18(1): 49–58.

Resnik, D., 1996c. Ethical Problems and Dilemmas in the Interaction between Science and the Media. In Ethical Issues in Physics: Workshop II Proceedings, M. Thomsen, and B. Wylo (eds.), Eastern Michigan University, Ypsilanti, MI, pp. 80–112.

Resnik, D., 1997. A Proposal for a New System of Credit Allocation in Science. Science and Engineering Ethics 3: 237–43.

Resnik, D., 1998a. The Ethics of Science. Routledge, New York.

*Resnik, D., 1998b. Conflicts of Interest in Science. Perspectives on Science 6(4): 381–408.

Resnik, D., 1998c. The Ethics of HIV Research in Developing Nations. Bioethics 12(4): 285–306.

Resnik, D., 1999a. Privatized Biomedical Research, Public Fears, and the Hazards of Government Regulation: Lesson from Stem Cell Research. Health Care Analysis 23: 273–87.

Resnik, D., 1999b. Industry-Sponsored Research: Secrecy Versus Corporate Responsibility. Business and Society Review 99: 31–34.

Resnik, D., 2000. Statistics, Ethics, and Research: An Agenda for Education and Reform. Accountability in Research 8: 163–88.

*Resnik, D., 2001a. DNA Patents and Scientific Discovery and Innovation: Assessing Benefits and Risks. Science and Engineering Ethics 7(1): 29–62.

*Resnik, D., 2001b. Financial Interests and Research Bias. Perspectives on Science 8(3): 255–85.

Resnik, D., 2001c. Ethical Dilemmas in Communicating Medical Information to the Public. Health Policy 55: 129–49.

*Resnik, D., 2001d. Bioethics of Gene Therapy. In Encyclopedia of Life Sciences, Nature Publishing Group, Macmillan, London.

Resnik, D. and Langer, P. 2001. Human germline gene therapy reconsidered. Human Gene Therapy, 12: 1449–1458.

Resnik, D., and Shamoo, A.E., 2002. Conflict of Interest and the University. Accountability in Research, 9: 45–64.

Resnik, D., et al., 1999. Human Germline Gene Therapy: Scientific, Moral, and Political Issues. RG Landes, Austin, TX.

Rifkin, J., 1983. Algeny. Viking Press, New York.

Rifkin, J., 1998. The Biotech Century. Tarcher/Putnam, New York.

Robert, L., 2001. Controversial from the Start. Science 291: 1182–88.

Roberts, R.J., 1992. The Societal Impact of DNA Fingerprinting Data. Accountability in Research 2: 87–92.

Robertson, H., and Gorovitz, S., 2000. Pesticide Toxicity, Human Subjects, and the Environmental Protection Agency's Dilemma. Journal of Contemporary Health Law and Policy 16: 427–58.

Robertson, J., 1994. Children of Choice. Princeton University Press, Princeton, NJ.

Rochon, P.A., et al., 1994. A Study of Manufacturer-Supported Trials of Nonsteroidal Anti-inflammatory Drugs in the Treatment of Arthritis. Archives of Internal Medicine 154: 157–63.

Rollin, B., 1989. The Unheeded Cry: Animal Consciousness, Animal Pain, and Science. Oxford University Press, New York.

Rollin, B., 1992. Animal Rights and Human Morality, 2nd ed. Oxford University Press, Oxford.

Rollin B., 1995. The Frankenstein Syndrome. Cambridge University Press, Cambridge.

Ronan, C., 1982. Science: Its History and Development among the World Cultures. Facts on File, New York.

Rooyen, S., et al., 1998. Effect of Blinding and Unmasking on the Quality of Peer Review. JAMA 280: 234–37.

Rose, M., and Fischer, K., 1995. Policies and Perspectives on Authorship. Science and Engineering Ethics 1: 361–70.

Rosenberg, S.A., 1996. Sounding Board—Secrecy in Medical Research. New England Journal of Medicine 334: 392–94.

Ross, W., 1930. The Right and the Good. Clarendon Press, Oxford.

Rothenberg, K., et al., 1997. Genetic Information and the Workplace: Legislative Approaches and Policy Challenges. Science 275: 1755–57.

Rothstein, P. (ed.), 1997. Genetic Secrets. Yale University Press, New Haven, CT.

Roy, R., 1993. Science Publishing Is Urgently in Need of Reform. The Scientist, September 6, 11, 22.

Rudner, R., 1953. The Scientist Qua Scientist Makes Value Judgments. Philosophy of Science 20: 1–6.

Rule, J.T., and Shamoo, A.E., 1997. Ethical Issues in Research Relationship between Universities, and Industry. Accountability in Research 5: 239–50.

Russell, W., and Birch, R., 1959. Principles of Humane Animal Experimentation. Charles C. Thomas, Springfield, IL.

Schaffner, K., 1986. Ethical Problems in Clinical Trials. Journal of Medicine and Philosophy 11(4): 297–315.

Schmaus, W., 1990. Honesty and Method, Accountability in Research 1: 147–53.

Schuklenk, U., 1998. Access to Experimental Drugs in Terminal Illness. Pharmaceutical Products Press, New York.

Shamoo, A.E., 1988. We Need Data Audit. AAAS Observer November, 4, p. 4.

Shamoo, A.E., 1989. Principles of Research Data Audit. Gordon and Breach, New York.

Shamoo, A.E., 1991a. Quality Assurance. Quality Assurance: Good Practice, Regulation, and Law 1: 4–9.

Shamoo, A.E., 1991b. Policies and Quality Assurance in the Pharmaceutical Industry. Accountability in Research 1: 273–84.

*Shamoo, A.E., 1992. Role of Conflict of Interest in Scientific Objectivity—a Case of a Nobel Prize. Accountability in Research 2: 55–75.

Shamoo, A.E., 1993. Role of Conflict of Interest in Public Advisory Councils. In Ethical Issues in Research, D. Cheney (ed.), University Publishing Group, Frederick, MD, pp. 159–74.

Shamoo, A.E., 1994. Editors, Peer Reviews, and Ethics. AAAS Perspectives 14: 4–5.

Shamoo, A.E., 1995. Scientific Evidence and the Judicial System. Accountability in Research 4: 21–30.

Shamoo, A.E., 1997a. Brain Disorders—Scientific Facts, Media, and Public Perception. Accountability in Research 5: 161–74.

Shamoo, A.E., 1997b. The Ethical Import of Creation. Baltimore Sun, March 2, F1, F7.

Shamoo, A.E., (ed.), 1997c. Ethics in Neurobiological Research with Human Subjects. Gordon and Breach, Amsterdam.

Shamoo, A.E., 1997d. The Unethical Use of Persons with Mental Illness in High Risk Research Experiments. Testimony to National Bioethics Advisory Commission, January 9, 1997. NBAC, Washington, DC.

Shamoo, A.E., 1999. Institutional Review Boards (IRBs) and Conflict of Interest. Accountability in Research 7: 201–12.

Shamoo, A. E., 2000. Future Challenges to Human Subject Protection. The Scientist, June 26, 35.

Shamoo, A.E., 2001. Adverse Events Reporting—the Tip of an Iceberg. Accountability in Research 8: 197–218.

Shamoo, A.E., and Annau, Z., 1987. Ensuring Scientific Integrity [correspondence]. Nature 327: 550.

Shamoo, A.E., and Annau, Z., 1989. Data Audit—Historical Perspective. In Principles of Research Data Audit, A.E. Shamoo (ed.), Gordon and Breach, New York, pp. 1–12.

Shamoo, A., and Davis, S., 1989. The Need for Integration of Data Audit Research and Development Operations. In Principles of Research Data Audit, A. Shamoo (ed.), Gordon and Breach, Amsterdam, pp. 119–28.

Shamoo, A.E., and Davis, S., 1990. The Need for Integration of Data Audit into Research and Development Operation. Accountability in Research 1: 119–28.

Shamoo, A.E., and Irving, D.N., 1993. Accountability in Research Using Persons with Mental Illness. Accountability in Research 3: 1–17.

*Shamoo, A.E., and Keay, T., 1996. Ethical Concerns about Relapse Studies. Cambridge Quarterly of Health Care Ethics 5: 373–86.

Shamoo, A.E., and O'Sullivan, J.L., 1998. The Ethics of Research on the Mentally Disabled. In Health Care Ethics—Critical Issues for the 21st Century, J.F. Monagle, and D.C. Thomasma (eds.), Aspen Publishers, Gaithersburg, MD, pp. 239–50.

Shamoo, A.E., and Teaf, R., 1990. Data Ownership. CBE Views 13: 112–14.

Shamoo, A.E., et al., 1997. A Review of Patient Outcomes in Pharmacological Studies from the Psychiatric Literature, 1996–1993. Science and Engineering Ethics 3: 395–406.

*Shamoo, A., and Dunigan, C., 2000. Ethics in Research. Proceedings of the Society for Experimental Biology and Medicine 224: 205–10.

Sharav, V.H., and Shamoo, A.E., 2000. Are Experiments That Chemically Induce Psychosis in Patients Ethical? BioLaw 2(1): S1–S36.

Shenk, D., 1999. Money & Science = Ethics Problems on Campus. The Nation, May 22, 11–18.

Shrader-Frechette, K., 1994. Ethics of Scientific Research. Rowman and Littlefield, Boston.

Sideris, L., et al., 1999. Roots of Concern with Nonhuman Animals in Biomedical Ethics. ILAR Journal 40: 3–14.

Sigma Xi, 1986. Honor in Science. Sigma Xi, Research Triangle Park, NC.

*Singer, P., 1975 [1990]. Animal Liberation, 2d ed. Random House, New York.

Singer, P., 1985. In Defense of Animals. Harper and Rowe, New York.

Smith, A., cited in Fleishman, 1982, p. 34.

Sneed, D., and Riffe, D., 1991. The Publisher–Public Official—Real or Imagined Conflict of Interests? Praeger, New York.

Snow, C., 1964. The Two Cultures and the Scientific Revolution. Cambridge University Press, Cambridge.

Sobel, A., 1978. Deception in Social Science Research: Is Informed Consent Possible? Hastings Center Report 8(5): 40–45.

Society of Professional Journalism, Code of Ethics, cited in Sneed and Riffe, 1991, p. 14

Solter, D., and Gearhart, J., 1999. Putting Stem Cells to Work. Science 283: 1468–70.

Spece, R., et al. (eds.), 1996. Conflicts of Interest in Clinical Practice and Research. Oxford University Press, New York.

Spier, R., 1995. Ethical Aspects of the University-Industry Interface. Science and Engineering Ethics 1: 151–62.

Sprague, R., 1991. One Man's Saga with the University Federal System. Paper presented at the Second Conference on Research Policies and Quality Assurance, Rome, May 6–7.

Sprague, R.L., 1993. Whistblowing: A Very Unpleasant Avocation. Ethics and Behavior 3: 103–33.

Stelfox, H.T., et al., 1998. Conflict of Interest in the Debate over Calcium-Channel Antagonists. New England Journal of Medicine 338: 101–106.

Steneck, N., 1999. Confronting Misconduct in Science in the 1980s and 1990s: What Has and Has Not Been Accomplished. Science and Engineering Ethics 5: 161–76.

*Steneck N., 2000. Assessing the Integrity of Publicly Funded Research. In Proceedings from the ORI Conference on Research Integrity, ORI, Washington, DC, pp. 1–16.

Stewart, W.W., and Feder, N., 1991. Analysis of a Whistle-blowing. Nature 351: 687–91.

Stokstad, E., 1999. Humane Science Finds Sharper and Kinder Tools. Science 286: 1068–71.

Stokstad, E., 2000. Stephen Straus's Impossible Job. Science 288: 1568–70.

Sundro, L., 1993. Keynote Address. Accountability in Research 3: 73–76.

Swazey, J., 1993. Teaching Ethics: Needs, Opportunities, and Obstacles. In Ethics, Values, and the Promise of Science. Sigma Xi, Research Triangle Park, NC, pp. 233–42.

Swazey, J., and Bird, S., 1997. Teaching and Learning Research Ethics. In Research Ethics: A Reader, D. Elliot, and J. Stern (eds.), University Press of New England, Hanover, NH, pp. 1–19.

Swazey, J.P., et al., 1993. Ethical Problems in Academic Research. American Scientist 81: 542–53.

Swisher, K., 1995. What Is Sexual Harassment? Greenhaven Press, San Diego.

Tagney, J.P., 1987. Fraud Will Out—or Will It? New Scientist, August 6, 62–63.

Taylor, P., 1986. Respect for Nature. Princeton University Press, Princeton, NJ.

*Tauer, C.A., 1999. Testing Drugs in Pediatric Populations: The FDA Mandate. Accountability in Research 7: 37–58.

Teitelman, R., 1994. The Profits of Science. Basic Books, New York.

*Thompson, D., 1993. Understanding Financial Conflict of Interest. New England Journal of Medicine 329: 573–76.

U.K. Patent Office, 2001. http://www.patent.gov.uk. Accessed March 16, 2001.

U.S. Congress, Committee on Government Operations, 1990. Are Scientific Misconduct and Conflict of Interests Hazardous to Our Health? Report 101-688, U.S. Government Printing Office, Washington, DC.

US Constitution, 1787. Article 1, Section 8.

U.S. Copyright Office, 2001. http://lcweb.loc.gov/copyright/. Accessed March 16, 2001.

U.S. Department of Health, Education, and Welfare (DHEW), 1973. Final Report of the Tuskegee Syphilis Study Ad Hoc Advisory Panel, DHEW, Washington, DC.

U.S. General Accounting Office (GAO), 1994. Peer Review—Reforms Needed to Ensure Fairness in Federal Agency Grant Selection. GAO/PEMD-94-1. GAO, Washington, DC.

U.S. Patent and Trade Office, 2001. http://www.uspto.gov/. Accessed March 16, 2001

U.S. Public Health Service (PHS), 2000a. Draft Interim Guidance: Financial Relationships in Clinical Research. PHS, Washington, DC.

U.S. Public Health Service (PHS), 2000b. Policy on the Humane Care and Use of Laboratory Animals. PHS, Bethesda, MD.

University of Maryland, Baltimore (UMB), 1997. Policies and Procedures concerning Misconduct in Scholarly Work. UMB, Baltimore.

VandenBerg, J.L., et al., 1999. U.S. Laws and Norms Related to Laboratory Animals. ILAR Journal 40: 34–37.

Varmus H., 1997. The View from the National Institutes of Health. In The Future of Biomedical Research, C. Barfield, and B. Smith (eds.), American Enterprise Institute, Washington, DC, pp. 9–16.

Varmus, H., and Satcher, D., 1997. Ethical Complexities of Conducting Research in Developing Countries. New England Journal of Medicine 337: 1000–1005.

Veatch, R., 1987. The Patient as Partner: A Theory of Human Experimentation Ethics. Indiana University Press, Bloomington.

Venter, C. et al., 2001. The Sequence of the Human Genome. Science 291: 1304–51.

Ville, C., 1977. Biology, 7th ed. Saunders, Philadelphia.

Von Hippel, F., 1991. Citizen Scientist. American Institute of Physics, New York.

Wade, N., 1981. The Rise and Fall of a Scientific Superstar. New Scientist 91: 781–82.

Wade, N., 2001. Genome Feud Heats Up as Academic Team Accuses Commercial Rival of Faulty Work. New York Times, May 2, A15.

Wadman, M., 1996. Drug Company Suppressed Publication of Research. Nature 381:4.

Wadman, M., 1999. NIH Strives to Keep Resources Sharing Alive. Nature 399: 291.

Walsh, M.E., et al., 1997. University-Industry Relationships in Genetic Research: Potential Opportunities and Pitfalls. Accountability in Research 5: 265–82.

*Walters, L., 1986. The Ethics of Human Gene Therapy. Nature 320: 225–27.

Walters, L., 1989. Genetics and Reproductive Technologies. In Medical Ethics, Robert M. Veatch (ed.), Jones and Bartlett Publishers, Boston, pp. 201–31.

Walters, L., and Palmer J., 1997. The Ethics of Human Gene Therapy. Oxford University Press, New York.

Warsh, D., 1989. Conflict-of-Interest Guidelines on Research Projects Stir Up a Hornets Nest at NIH. Washington Post, December 27, F3.

Watson, A., 2000. A New Breed of High-Tech Detectives. Science 289: 850–54.

Waugaman, P.C., and Porter, R.J., 1992. Mechanism of Interactions between Industry and the Academic Medical Center. In Biomedical Research: Collaboration and

Conflict of Interest, R.J. Porter and T.E. Malone (eds.), Johns Hopkins University Press, Baltimore, MD, pp. 93–118.

Weaver, D., et al., 1986. Altered Repertoire of Endogenous Immunoglobulin Gene Expression in Transgenic Mice Containing a Rearranged mu Heavy Chain Gene. Cell 45: 247–59.

Weil, V., 1993. Teaching Ethics in Science. In Ethics, Values, and the Promise of Science, Sigma Xi, Research Triangle Park, NC, pp. 242–48.

Weil, V., and Arzbaecher, R., 1997. Relationships in Laboratories and Research Communities. In Research Ethics: A Reader, D. Elliott and J. Stern (eds.), University of New England Press, Hanover, NH, pp. 69–90.

Weiner, T., 1994. Inquiry Finds Star Wars Plan Tried to Exaggerate Results. New York Times, July 22, A1, A26.

Weiss, R., 1997. Thyroid Drug Study Reveals Tug of War over Privately Financed Research. Washington Post, April 16, A3.

Welsome, E., 1999. The Plutonium File. Dial Press, New York.

Wenger, N., et al., 1999. Reporting Unethical Research Behavior. Evaluation Reviews 23: 553–70.

Westrum, R., 1991. Technologies and Society. Wadsworth, Belmont, CA.

Whitbeck, C., 1998. Ethics in Engineering Practice and Research. Cambridge University Press, Cambridge.

Wilcox, B.L., 1992. Fraud in Scientific Research: The Prosecuters Approach. Accountability in Research 2: 139–51.

Wilcox, L., 1998. Authorship: The Coin of the Realm, The Source of Complaints. JAMA 280: 216–17.

Williams, S., 1985. Conflict of Interest: The Ethical Dilemma in Politics. Gower, Brookfield, VT.

Williams, T., 1987. The History of Invention. Facts on File, New York.

Wilmut, I., 1997. Cloning for Medicine. Scientific American 279(6): 58–63.

Woolf, P. 1986. Pressure to Publish and Fraud in Science. Annals of Internal Medicine 104: 254–63.

Wyatt, R.J., 1986. Risks of Withdrawing Antipsychotic Medication. Archives of General Psychiatry 52: 205–208.

Wyatt, R.J., et al., 1999. The Long-term Effects of Placebo in Patients with Chronic Schizophrenia. Biological Psychiatry 46: 1092–105.

Ziman, J., 1984. Introduction to Science Studies. Cambridge University Press, Cambridge.

Zolla-Parker, S., 1994. The Professor, the University, and Industry. Scientific American 270(3): 120.

Zuckerman, H., 1977a. Deviance Behavior and Social Control in Science. In Deviance and Social Change, E. Sagrin (ed.), Sage, Beverly Hills, CA, pp. 87–138.

Zuckerman, H., 1977b. Scientific Elite: Nobel Laureates in the United States. Free Press, New York.

Zuckerman, S., 1966. Scientists and War. Harper and Row, New York.

Zurer, P., 1990. Conflict of Interest: NIH Rules Go Back to Drawing Board. Chemical and Engineering News, January 8, 4–5.

Zurer, P., 1993. NIH Peer Reviewers to Watch for High-Risk, High-Payoff Proposals. Chemical and Engineering News, June 7, 25–26.

Index